DEATHTEXT
A CORONER'S HANDBOOK

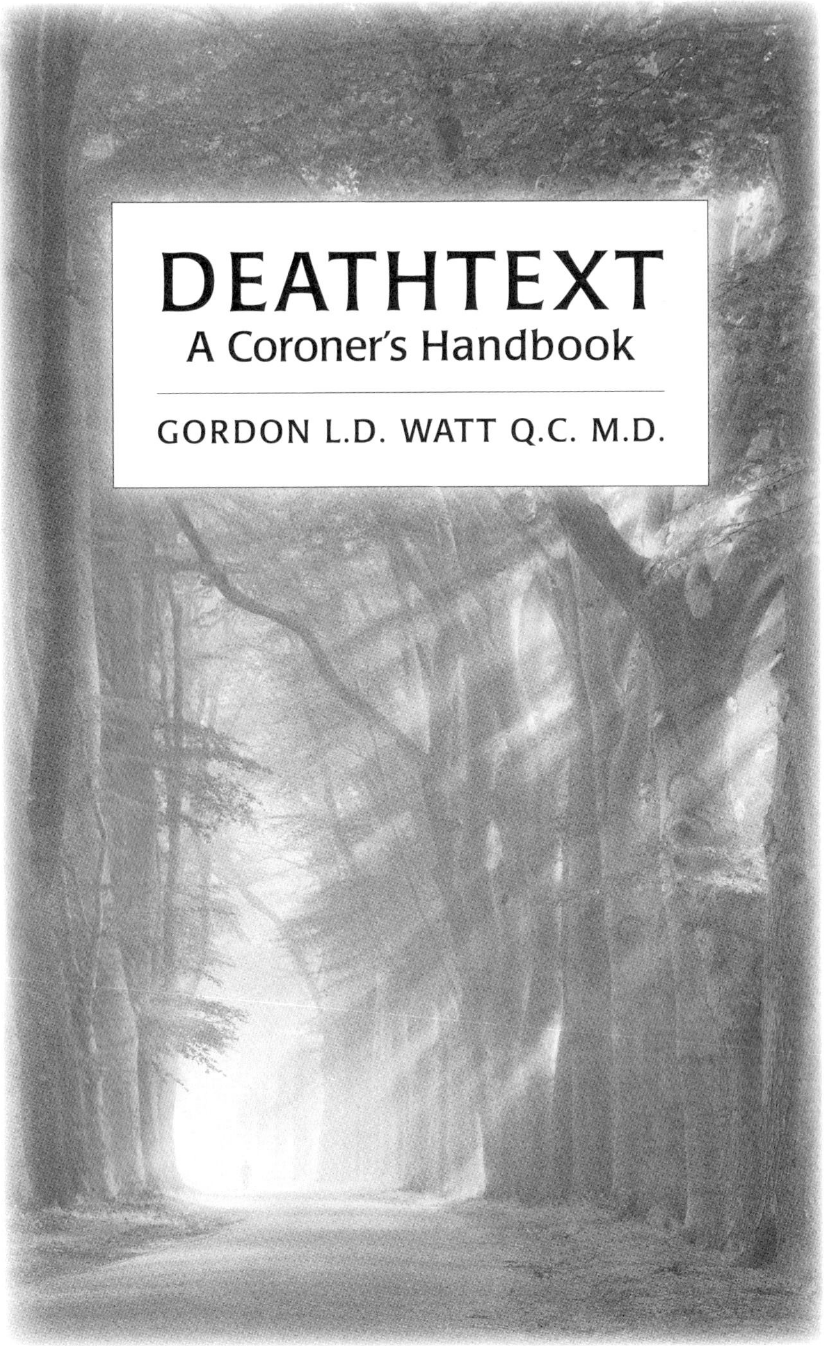

DEATHTEXT

A Coroner's Handbook

GORDON L.D. WATT Q.C. M.D.

www.deathtextbook.com

ISBN-13: 978-1-7778136-0-4

Printed and Bound in Canada.

Editor: Linda Jenkins, Red Pen Services
Illustrations: John Rey Dado
Indexing: Frances Curry
Cover photo: Rob Visser
Cover and interior design: Magdalene Carson RGD, New Leaf Publication Design

DEATHTEXT
A CORONER'S HANDBOOK

Table of Contents

List of Figures

List of Tables

Introduction

Some readers of this book may have little familiarity with the role and functions of coroners. Coroners' duties will differ depending on the jurisdiction in which they work, but there is one common responsibility: death investigation. This responsibility is the focus of this book.

Throughout the world the task of investigating deaths is the responsibility of people of varying occupations. In some territories, all death investigation is always the job of the police. In other jurisdictions deaths are examined by pathologists; when functioning in this role, pathologists are called medical examiners. Police have been around at least since the Bow Street Runners in the mid-eighteenth century in London, England. The role of medical examiner was created at the end of the nineteenth century. The oldest type of death investigator, who preceded them by centuries, is the coroner. That position can be traced back to William the Conqueror, who created the position of coroner as a death investigator over a thousand years ago.

Most death investigations are carried out by a single responsible person, or a group of designated individuals—without any publicity attached to the task. However, in some places where some social good will come of it, members of the public may be given that responsibility. Public involvement in death determinations has a long history. At the start of the last millennium, mediaeval coroners became the first people to hold public inquiries into deaths when they held an inquest, and coroner's juries continue to this day. An inquest is a hearing that usually includes a jury that takes over the coroner's responsibility in investigating a death. An inquest jury and a coroner have identical responsibilities.

So what exactly must a coroner or a coroner's jury do? A coroner's principal responsibility is to determine answers to the following questions:

1. What is the name of the deceased person?
2. When did death occur?
3. Where did death take place?
4. What is the medical cause of this death?
5. By what means did the person die? Was it natural, accidental, suicide, homicide, or undetermined?

Most statutes under which coroners are appointed require that these five questions be answered for every investigation as the bare minimum. They are also five of the questions that every family of a dead person wants answered. Invariably, families also want to know

6. How did the person feel while dying?

Coroners are quite good at answering the first five questions. There is extensive professional literature available to help them do so. Coroners' offices may provide courses prior to their appointment or after their election. These courses are directed at ensuring coroners are able to answer questions 1 through 5 correctly. In some jurisdictions – including Ontario, where I work – continuing education courses are offered annually to help coroners stay up to date. However, the government doesn't help coroners answer questions about the dying process or about the dead person's suffering. Coroners are left to muddle through when answering queries on these topics.

Coroners may be either physicians or laypeople, depending on the requirements of the jurisdiction in which they work. Many coroners without a lot of clinical experience in dealing with dying people find it difficult to give informed answers when questioned about dying, pain or suffering. This problem is not limited to just non-physician coroners. Many physicians deal with dying people only occasionally. Simply being a physician does not mean a coroner can accurately explain what likely happened. Most coroners have gaps in their knowledge about how people actually die and the discomfort felt while dying. Nobody teaches that. A lot has to be learned on the job.

This handbook tries to remedy that deficit. Nobody can ever be sure exactly what people feel while they are dying, but it is possible to make some educated guesses. Doctors have long observed and recorded the process by which their patients die of different diseases or injuries. Many observers, be they co-workers, nurses, family members, passers-by or simply the discoverers of dying people, have described what they saw as a person died. With their experiences as a basis, a reasonably intelligent hypothesis can be created to explain a dying process.

In addition, the internet makes much information about dying widely available, although not necessarily easy to find. Many family members know quite a bit about any condition affecting a relative but lack information about the actual dying process. Answering a question about the pathophysiological process that led to death is beyond the limits of most coroners' knowledge. They lack the basic understanding of anatomy, physiology and disease that they need to answer questions like "How did he actually die?", "Was it quick?", and "Do you think she suffered a lot?"

Even with some knowledge about the cause of death, a coroner needs to discern how informative an answer is needed. If a simple explanation will suffice, by all means give it. Only a foolhardy coroner would try to explain to a cardiac physiologist how a person with coronary artery disease died. Experienced coroners know that a great many people in the world are better informed about specific mechanisms of death than they are themselves.

When a coroner concludes that a questioner knows more about a mode of dying than the coroner, there is no shame in making that admission. People want some information, but nobody expects coroners to know everything. The honest answer "I don't know" is acceptable and wards off further questions.

This handbook is a guide to help provide answers to questions about common mechanisms of death, pain and suffering. It is not exhaustive but covers the usual types of death coroners investigate. It contains enough information to adequately answer most questions likely to be asked. If you can't find the answer to a relative's question here, apologize. Then suggest consulting the family physician, an appropriate specialist or a reliable internet source.

DEATHTEXT
A CORONER'S HANDBOOK

1

Brain Deaths

Brain death occurs once so many of the brain's nerve cells die that the brain can no longer instruct vital organs how to keep working. Over the past two hundred years, physiologists have learned more and more about the function of neurons — the brain's nerve cells. Today's scientists know quite a bit about how neurons live, function and die, but more is discovered every year. The brain's neurons are quite unique.

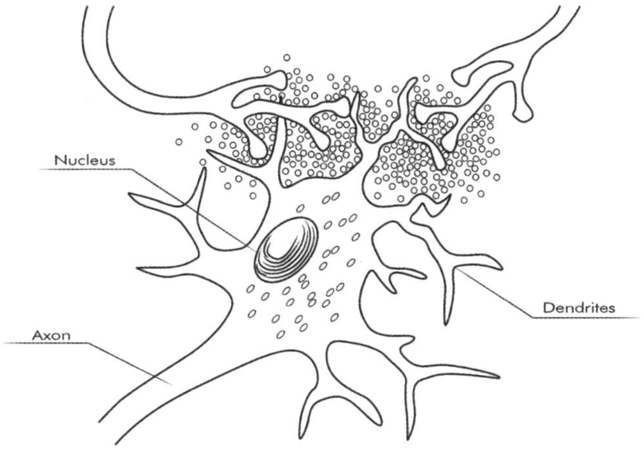

Figure 1.1: Neuron

At birth, an infant's brain has more nerve cells than it needs. As neurological functions sort themselves out during infancy, the excess, unneeded neurons self-destruct.[1] Barring a brain injury, all remaining neurons last throughout childhood, the teenage years and into early adulthood. Only then do some start to die. Once dead, a nerve cell is lost forever. Unlike other types of cells, these neurons do not regenerate. With each neuronal death brain functions continue, but with one fewer nerve cell to operate them.

All neurons die the same way. At first a dying cell swells a lot. Once it stops expanding, the bloated neuron stays enlarged for a while before starting to shrink, waste away and finally shrivel up. Nobody dies after losing just a few of their brain's nerve cells. Destruction of a brain's neurons only becomes lethal once so many nerve cells die that at least one vital body part can no longer function.

For decades, neurophysiologists were the sole people interested in the death of neurons. Brain cell death only started to catch the attention of physicians and the general public in the 1950s. That was the decade in which ventilators started appearing in hospitals and organ transplants began. Prior to that time the question of exactly when the brain died had little clinical importance.[2]

Even today, most physicians certify death without paying any attention to the brain. Usually doctors just look for functions in organs other than those of the brain itself, such as checking for a heart beat, feeling for a pulse, and placing one hand over a patient's mouth to try to detect a breath. Sometimes they touch the cornea of one eye looking for a blink. When none of these tests elicits any response, death is declared.

These tests don't work on a ventilated person whose brain has stopped working though. A ventilator keeps blowing air in and out of the lungs. This action ensures the lungs keep the heart pumping well-oxygenated red blood cells throughout the body to produce a pulse and heartbeat. So long as the body's tissues continue to receive oxygen they function perfectly well. Organs and other body tissues don't know or care whether it's a brain or a ventilator that causes a body's lungs to deliver oxygenated blood to them.

Ensuring that a ventilated person's heart muscle continues beating has become routine. Long after her ventilated patient's brain death, a nurse can ensure that all other body tissues are doing well by simply watching a cardiac monitor to make sure the heart keeps beating normally. Cardiac monitoring of ventilated patients can go on for days.

Remove the ventilator and fresh oxygen flow to the body's tissues stops immediately. Over the next few hours all cells will die. A patient with no functioning brain is dead. Yet apart from the brain, all other tissues in the body continue to function until the ventilator is removed. For that reason, ventilators are colloquially referred to as "life support."

"Life support" is a popular journalistic term that is technically incorrect since, with the brain dead, there is no life to support. Brain death means no "person" exists to direct the body's actions. A ventilator does not maintain life in the dead brain. It simply maintains a basic level of function of the rest of the body's tissues by providing them with oxygen. These tissues' ability to continue functioning normally is what makes it very hard to determine that death has actually occurred.

To declare a ventilated patient dead, physicians need to be certain that all brain function has stopped. Only then can a body be used for organ donation. To determine a ventilated patient's brain is dead the ventilator must be disconnected. Yet ventilatory support cannot be removed for very long lest tissues degenerate and become unsuitable for transplantation. For that reason, the time during which a ventilator is unhooked to determine death must be minimised.

Canada and a number of other countries, including the United States, call the neurological death of a ventilated person "brain death."[3] The United Kingdom and several other jurisdictions call it "brainstem death."[4] Regardless of how it is termed, confirmation of neurological death in ventilated patients is so important that elaborate procedures, gradually refined over time, are now undertaken before death can be said to have occurred.

Different protocols are used to determine brain death. One that is widely used and simple to understand, though complicated to perform, is the "five minutes apnea test." At some point after the death of a ventilated patient is suspected and following extensive preparations for monitoring, the supporting ventilator is disconnected for five minutes. Staff watch the patient carefully, looking for any sign of a spontaneous breath. Once five minutes or more have passed without a breath being detected, death is formally declared.

The ventilator must then be hooked up again quickly. Vital organs and other body tissues easily survive oxygen starvation for five minutes, but they are damaged if oxygen deprivation lasts much longer. Once resupplied with oxygen, tissues and organs continue to function for days on end. This is fortunate, or organ transplantation would never have become possible. Brain death is usually declared many hours or even days before the organs or tissues can be removed and transplanted. A ventilator will be needed for many hours after it was unhooked for the five minutes needed to confirm brain death.

Doctors created this test. It received legal sanction in the United States through the Uniform Determination of Death Act, 1981, which has now been adopted by most states. While other countries may not have such legislation, most of the developed world now accepts and uses this or a similar method of brain death determination to ensure a person is dead before their organs are harvested for transplantation.

The common causes of brain death are discussed below, after some information on skull and brain anatomy that makes it easy to understand the ways the brain dies.

The Skull and Brain

Most people know some cranial anatomy and neuroanatomy. Almost everyone knows a skull is made of bones and has seen pictures of skulls at one time or another. Some people even know the large space at the bottom of a skull is called the *foramen magnum* (Latin for "big hole"). Through the foramen magnum passes the spinal cord, which transmits the brain's messages to every organ and tissue in the body below. The foramen magnum is an important name to remember because of its frequently critical role in brain death.

A number of people also know the two halves of the brain are called the cerebral hemispheres. A band of brain tissue, the corpus callosum, hooks them together at their base. Some people are also able to position the cerebellum behind the cerebral hemispheres. This is the limit of most laypeople's knowledge of neuroanatomy, and it is set out in Figure 1.2. That knowledge is almost, but not quite, enough to understand brain death.

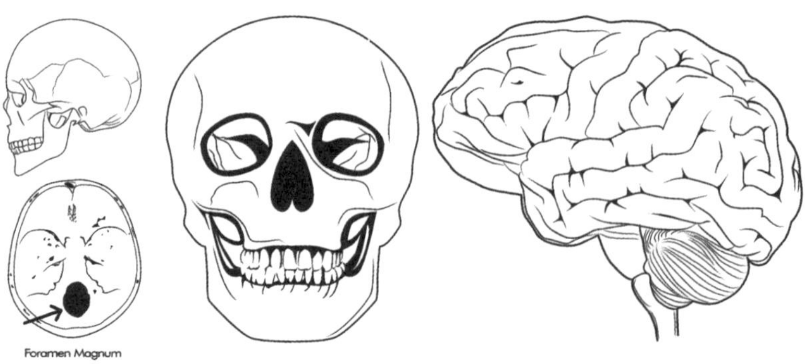

Figure 1.2: Major structures of the skull and brain

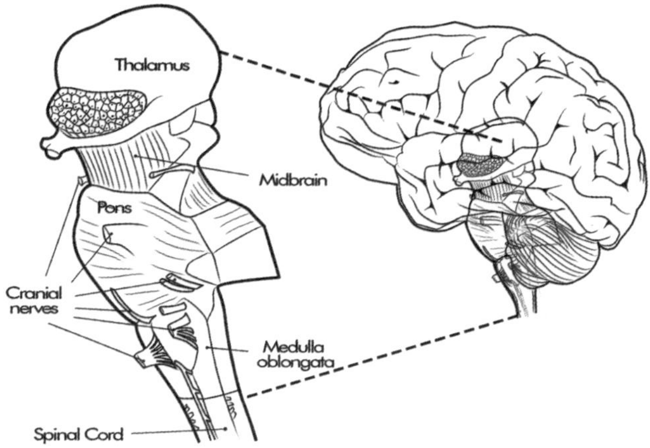

Figure 1.3: The brainstem

One missing piece of neuroanatomy needed to understand brain death is the brainstem, a part of the brain that sits below the cerebral hemispheres. Figure 1.3 shows the brainstem's relationship to the cerebral hemispheres, the cerebellum, and the spinal cord. Coroners need not know the brainstem's constituent parts.

The cerebellum sits behind the brainstem. Both of these parts of the brain are connected to the spinal cord and serve different functions. The cerebellum initiates movement and sensory activity. The brainstem maintains life by regulating the heart rate, breathing, eating, sleeping and consciousness. Nerve tracts that control movement, touch, pain, itch, vibration sensations, and other bodily functions pass through the brainstem. When the brainstem stops functioning, death follows rapidly.

Even most doctors find learning neuroanatomy and neurophysiology hard. Luckily, not much is needed to understand what is termed "brain death" throughout this chapter. The one necessary but easily understandable physiological fact needed is that blood must continually deliver an adequate amount of oxygen to the body's organs to keep them alive. Oxygenated blood flows from the heart toward the brain through the neck's internal carotid and basilar arteries. Once inside the skull, blood delivers oxygen to each of the brain's nerve cells (neurons) through a pipeline of increasingly smaller blood vessels.

Complete blockage of both basilar arteries is lethal because it stops all blood flowing to the brainstem. Decreased oxygen from partial blockage damages the brainstem. With severe enough damage, the brainstem stops instructing the lungs to breathe or the heart to beat. Once heart and lungs stop working, the rest of the body dies shortly afterwards.

Dying brain neurons don't cause pain. These nerve cells die once their environment changes to become neurotoxic. Neurotoxicity frequently results from inadequate oxygen, but other biochemical processes can also kill the brain's nerve cells. A neuron's complicated dying process has now been well described. It starts sixty to ninety seconds after inadequate oxygen triggers a glutamate cascade within the brain's nerve cells.

Coroners need never discuss this very technical process, which involves many long scientific names that are hard for anyone but a biochemist to remember. Any coroner lacking a PhD in neurophysiology should avoid discussing the physiology of neuronal death with anyone. If pushed for information, a coroner can say that after three hours of insufficient oxygen, brain cells will have died in several brain regions. Any questioners who want more detailed information explanation can be referred to Wikipedia or any trusted source of medical information.

Coroners should concentrate on the gross mechanics of brain death that are easy to understand and explain. Many people have heard of them, and general explanations should provide satisfactory answers to most questions that family members ask about brain death. One common brain death mechanism that coroners will need to understand is coning.

Coning

When pressure builds up within the skull, the brain's uppermost neurons push against the inside of the top of the skull. Its lower-most neurons are pushed downward against the skull's floor and the foramen magnum. Pressure within the skull is called intracranial pressure. When the intracranial pressure builds up enough to force part of the

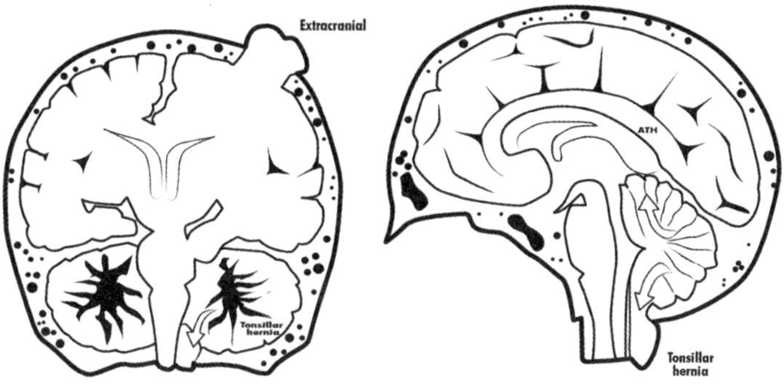

Figure 1.4: Coning

brainstem or the lower part of the cerebellum through the foramen magnum, coning occurs, as shown in Figure 1.4. Death follows.

A skull is a hard, bony, structure that is designed to contain one specific brain surrounded by its coverings and fluid. An adult skull's bones are tightly adherent or fused together, so they cannot move. This means that whenever tissue or liquid volume increases within an adult's skull something must give. When the total volume of matter within the cranium increases, the volume of brain tissue inside the skull must decrease. Increased intracranial pressure forces brain tissue out of the skull in an effort to lessen the pressure. Unless another hole has formed in the skull, the only direction the brain can move is downward through the foramen magnum.

The brainstem is the first part that passes through the foramen magnum. Its transit downward, squashed against the rim of the foramen magnum, may cause enough bleeding within the brainstem to stop it from functioning. The other way the brainstem's downward trajectory causes death is when its new position, wedged tightly against the edges of the foramen magnum, cuts off arterial blood flow to the brain above. The downward movement of the brainstem, with or without the cerebellum accompanying it through the foramen magnum, is a herniation called coning.

It takes a while to die from coning. Once oxygen flow to the brainstem and the cerebral hemispheres stops, brain cells die, neuron by neuron. Brain death occurs once a critical mass of dead neurons is reached. Coning occurs while comatose.

Death from Coning

Four common problems increase intracranial pressure enough to cause coning.

1. Malignant cancerous growths in the brain increase the volume of both tissue and fluid within the skull.
2. Brain diseases or infection may cause large numbers of neurons to swell and the volume of fluid within the skull to increase. Inflammation of the brain linings (called meninges) causes them to swell and extra fluid develops in the spaces between them. Coning follows.
3. Extra blood collects in the skull when any artery or vein within it leaks. Bleeding may be localized or spread diffusely around the brain. In either case, increased fluid volume caused by extra blood in the skull raises intracranial pressure so high that coning starts.
4. Inadequate blood supply to the brain usually arises from a mechanical blockage in one of the arteries leading to the brain. At other times something decreases the ability of the heart muscles to pump enough oxygenated blood to the brain. In both cases, the swelling of the brain's dying neurons raises the intracranial pressure enough to cause coning.

Coning Caused by Brain Cancer

Most brain cancers develop over a period of many months without anyone becoming aware of their existence. As tumour cells increase in size and number the intracranial pressure goes up. Steadily worsening headaches begin, followed by nausea and vomiting. Many people live with these symptoms for quite a while before their brain cancer is finally diagnosed.

Headache, nausea and vomiting are not brain cancer's only symptoms. Others occur varying with the tumour's location within the brain. Depending on which part of the brain develops a malignancy, sight, hearing, smell or taste can be affected. Confusion is common. Differing locations of brain cancer can cause muscle weakness, numbness or pains to develop virtually anywhere in a person's body.

Close relatives of people dying from brain cancer observe worsening symptoms as the disease progresses. They well understand the suffering experienced by their dying relative whom they watch decline over days, weeks or, more often, months. These people never ask about what their relative experienced while dying from brain cancer. They have first-hand knowledge.

Relatives out of contact with a person who died from brain cancer will likely know little about the illness. Those are the people with whom coroners may have to discuss the dying process. Any estimate of how much suffering a tumour causes is always a guess. Inpatient hospital records sometimes, if not always, describe the severity of symptoms that led to the terminal admission. When available, that information can somewhat inform the estimate of suffering.

Unfortunately, nowadays most hospital records provide only a blurry snapshot of a patient's terminal days. Entries are short, template-based and less frequent now that most hospital records have become electronic. Generally, these records minimize descriptions of pain severity and duration, leaving the dying experience to the imagination.

Modern medical records avoid literary flair in favour of summarizing events. Brevity saves time, keeps the reader focused, maximizes understanding, minimizes transcription and storage costs, and generally records the minimum hospital experience needed to satisfactorily understand the outcome. A coroner could perhaps estimate the degree of pain suffered by reviewing the type and quantity of pain medicines dispensed during the terminal hospital admission, but that review would never be made as a matter of course.

Brain death from cancer is preceded by weakness, drowsiness and then a comatose state that can last for hours or even days. When talking to relatives who don't know the course of a brain tumour–induced death, it is kindest to avoid speculating on the extent of the misery that might have been experienced in the months before death. Focus on the painless comatose period. Reassurance that, in the end, death came while unconscious leaves relatives happier.

Coning Caused by Inflammation of the Brain

Meningitis

Meningitis, which is essentially an inflammation of the tissues (meninges) that cover the brain, is sometimes fatal. All meningitis progresses toward death in a similar fashion regardless of its origin. Viruses or bacteria are the usual causes, but in rare cases meningitis can arise from a fungal infection or a parasitic infestation. Chemical meningitis is an uncommon type of meningitis that occasionally follows a neurosurgical procedure.

Regardless of the type of fatal meningitis most people die after hospital stays of varying lengths. Deaths from meningitis in hospital are considered natural, unfortunate outcomes of a serious disease and are usually not investigated by coroners. For this reason most meningitis deaths investigated by coroners will not have been diagnosed or treated in hospital. A coroner only investigates a meningitis death when (a) there is a complaint about the disease's treatment in hospital or (b) when it occurs in a recluse who has avoided medical treatment and is found dead at home. In the latter case, meningitis is almost always discovered during an autopsy by a pathologist.

If coroners need to talk to a relative about meningitis before its causative organism has been identified, mention only viruses or bacteria. Should the meningitis eventually turn out to be due to something else the family can be told later. Simply knowing death was due to meningitis satisfies most relatives.

But not all. For example, when an epidemic of bacterial meningococcal infections strikes high school students in a municipality, any teenage meningitis death achieves a very high profile. The local public health authorities want and get the lab test results quickly so they can trace and vaccinate everyone in contact with those who have died. Fortunately, most of the time a coroner is not involved with these deaths.

Regardless of the type of meningitis, symptoms develop in the same way. Early symptoms include severe headache, stiffening of the neck and, perhaps later, seizures. Meningitis also makes a person feel quite hot – sweats and chills accompany a high fever. The first outward sign that relatives usually see is that the person with meningitis becomes hot and cranky.

Meningitis may lead to such acute neuronal swelling and fluid production inside the skull that death from coning comes quickly. At other times, death arises from sepsis when the infecting germ spreads into the blood stream and causes septic shock. Clotting within multiple blood vessels sometimes accompanies these septic deaths.

Fatal meningitis may develop rapidly, but usually symptoms begin at least a couple of days before death. Thankfully, nature ends the dying process painlessly. People invariable lose consciousness some time before dying. All suffering is confined to those days before becoming comatose.

In urban areas of the developed world, most people (other than recluses) are hospitalized for meningitis treatment before death. Coroners usually only investigate meningitis deaths of the solitary. In these cases, there are few questions about suffering prior to death. These people are quite isolated and often forgotten. Other than those who didn't know that their relative was ill, family members fully understand how much suffering dying with meningitis caused because they watched it. They usually won't ask questions either.

Encephalitis

Failure of the blood to deliver adequate oxygen to the brain's neurons is not the only cause of fatal brain swelling. Inflammation of the brain itself, called encephalitis, can be fatal too. One way encephalitis occurs is when brain cells that are infected with a virus or bacteria swell, sometimes to the point of death. The polio, rabies, West Nile and herpes simplex (cold sore) viruses can all make the brain's neurons swell lethally. Syphilis, toxoplasmosis and Lyme disease are illnesses caused by bacteria that can do the same thing.

Up to 20% of encephalitis cases are autoimmune and occur without any infection.[5] Half the time the cause of encephalitis is never clearly determined. Regardless of the precise cause of encephalitis, death from this condition follows the same course. Brain neuron swelling is accompanied by fever, headache, seizures, confusion and muscle spasms, followed by a comatose period prior to death. In most cases, the patient takes weeks to die.

Nobody can accurately describe the course of encephalitis without seeing it. If asked about what happened regarding a death due to encephalitis, don't duck the question. Slide over the likely early symptoms. Concentrate on the fact that the person at some point became comatose before death. A frank explanation that nobody can estimate the time or extent of suffering before dying usually suffices. As with meningitis deaths, coroners are only occasionally involved with cases of encephalitis.

Coning Caused by Intracranial Bleeding

Bleeding within the skull is described in its relationship to either the brain or the meningeal linings around the brain. Two of these linings, called the dura and the arachnoid maters, are reference points used to describe these haemorrhages. The dura lies adjacent to the undersurface of the skull. The arachnoid mater is another covering that floats between the dura and the brain itself. See Figure 1.5.

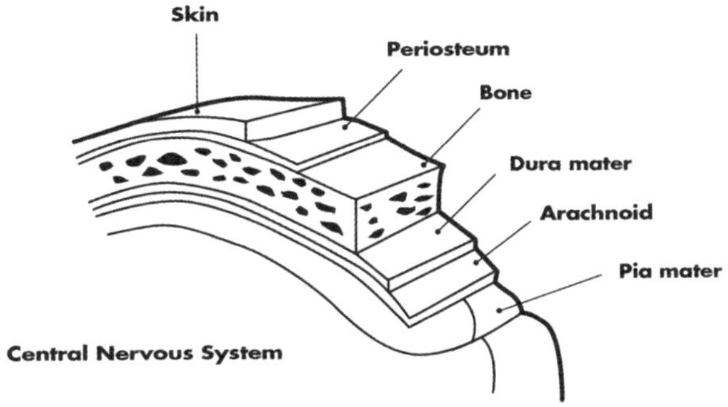

Figure 1.5: The meninges lining around the brain is made up of the pia mater, the arachnoid layer, and the dura mater.

Though virtually all coning deaths end painlessly, they frequently don't start out that way. This is certainly true of intracranial haemorrhage. Bleeding inside the skull often starts when a person is awake. Its cause can be either natural or some sort of accident. A large, sudden bleed causes an immediate severe headache. A blow to the head that causes intracranial bleeding also always leads to a severe headache, or to the person being rendered instantly unconscious.

Any blow to the head has the potential to cause painful bleeding in the skull. The pain experienced varies. A faint tap on the head causes virtually no pain at all. A blow from a crowbar hurts a lot. The pain from the blood building up inside the skull is much worse than any discomfort caused by striking the head.

The blow does not have to fracture the skull to cause intracranial bleeding. Often, blows have enough force to bruise the brain, tear fragile blood vessels, and cause profuse bleeding inside the skull and yet not actually crack any part of the skull. Regardless of its cause, bleeding in the substance of the brain, or from torn blood vessels that surround it, can increase the intracranial pressure. The swelling of bruised neurons may increase the pressure to a lethal point. In most cases that coroners investigate, some period of headache will have preceded death. Coroners can guess that if consciousness was not quickly lost a period of nausea likely preceded the onset of coma.

Still, bleeding within the skull is frequently associated with skull fractures, which relatives tend to focus on when they hear about them. Though fractures are rarely the cause of death it is useful to know a few facts about them.

Subdural Haemorrhage (Haematoma)

In a subdural haemorrhage, bleeding occurs between the dura and arachnoid maters. These bleeds are quite common and sometimes fatal. Most subdural haemorrhages investigated by a coroner result from the head striking something when falling. These cases are almost always caused by an accident or suicide. Less commonly a blow to the head triggers the lethal bleed. These cases are almost always caused by an accident or homicide. In either case the skull need not fracture

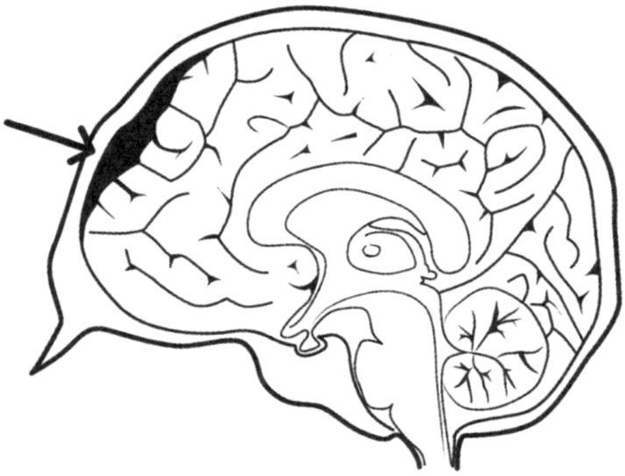

Figure 1.6: Location of a subdural haemorrhage

for such bleeding to be fatal. Force delivered to the skull simply tears small bridging veins crossing the space between the dura and the arachnoid maters.

In fact, these bridging veins are fragile enough to tear even without a blow to the head. Any action forcefully whipping the head back and forth might rupture them. The resultant bleed is usually accompanied by some sort of headache. When a large enough pool of blood collects in one discrete area between the dura and arachnoid to raise the intracranial pressure enough to lead to coning, the subdural haemorrhage becomes fatal.

Since it doesn't take much force to make a bridging vein leak, physicians are able to identify the precise cause of only about half of the subdural bleeds they see. For coroners, identifying the cause is not usually a problem. Most of the subdural haemorrhage deaths they investigate are caused by an elderly person falling in a seniors' facility or in their own home. As examples, let's look at two cases.

Frail, elderly Person A falls and cannot get back up. Person A is then taken to hospital, where a CT scan reveals a fatal subdural haemorrhage.

Now let's look at frail, elderly Person B, who is able to get up after the initial fall. Person B is likely to complain of a sore head and/or a headache, but nothing else. Person B's caregivers believe that this indicates the bump to the head was trivial. Life goes on and the headache goes away. At this point, no one is aware that Person B's fall actually caused a subdural haemorrhage. Then, weeks or months later, Person B falls again. This time (and in most such cases), the headache is worse, which leads to a medical investigation. The radiologist can see via a CT scan that the old subdural haemorrhage caused by Person B's first fall has now clotted and become a subdural haematoma. The radiologist can also see the new bleeding around the margins of the old clot. The combination of the old haematoma and the new bleeding is enough to cause fatal coning in Person B. However, it is impossible to accurately estimate how much the first injury contributed to Person B's death. There is certainly a connection between the first bleed and eventual death, when the second bout of bleeding recurred on the clot's margins. From the coroner's point of view, death was caused by the second, lethal fall.

Subarachnoid Haemorrhage

A subarachnoid haemorrhage is the second potentially fatal type of bleeding that occurs in the space between the arachnoid mater and the brain. About half of all these haemorrhages are fatal.[6] Survivors of subarachnoid bleeding usually remember every detail about the event. At the start of a fatal subarachnoid haemorrhage, a dying person has the same experience as a survivor.

Subarachnoid bleeding initiates a sudden, extraordinarily painful,

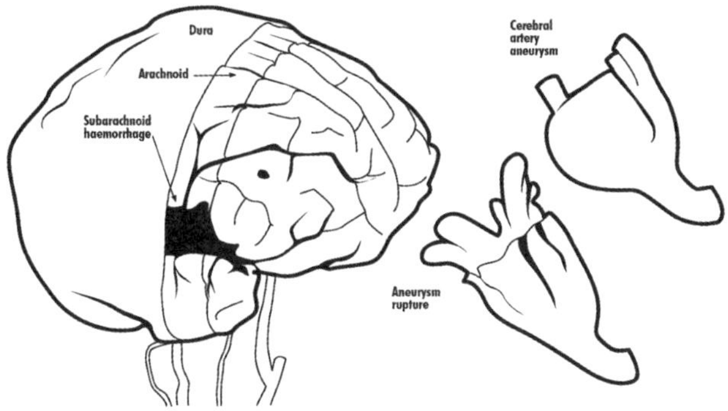

Figure 1.7:
A ruptured aneurysm can cause a subarachnoid haemorrhage.

headache typically described as a "thunderclap." Vomiting often follows. Lights bother the eyes. Neck muscles stiffen. Sometimes one side of the body weakens and goes limp. Seizures and a subsequent state of confusion may follow. Even without a seizure, lots of people still become confused. When subarachnoid haemorrhages are lethal, these symptoms don't last long before coma develops.

Blows to the head can cause subarachnoid haemorrhages, but more often bleeding arises without much trauma. Frequently a bulge (aneurysm) in a cranial arterial wall spontaneously ruptures. The aneurysm's wall is much thinner than the walls of the adjacent artery. Quite minor head movements may be enough to rupture a paper-thin aneurysm.

Most people have no idea they have an aneurysm until it bursts. In fatal cases, the rupture causes heavy bleeding. When enough blood accumulates within the skull to raise the intracranial pressure high enough, coning follows.

People who witness the onset of someone else's subarachnoid haemorrhage don't forget what happened. They never ask questions about suffering.

Subarachnoid haemorrhages are one form of haemorrhagic stroke. Another type occurs when a blood vessel in the brain ruptures into either the substance of the brain or the fluid-filled spaces that exist inside the brain. These spaces are called the cerebral ventricles. (See Figure 1.8.)

If required to talk about an unwitnessed fatal subarachnoid haemorrhage, a coroner should describe typical symptoms and the usual

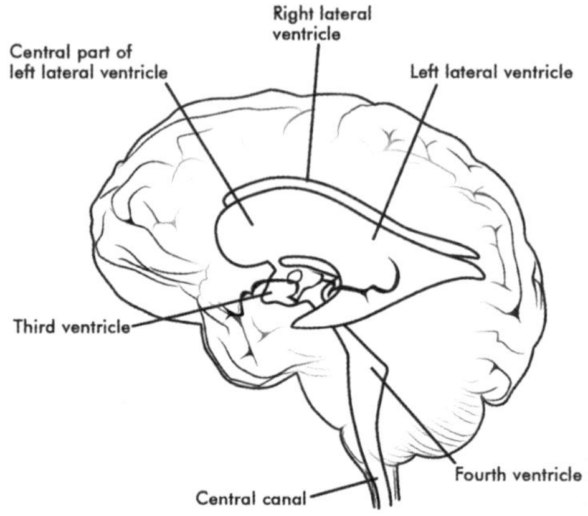

Figure 1.8: The cerebral ventricles.

course of dying. It is kindest to suggest that coma usually follows shortly after the onset of headache, which is the best-case scenario. Adding that this is not a guarantee but an optimistic, educated guess usually ends questioning on a relatively happy note.

Intracerebral Haemorrhage

Fatal bleeding also occurs in the substance of the brain itself. Its most common cause is high blood pressure. Bleeding will more likely be fatal when a person has an arteriovenous malformation (AVM) of blood vessels in the brain that disrupts normal blood flow. Equally lethal contributors to a fatal hypertensive bleed are the use of blood thinners or the existence of bleeding disorders such as haemophelia or sickle-cell anaemia. At other times brain tumours terminally rupture an artery within the substance of the brain. Most of these cases never involve a coroner.

Two types of intracerebral bleeds do come to the attention of coroners. One occurs when people develop a fatal hypertensive haemorrhage after or while they consume cocaine or methamphetamine. The other, more common, cause is trauma to the head. (See the section on Skull Fractures below.)

Regardless of the cause of the intracerebral haemorrhage, death results from coning when increased intracranial pressure eventually forces the brainstem through the foramen magnum. It is the bleed that is fatal. However, the same force that fatally tore the artery will quite often have also fractured the skull.

Families are always impressed by skull fractures, so it is important to know how to talk about cracks in the skull. Emphasize that the broken bones are associated injuries rather than the actual cause of death in most cases.

Skull Fractures

Many people believe that every skull fracture is a severe injury. In reality, most are not, and they heal with no residual complications. Coroners view skull fractures as just one component of a fatal head injury — the fracture itself is not the lethal part.

Injuries to the brain and blood vessels within the skull are what lead to death. Bits of bone from a depressed fracture may tear a blood vessel and cause bleeding. When this haemorrhage is fatal, the increasing volume of blood collecting within the skull raises the intracranial pressure. Once it rises high enough, coning starts, and death is its inevitable consequence.

The skull's bones can fracture in two different ways, both of which cause a sudden sharp headache. The more common type of fracture is a continuous linear skull fracture, which often results from the head striking a wall or the ground when falling. A similar type of fracture can be produced when any wide flat object forcefully strikes a person's head.

While most skull fractures do not cause death, coroners usually investigate the deaths in which skull fractures have occurred. Linear skull fractures (see Figure 1.9) usually become fatal when they cross an underlying blood vessel. The vessel wall is torn either by transmitted force from the blow or by the movement of a sharp cracked bone edge that cuts the blood vessel. Leakage of blood from the lacerated blood vessel into the space around the brain lethally raises the intracranial pressure.

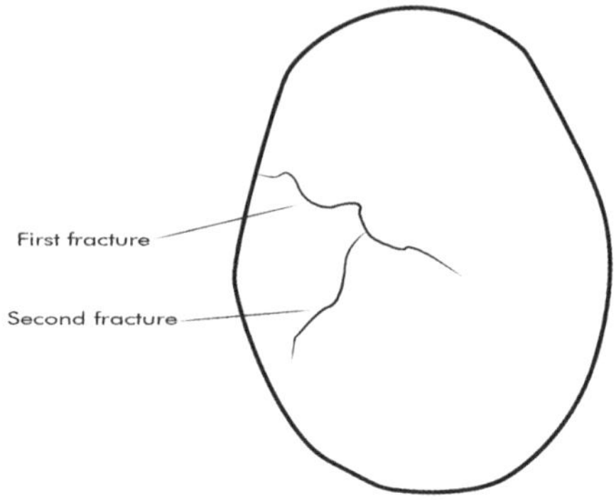

Figure 1.9: Linear skull fracture

A hard blow by a small hard object, such as a hammer, causes a depressed skull fracture. Its force cracks a ring of bone where the striking object meets the skull. The broken bits of skull push downward, frequently into the brain itself.

Bleeding is not always limited to the site of the blow. When a blow's force is transmitted to another part of the brain, bleeding occurs far

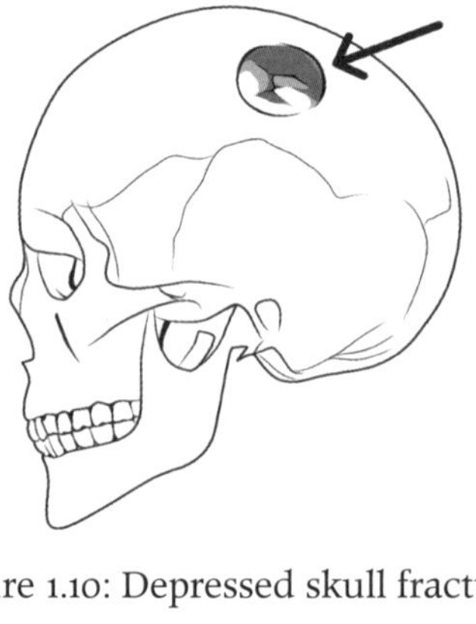

Figure 1.10: Depressed skull fracture

from the injury site. Both cases result in immediate and excruciating headaches.

Bleeding within the brain is always problematic and often fatal. When a haemorrhage does not result from a blow to the head, the blood may remain within the brain tissue itself or it may seep into the brain's surroundings. About 25% of people who experience a spontaneous intracranial haemorrhage die within two days. Another 25% die within the twenty-eight days that follow.

Coning Caused by Inadequate Blood Supply

Strokes

Haemorrhage is one way that brain death can arise from a stroke. But it is only one of three categories, two of which – haemorrhagic and ischaemic – coroners need to think about. When blood delivered to the brain lacks enough oxygen to keep the brain's neurons alive and functioning, an ischaemic stroke occurs. This can happen when a clot, called a thrombus, forms in one of the arteries that supplies oxygenated blood to some part of the brain.

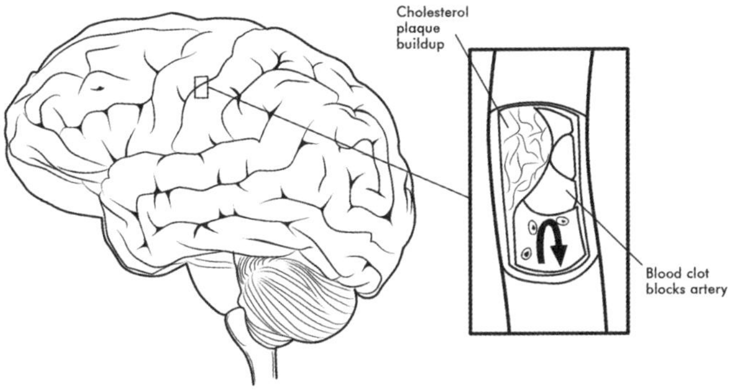

Figure 1.11: An ischaemic stroke occurs when a blood clot (thrombus) blocks an artery in the brain.

Clots can occur anywhere in the body. Should one break loose from the arterial wall where it formed in the neck, for example, the clot will be carried by the blood to a point where it wedges in an artery supplying the brain. A mobile clot is called an embolus. It has an identical make-up to a thrombus. Both stop blood flow and prevent delivery of oxygen to the brain the same way. Most ischaemic strokes do not cause headaches. Roughly 15% of ischaemic strokes cause death within thirty days of onset.

All fatal strokes are the result of the brain's nerve cells dying because of oxygen starvation. Neurologists describe the 30% to 40% of cases where no clinical cause for a stroke can be found as cryptogenic. Coroners need not worry about cryptogenic strokes — any autopsy report received will always describe a fatal stroke as either ischaemic or haemorrhagic.

Stroke symptoms start suddenly. What a person experiences between the stroke's onset and death depends on the part of brain affected. Different strokes may cause loss of movement, loss of use of an arm or leg, problems in comprehension, difficulty speaking, loss of sight, or dizziness.

How strokes produce symptoms varies. Dying brain neurons cause no pain. That is why some people experience "silent" strokes. These are likely ischaemic, but we can never know for sure since they are usually discovered long after they happen. Silent strokes occur frequently. In fact, one form of dementia occurs when multiple little silent strokes impair a brain so much that it stops functioning properly.

Ischaemic strokes frequently result from a clot developing in an area where a lump of cholesterol, called a plaque, has formed in a wall of one of the cerebral arteries (shown in Figure 1.11). At other times these strokes can also arise from emboli. As mentioned above, an embolus is a blood clot (or part of one) that originated outside the skull.

Malfunctioning chambers of the heart cause many ischaemic strokes. Atrial fibrillation commonly causes clot formation in one of the upper chambers of the heart, which will be discussed in more detail in the next chapter. A fibrillating atrium wall simply flaps instead of squeezing rhythmically. The blood in the chamber becomes turbulent and clots form. The heart's left ventricle then pumps these clots out of the heart through arteries of decreasing diameter until they can go no further and end up stuck in an artery leading to or within the brain. Many other problems, both cardiac and non-cardiac, can send emboli to the brain too.

It cannot be overemphasized that most fatal intracranial bleeds start with a terrible headache, followed by nausea, vomiting, collapse, coma and death. But in most coroners' cases, the specifics of these symptoms are not actually known, just surmised. Many stroke cases coroners investigate result from a neighbour or relative coming over for a visit discovering a dead body. This type of death is always unexpected. When the person died at home, the only way a stroke can be diagnosed is by autopsy. When the person died in hospital, in most cases the stroke will have been well delineated by a CT scan of the head.

When talking to surviving relatives about death from an intracranial haemorrhage, a coroner can honestly say that there is a good chance that the headache did not last very long. Perhaps just seconds, or minutes at most, elapsed before the person became comatose. The odds are that the decedent did not lie alive on the floor for more than a day or two — probably a much shorter time than that.

Global Brain Ischaemia

Not only localized events lead to ischaemic brain death. Diffuse brain injury or illness causes death when the whole brain, or its coverings, swell uniformly. Generalized brain swelling is called cerebral oedema and usually arises from lack of adequate blood supply (ischaemia) to the brain. In both cases the tissue and fluid volume increase within the skull resulting in death by coning. This global brain ischaemia occurs when a person's blood pressure drops so much that insufficient blood flows to the brain to keep its cells alive. Coroners often become involved in cases of global ischaemia because it is usually the result of unsuccessful resuscitation following a cardiac arrest.

All medical professionals used to call global brain ischaemia "anoxic encephalopathy." Today that term still holds currency in coroners' circles, but pathologists and some neurologists prefer either "hypoxic-ischaemic brain injury" or "brain attack." All three of these terms refer to death that results once so many neurons in the brain's areas controlling respiration and cardiac function have become so oxygen-deprived that they can no longer continue to function.

Coroners also see anoxic encephalopathy when a hanging is only partially successful. The suspended man (usually) is initially awake.

Subsequently he loses consciousness but unluckily does not die before his dangling body is discovered and cut down. The noose has deprived his brain of enough oxygen to partially asphyxiate him and kill so many neurons that death will inexorably follow.

All types of incomplete asphyxia, including near drowning, produce brain damage. Anoxic encephalopathy can also arise from exposure to a quantity of carbon monoxide or other poisonous gas that is sufficient to destroy enough brain neurons to almost — but not completely — stop most vital brain functions at the time of discovery.

The earliest time when asphyxia can happen is at birth. Too long a time elapsing between the placenta separating from the mother's uterus and a baby drawing his or her first breath causes brain damage and is termed "perinatal asphyxia." In cases coroners investigate, resuscitation usually was partially effective. Breathing, pulse and circulation may have been restored for some period of time, but consciousness was never regained.

Dying from anoxic encephalopathy triggers seizures in 50% to 70% of neonatal deaths.[7] A lack of oxygen can also produce such muscle spasms that a dying person's body contorts itself into abnormal postures. As brain damage worsens, wrists, elbows and fingers start tightly flexing while feet extend downward. This initial posture is termed "decorticate." Later on, the head arches backwards. Arms and feet become extended. This latter state, called "decerebrate rigidity", usually means that coning has started. Observers may see this shortly before the person's death, but coroners never will because death relaxes all the muscles that were in spasm.

Most coroners' investigations of anoxic encephalopathy deaths start in the intensive care unit of a hospital. Death will have been pronounced hours or days after the event that led to the coma. During the period between the incident and death, some of the brain's neurons functioned enough to barely allow vital functions to continue.

On the path to a slow death from cerebral anoxia, muscles slowly weaken. Paralysis of any sort can occur — ranging from as little as a finger that won't work properly up to and including quadriplegia (the inability to move either arms or legs). Before brain death occurs, some people experience a stage with tremors or Parkinson's-like shakes or shuffles. Others may have difficulty speaking or find themselves involuntarily flailing around.

Apart from problems finding words, almost any other conceivable cognitive abnormality could precede loss of consciousness. Some people become delirious, delusional or hallucinatory before slipping into a terminal coma.

The third uncommon type of ischaemic brain death can occur when clots arise in central veins rather than arteries. Such a death is natural and virtually never investigated by a coroner. For that reason, it is not discussed here — just mentioned for completeness.

NOTES

1 Hutchins, J. B. & Barger, S. W. (1998). Why neurons die: Cell death in the nervous system. *Anatomical Record, 253*(3), 79–90.

2 Machado, C., Korein, J., Ferrer, Y., Portela, L., de la C Garcia, M.,& Manero, J. (2007). The concept of brain death did not evolve to benefit organ transplants. *Journal of Medical Ethics, 33*(4), 197–200.

3 Guidelines for the diagnosis of brain death. (1987). *Canadian Medical Association Journal, 136*(2), 200A–200B.

4 Pallis, C. (1982). ABC of brain stem death: From brain death to brainstem death. *British Medical Journal, 285*(6353), 1487–1490.

5 Teunissen, L. L., Rinkel, G. J., Algra, A., & van Gijn, J. (1996). Risk factors for a subarachnoid hemorrhage: A systemic review. *Stroke 27*(3), 544–549.

6 Vannucci, R. C. (2000). Hypoxic-ischemic encephalopathy. *American Journal of Perinatology, 17*(3), 113–120.

7 Macher, S., Zimprich, F., De Simoni, D., Hoftberger, R., & Rommer, P. S. (2018, November 22). Management of autoimmune encephalitis: An observational monocentric study of 38 patients. *Frontiers in Immunology.*

2

Cardiac Deaths

"Heart" in day-to-day conversation is more often used as a metaphor than a reference to the living organ. The symbolic meanings related to importance, bravery and love are now so trite that people don't even perceive *heart* as a metaphor. Its wide use simply reflects the fact that everyone understands the heart is very important.

At home, health-care workers use cardiac metaphors too, but in their conversations on the job, *heart* refers only to the functioning human organ. To coroners, the word refers to an electronic pump that stopped. Among a coroner's responsibilities are figuring out how, when, where and why the heart ceased its pumping.

A heart's last beat has traditionally signalled the end of life and the starting point for a coroner's investigation. To answer the how and the why in that investigation, a coroner considers two different scenarios. In one, the heart is the principal organ that is fatally diseased or injured. In the other, heartbeats stop at the end of a cascade of events arising elsewhere in the body. Any problems of concern to coroners in this latter group are dealt with elsewhere in this book. This chapter deals only with deaths arising within the heart itself.

Cardiac Anatomy and Physiology

Savants have pondered the workings of the heart for millennia. Much has been learned, though mysteries remain. Cardiac anatomy has been understood for centuries, and now much of its physiology has also become well known. Fortunately, coroners need only know a smattering of details of the heart's anatomy and physiology to understand cardiac death.

A heart must be properly structured to ensure survival. All human hearts need four chambers. Roughly 95% of babies born missing one don't survive a month without immediate surgery to remedy the defect.[1] The heart's two upper chambers are called atria (singular atrium); the two lower two chambers are termed ventricles. These chambers momentarily store blood as it passes through the heart en route to other parts of the body.

Heart muscle fibres are unique. They synchronously contract and relax, never stopping until death. Cardiac muscle repeatedly pumps blood from an atrium through a ventricle either toward the lungs to replenish red blood cells with oxygen or into the aorta to deliver freshly oxygenated blood to the rest the body. Electricity flows through the heart to ensure muscle fibres alternately contract and relax in rhythmical fashion.

The heart's continual pumping ensures adequate freshly oxygenated blood throughout the body. This is vital. Any body part lacking oxygen will die. A normal, continual blood flow through the arteries ensures that all the body's tissues receive enough fresh oxygen to function properly.

Blood enters the heart by flowing into the right atrium, through the tricuspid valve into the right ventricle. That ventricle's contraction pumps blood through the pulmonary valve into the lungs. After its pulmonary reoxygenation, blood flows out of the lungs into the left atrium. The next heartbeat pumps newly refreshed blood through the mitral valve into the left ventricle. From there it flows through the aortic valve into the aorta and then on to the rest of the body. Thus, the four cardiac valves lead into and out of the ventricles. Valve damage can cause death. This is a less common cause than when the heart's muscle fibres die or its electrical system malfunctions.

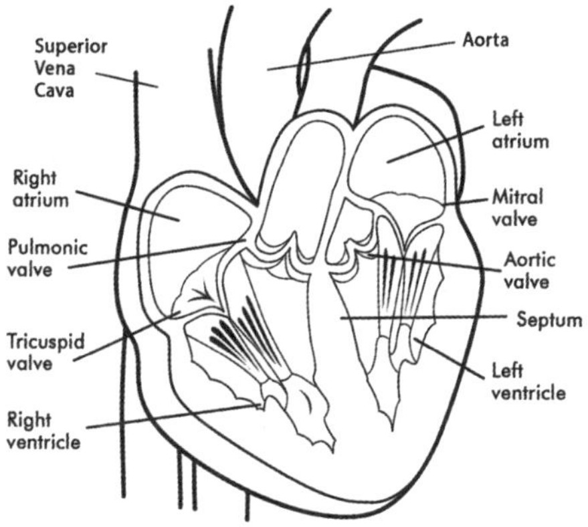

Figure 2.1: The major structures of the heart

The left ventricle is the heart's biggest chamber; it contains many more muscle fibres than the other three chambers. The reason for its size is that extra muscle power is needed to pump freshly oxygenated blood around the whole body. Regular electric impulses control this pumping process. Disturbing continuous electrical flow to the left ventricle can be fatal.

Fortunately for human survival, the heart beats involuntarily. Alternating electrical flows repeatedly cause heart muscle fibres to contract and relax throughout a lifetime. The conscious mind has little or nothing to do with starting or stopping a heartbeat. People normally do not even think about their heart beating.

But both voluntary and involuntary activities do speed up or slow down the heart. Running in a race is a voluntary, stressful activity that increases the body's need for oxygen. A sprinter arising from the starting blocks quickly develops a "racing" heart that beats rapidly until hitting the finish line slows the pace from a run to a walk. Athletes consider their race-long pounding heartbeats quite normal.

People who are experiencing a panic attack also become aware that their hearts are beating and tend to think that their rates have sped up too. This is sometimes true, but often not. Though a panic attack is unexpected and an involuntary activity, some of its sensations are similar to those felt by a sprinter.

Relaxation involuntarily slows heartbeats. When exercise stops, the heart rate slows automatically without any need to think about it. However, control of the heart rate is not totally unconscious. Through centuries of meditation Tibetan lamas have learned to temporarily slow beating hearts.[2] Even lamas can only pause heartbeats momentarily though, or life will end very quickly.

The heart's initial controlling electrical impulse arises from a clump of nervous tissue called the sinoatrial node (see Figure 2.2). From there electricity travels across the atria contracting their muscle fibres along the way. The bulk of the current proceeds to the atrioventricular node, another clump of nervous tissue located where the four heart chambers meet. Then the current moves down the septum — the muscular divider between the two ventricles. From there it proceeds around the bottom of the heart up the outer walls of the ventricles.

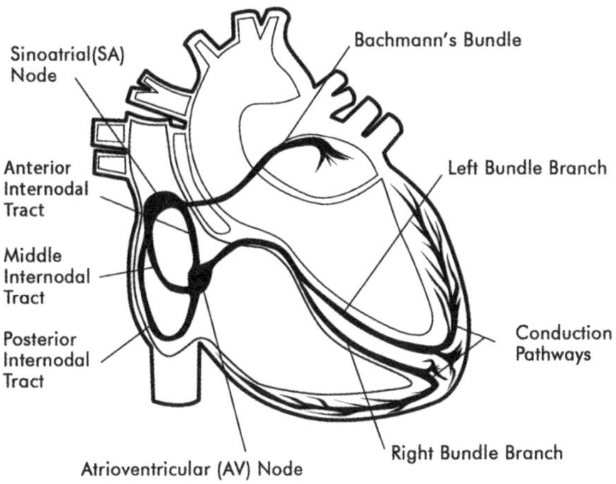

Figure 2.2: The heart's electrical conduction system

The resultant jolt of electricity makes cardiac muscle fibres contract and pump blood out of the ventricles. Once a ventricle has pumped out all its blood and the electrical impulse is spent, cardiac muscle fibres relax. The chambers fill up with blood again and the process repeats itself.

Life goes on uneventfully provided these electrical currents regularly contract and relax the heart's muscle fibres. Should the current become very irregular or cease completely, pumping stops and the heart becomes still. Cardiac standstill is always the terminal event in any death. When the cause arises within the heart the reason is usually malfunction in the heart's electrical system.

All human tissues, including the heart, need arteries to continually deliver blood containing adequate oxygen to them to keep them functioning. Since the coronary arteries (see Figure 2.3) are nature's vehicles for delivering oxygen to heart muscle fibres, these arteries are very important. They are wrapped around the heart's outer wall to deliver oxygen to the heart's muscle fibres. Without adequate oxygen in the blood delivered by these vital coronary arteries, cardiac muscle fibres will die.

The heart's electrical conducting system is outlined in dashes in Figure 2.3.

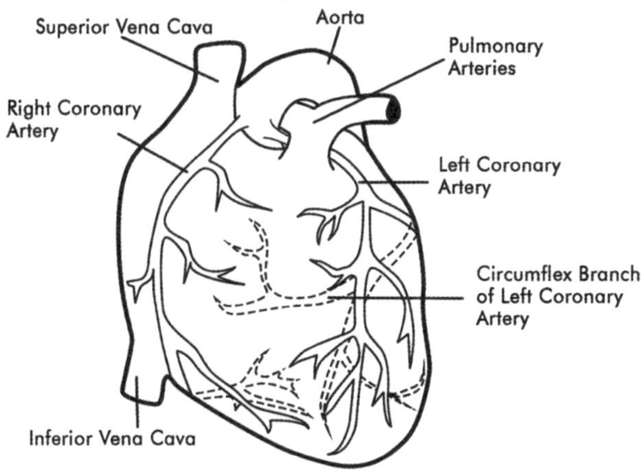

Figure 2.3: The arteries of the heart. The dashed lines show the heart's electrical conducting system.

That is all the cardiac anatomy and physiology you need to know to understand cardiac death.

Methods of Dying

Though there are many sources of detailed information about different cardiac ailments, coroners are repeatedly asked questions about cardiac deaths. Each lethal heart condition follows a different pathway to death, but all result in cardiac standstill once heartbeats stop. Symptoms felt by those who survive a major cardiac incident are likely the same as felt by those who did not make it. Luck is often the only difference between life or death.

Most people colloquially refer to any type of cardiac death as a heart attack. Coroners sometimes use that term in speaking to relatives about deaths arising from coronary artery disease, but they do not use it when talking with their colleagues. Physicians and coroners talk to each other about a myocardial infarction. The terms *heart attack* and *myocardial infarction* can sometimes be synonymous, but that is not always the case in public colloquial discourse.

Myocardial Infarction

Myocardial infarctions (MIs) are common in Europe and North America. About 30% are fatal.[3] Many are totally unexpected. Sudden death may be the first sign of any heart problem, although that's not the usual case. MIs arise in people with diseased coronary arteries. Warning signs of the underlying coronary artery disease frequently precede an MI's onset for quite a long time.

Long before it comes, many people destined for a fatal MI develop fatigue, become short of breath, or feel some form of mild discomfort in their chest, back, abdomen or jaw. Many people do not connect these sensations to the heart. In other cases, either consciously or subconsciously, people deny that a cardiac cause for these symptoms could be possible.

For example, let's look at fatigue. Most people do not connect fatigue with heart disease. More often it's the result of working too hard, not getting enough sleep or feeling a bit depressed. These types of problems occur much more frequently than a myocardial infarction. In addition, people know from experience that fatigue is usually inconsequential. Rest or changing activity make it go away. People who are overweight frequently attribute fatigue to their excess weight or to their being out of shape. Though people don't connect feeling tired with a future fatal MI, fatigue commonly precedes one at some point.

Now consider shortness of breath. When an MI impairs the heart's ability to pump, fluid backs up in the lungs and breathing becomes very difficult. Severe breathlessness isn't easily forgotten, but mild shortness of breath is easily misinterpreted or ignored. Older people or diabetics frequently initially attribute their shortness of breath to their age or to having diabetes. Yet doctors equate shortness of breath to anginal heart pain when assessing the severity of coronary artery disease.[4] With fatal myocardial infarctions, respiratory distress commonly precedes death.

Severe pain is one heart attack symptom people usually don't ignore. Both metabolic by-products of oxygen-starved or dying cardiac muscle fibres and spasms of the coronary arteries trigger a pain called angina. Though angina may quickly come and go leaving no significant damage to the heart musculatures, it portends a future fatal heart attack. Angina does not precede every MI, but some variant of its pain commonly accompanies dying from one.

The sensations angina produces vary. Sometimes it is indigestion-like or a bloated feeling. At other times the front of the chest hurts, or perhaps the back. Angina can radiate to the jaw, either arm, or the abdomen. The discomfort may resemble mild indigestion, making spicy food, constipation or a muscle strain seem a more likely cause than a cardiac problem.

Other than immediately before an MI, anginal pain is transient. Should a visit to a doctor's office reveal coronary artery disease to be the cause of angina, a future fatal heart attack becomes a real possibility. Intermittent anginal pain is the transient version of the steady pain dying cardiac muscle produces during an MI. The more muscle fibres that die during the myocardial infarction the more severe the pain is likely to be.

Improved medical care in the developed world has greatly increased heart attack survival once in hospital. The experiences of MI survivors tell us that the quality and intensity of a heart attack's discomfort varies enormously. Most myocardial infarctions hurt — but not all. Nobody forgets severe pain, yet some people have no inkling that part of their heart muscle is dying.

Many people expect the pain of an MI to resemble the classical description taught to every medical student. It goes something like this: a dull, heavy, squeezing pain begins in the left side of the chest or behind the sternum (breastbone). The pain radiates into an arm, more often the left, but sometimes the right. It may spread into the back, the pit of the stomach and even into the jaw. Beads of sweat develop on the forehead. Breathing becomes fast, shallow and generally difficult. It often feels like a heavy weight pressing down on the chest.

When these symptoms come on but disappear without any muscle fibres dying, the pain is simply angina. The pain plus muscle death signifies a myocardial infarction.

This classical description of this type of heart attack is also accompanied by a classical description of its victim — an overweight, middle-aged male who smokes and gets no exercise. While many who experience an MI fit that bill, even more don't. Far from it. Heart attack pains can affect anyone. Women, especially those past child-bearing age, frequently experience far less discomfort than do men at the onset of an MI. Doctors investigating a post-menopausal woman's complaints of indigestion, bloating, burning, aches, or any upper abdominal sensation must always consider the possibility that the sensations arise from atypical angina or even an MI.

Women aren't alone in experiencing other-than-classical heart attack symptoms. Many a man's routine electrocardiogram has revealed a previously unknown myocardial infarction. Occasionally the MI's timing can be divined by reflecting on past unexplained symptoms. More often, when it happened remains a mystery. Cardiologists call these silent myocardial infarctions.

Before discussing the intensity of any pain experienced by someone who had any sort of a cardiac death, particularly due to MI, a coroner needs to let the questioner talk as much as possible before replying. The coroner's response should be carefully phrased.

Coroners draw on the experiences of myocardial infarction survivors to talk about the likely pain experienced when dying from an MI. A coroner should never, ever catastrophize. The type and intensity of MI pain varies widely. This allows a coroner to honestly mention that an MI is sometimes painless. A coroner needs to keep the questioner's emotional state in mind before commenting on the level of pain that might have been experienced while dying. Surviving relatives may be experiencing significant distress. Their upset tends to be greater the more sudden and unexpected the death.

Minimizing the pain experienced by the deceased while dying probably provides relatives with some solace. People create all sorts of mental scenarios to minimize their emotional discomfort. Anyone so inclined will seize on the coroner's words to imagine a relatively pleasant death. The coroner's words can help shape that mental image to be a comforting one. The person's subconscious is quite aware that nobody can prove the image in their mind wrong because only the dead person knew what was actually felt.

Words a coroner utters at the death scene are never forgotten. That's why it's best to avoid discussion about the pain experienced in dying when possible. If the topic can't be avoided, make it clear that any discussion must be hypothetical. If asked, by all means acknowledge myocardial infarctions may cause a person to sweat, grunt, wince or experience something much worse, but also emphasize that the degree of pain that preceded death might have been minimal.

Seeking a detailed pathophysiological path to death is sometimes part of a relative's grieving process. Nobody expects a coroner to know everything about a death, but all relatives want some information. An adequate answer needs only basic knowledge about myocardial infarctions. Talk simply and be wary of any protracted conversation. Some questioners will know more about the cause of death than the coroner. A coroner who cannot answer a question should freely admit it, change the topic, or end the conversation.

Any discussion about dying should be limited to the mechanical causes of cardiac death only. Even if you know some of the physiology, don't speculate on whether or how passage of ions (atoms lacking an electron) through cell membranes might lead to death. Coroners should stick to anatomy, simple physiology, and gross pathology. Molecular discussions about dying are outside a coroner's expertise. Any response is more credible when it includes an admission that an area is beyond the limit of your knowledge.

Families can be told that coronary artery disease arising from cholesterol accumulating in coronary arteries (see Figure 2.4) will cause death in young people occasionally. To convince doubting listeners, coroners can point out that autopsies on young American soldiers during the Korean War found that these previously healthy young men already had multiple cholesterol plaques in their coronary arteries.[5] Parents are usually only convinced after a pathologist proves coronary artery disease by autopsy.

They may ask, "Why does this occur?" It isn't only age that leads to plaque development. Bad genes, smoking, lack of exercise, and overeating fatty foods all speed atherosclerotic plaque development. People often identify one or more of these factors in their dead relative. Family members frequently tell coroners how they counselled stopping some behaviour they frowned upon or "It would be the death of

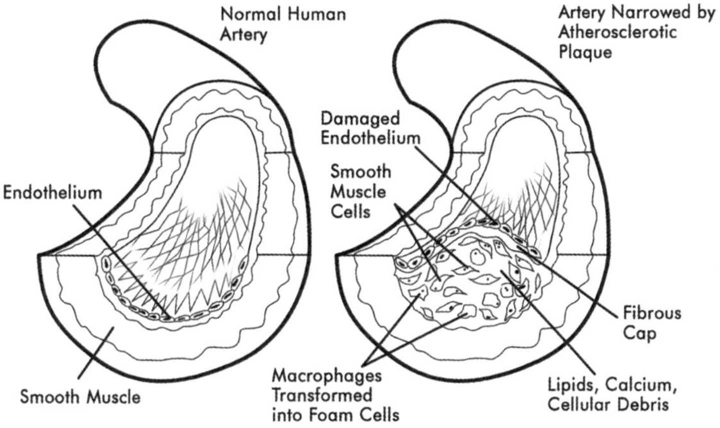

Figure 2.4: Cholesterol plaque builds up in arteries.

him." These relatives expected an atherosclerotic cardiac death. They ask no questions. Others need more explanation than just "death from atherosclerosis."

A coroner could safely say that cholesterol deposits in a coronary artery wall can lead to fatal cardiac massage in the following sequence of steps. They bulge the arterial wall and narrow a coronary artery's diameter, which allows less blood to flow past the deposits. The narrowed arterial lumen (the empty space in the tube) permits less oxygen-rich blood to flow to the cardiac muscle fibres. As their oxygen supply wanes, these heart muscle fibres start to die.

Red blood cells swirling around the cholesterol plaques form an eddy that create clots and stop arterial blood flow. Blood flow can also stop when cholesterol plaques rupture into the artery, as shown in Figure 2.5. A large enough plaque completely blocks blood flow right away. A smaller rupture causes turbulence that develops into a clot that then causes total blockage of arterial blood flow. When blood stops flowing through the artery cardiac muscle quickly becomes starved of oxygen. Eventually, all cardiac muscle fibres nourished by the blocked artery die.

Dying cardiac muscle ends life completely in three different ways. Sometimes the heart's electrical flow becomes irregular and then ceases, completely stopping the heart from pumping. In other cases, those cardiac muscle fibres that remain alive are too weak to circulate

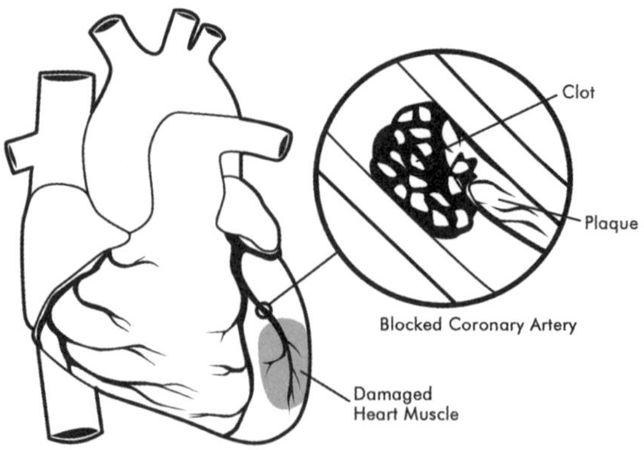

Figure 2.5: A ruptured cholesterol plaque may form a clot that blocks arterial blood flow.

enough oxygenated blood to keep the body's tissues operating. The third route to cardiac death is rupture of a dying heart's wall, which allows blood to pour out and disrupts the heart's electrical system at the same time.

Electrical Failure

During regular flow of an electrical current through the heart, cardiac muscle fibres alternately contract and relax in unison. During contraction blood is pumped from the heart into the aorta or into the lungs. When the heart muscle fibres relax, the heart's chambers simply refill with more blood.

There are many possible disturbances to regular electrical flow through the heart. A coroner need not know most of them because they are not lethal. They become fatal when the rhythm switches into ventricular fibrillation (see Figure 2.6). Pumping stops because instead of ventricular muscle rhythmically contracting and relaxing it simply flaps.

To compare the heart's action in ventricular fibrillation to a normal rhythm, carry out this demonstration. Cup one hand as though holding an orange. Make a fist. Then open and close it repeatedly. That movement represents the normal pumping function of a heart. Then hold one hand cupped while rapidly rotating the same wrist. The hand

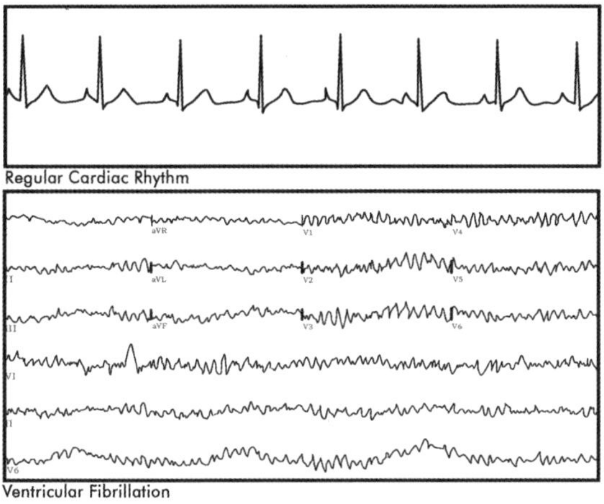

Figure 2.6: Regular cardiac rhythm and ventricular fibrillation appear quite different on an ECG.

appears to flap. An observer can see clearly that pumping has ceased and that anything that might have been contained in the cupped hand simply stays put. Explaining what the movements represent in the heart while going through the demonstration makes the effect of ventricular fibrillation quite clear to onlookers.

The reason for a heart's electrical failure is always speculative — nobody knows what causes ventricular fibrillation. The reason why the heart's electrical current stops is also often unknown. One trigger is certainly inadequate blood flow in a coronary artery that deprives some part of the heart of oxygen. Blocked coronary arteries somehow trigger ventricular fibrillation or other electrical rhythms that stop the heart from pumping when a myocardial infarction becomes fatal.

Scar tissue created by a healed myocardial infarction or cardiac surgery may block normal electrical flow, and this is sometimes fatal. Without extensive knowledge of prior cardiac investigations or a cardiac pathologist's autopsy of the heart, a coroner has no basis for a hypothesis about any electrical arrhythmia causing death. With that background information it may be possible, though inadvisable, to speculate about the mechanism of death. Without it, offer no opinion.

Coroners shouldn't really need a reminder not to discuss any possible roles serum electrolytes might play in a heart's electrical failure.

Electrolytes are salts. Sodium, calcium, magnesium and potassium salts that cross cell membranes facilitate electrical flow in the heart. Excess potassium ions, in particular, are often associated with fatal cardiac arrhythmias, but exactly why is uncertain.

It's widely known that the body's adrenaline increases when excited. Adrenaline, a word used colloquially, is the former name for a hormone in the catecholamine family that is now called epinephrine. When too many catecholamines overstimulate cardiac muscle fibres a fatal cardiac arrhythmia ensues.

Cocaine and various types of amphetamines bought for recreational abuse can trigger fatal cardiac rhythms. After ingesting these drugs, the heart continues to beat regularly as long as a single focus initiates the beats. When the drugs start to trigger electrical impulses from multiple points in the heart, the ventricular muscle starts to fibrillate and stops pumping. An immediate loss of consciousness is followed by death minutes later.

Coroners are rarely asked about exactly how substance abuse kills. Knowing death arose from drug abuse is usually enough for family members. If pursued about this rather esoteric subject, admit you don't know much about it. Direct the questioner to a physician for an answer. Wikipedia also provides accurate information.

A coroner should not attribute death to any specific cardiac electrical cause other than to talk about a fatal arrhythmia. Such an arrhythmia's most common cause is an as yet undiscovered process resulting from atherosclerotic heart disease. In a much smaller number of cases, fatal arrhythmias arise in people with a genetic predisposition to their development.* Some of the genes responsible have now been discovered, and whenever a genetic cause is suspect, such as a sudden teenage death, further investigation should be undertaken by a geneticist.

Longstanding high blood pressure is the second most common cause of fatal cardiac arrhythmias. The longer this hypertension lasts the harder it becomes for the heart to keep pumping blood around the body. Continual pressure from pushing blood against increasingly

* Family members may talk to you about Long QT syndrome, Short QT syndrome, Brugada syndrome, Catecholaminergic Polymorphic Ventricular Tachycardia, Wolfe Parkinson White syndrome, and Torsade de Pointe arrhythmias. They will probably know more about these arrhythmias than the coroner, so just listen.

stiff arterial walls enlarges the left ventricle's muscle wall. The larger the ventricle becomes, the more likely a fatal cardiac arrhythmia is to develop, though nobody knows why.*

Fatal cardiac arrhythmias arise in both congenital heart disease and a group of heart conditions called cardiomyopathies. Cardiomyopathies may have a genetic basis, but most follow a viral infection of the heart muscle. There is no explanation for why a fatal cardiac arrhythmia develops in either case.

Valvular heart disease also causes sudden cardiac death. This is particularly true of a disease called aortic stenosis. Theories exist why this condition causes death, but a coroner need not know them. There are four heart valves. Disease in any one of them could trigger a fatal arrhythmia, but aortic stenosis is the most common. Refer persistent questioners to a cardiologist for the latest theories.

In summary, while failures in the cardiac electrical system have no simple explanations, their consequences can be simply explained. Any time the heart's electrical system ceases to function for any reason, death follows within five minutes.

Pump Failure

Changes to the heart muscle alter the organ's ability to pump properly. To help explain to a family member how a relative died when the heart became unable to pump any longer, a coroner should talk about death arising from one of the following three changes in the heart:

1. The heart muscle became too thin.
2. The heart muscle became too thick.
3. One or more valves was damaged.

An autopsy clearly reveals whether one or more of these changes occurred. When there has been no autopsy, talk about these three common types of pump failure in general terms as possibilities.

---

* Some hypothesize a mechanism similar to the way a high potassium level in the blood causes ventricular fibrillation. However, that's not very helpful because that process is not yet really understood. Don't even talk about it. Just say large hypertensive hearts sometimes cause sudden death from ventricular fibrillation.

Ventricles that either thin or become thicker pump less well. Let's start with the ventricular muscle getting thinner. Thinning heart muscle leads to an enlarged heart, which is described as a dilated cardiomyopathy.

The most common reason for weakened (too-thin) heart walls is coronary artery disease. Diabetes mellitus and viral infections are other causes. Diseased valves, years of excessive alcohol consumption, hypothyroidism and hepatitis also can produce a dilated heart.

Thin cardiac muscle can't pump blood as well as when it has normal thickness. Heart walls that are little thicker than a piece of paper can still pump out just enough blood to keep body tissues alive.

High-pressured blood pushing against the walls inside heart chambers will dilate both atria and ventricles. The larger these chambers become the greater the volume of blood inside the heart. Pumping more blood makes the heart's muscle work harder. The muscle eventually weakens, which slows down the movement of oxygenated blood from the lungs into the left side of the heart and then into the aorta to circulate around the body. In turn, this causes the blood pressure in the arteries running through the lungs to increase. Components of the blood's plasma ooze out of the arteries into the air sacs (alveolae) of the lungs, as shown in Figure 2.7.

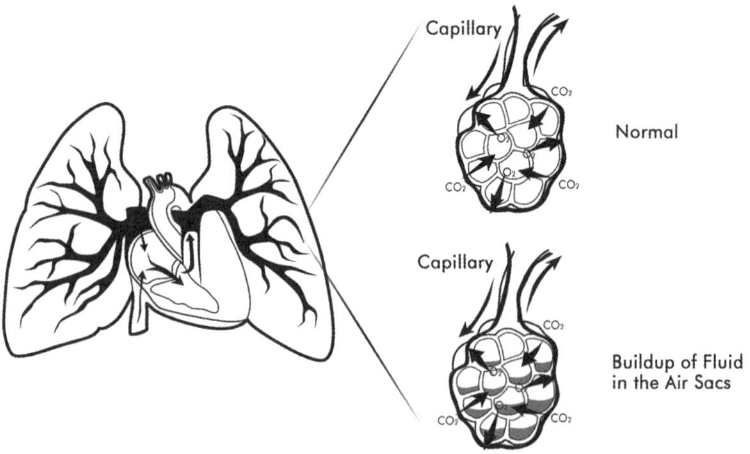

Figure 2.7: The shaded areas in the diagram at the bottom right represent fluid that has built up in the alveolae of the lungs.

At this point, the person has developed congestive heart failure. Fluid spreads throughout the alveolae, but gravity initially pulls it to the bottom of the lungs. As the heart's pumping weakens, fluid fills alveoli higher up the lungs and breathing becomes increasingly difficult.

Once most of the lungs' alveoli fill up with fluid, congestive heart failure turns into pulmonary oedema. Blood leaving the lungs contains so little oxygen that a person asphyxiates. This smothering creates great anxiety in a person who is still conscious, but it's not a particularly painful way of dying when consciousness is lost in a short time. People experiencing acute pulmonary oedema frequently seem aware they will shortly die.

Deaths from longstanding congestive heart failure are rarely investigated by coroners, whereas some cases of acute pulmonary oedema (a large, sudden fluid build-up in both lungs) are. In the absence of, and even with, appropriate medical attention, pulmonary oedema can lead to death within minutes. Coroners' cases usually involve deaths of people found at home or in the outdoors. Coroners who investigate these deaths often recognize pulmonary oedema from dried bubbles on the lips.

Since most of these deaths are unwitnessed, it is impossible to determine how long it took the person to die. The period of dying may have been relatively short and relatively painless. Pointing that out comforts some relatives. If a conversation gets into sensations felt before death, a coroner should focus on discomfort — dullness settling in the chest — and avoid talking about the fear of suffocation.

Congestive heart failure occurs when the heart weakens and thins, but it can also occur when the heart muscle gets larger, which is called hypertrophic cardiac myopathy. Large hearts develop in athletes; among non-athletes, sometimes their cause is genetic, but their origin is often a mystery. Enlarged heart muscle can cause death in different ways. Fatal cardiac failure may result from thickened cardiac muscle preventing blood flow through the aortic valve. Ventricles may become too stiff to properly pump blood out of the heart anymore, and people die of pump failure for that reason. Hypertrophic cardiomyopathy also put people at risk of arrhythmia and sudden death.

Stiff ventricles are not only found in hypertrophic cardiomyopathy. They also occur in a group of conditions that are called restrictive cardiomyopathies, the cause of which is usually unknown. Less common but known causes of fatally stiffened ventricles include scarring from prior cardiac disease, radiation, chemotherapy, and some heart transplants. Coroners usually only investigate these deaths in people discovered to have unexpectedly died at home.

Diseases such as sarcoidosis, haemochromatosis and amyloidosis deposit stiffening material into ventricular walls. Again, coroners only investigate these deaths when a death occurred unexpectedly outside hospital. Unless known to surviving relatives the diagnosis will be made by autopsy. People with one of these diseases die in a similar way to anyone afflicted with any other cardiomyopathy. Many will have been treated for congestive heart failure for a long time without knowing its reason.

When the stiffening deposit occurs in the papillary muscles attached to cardiac valves (see Figure 2.8), or even in the valves themselves, a person has valvular heart disease. Once stiffened aortic or mitral valves limit the flow of blood through them fatal congestive heart failure develops. But note that these diseases are not the most common causes of valvular heart disease — most valves simply degenerate with age.

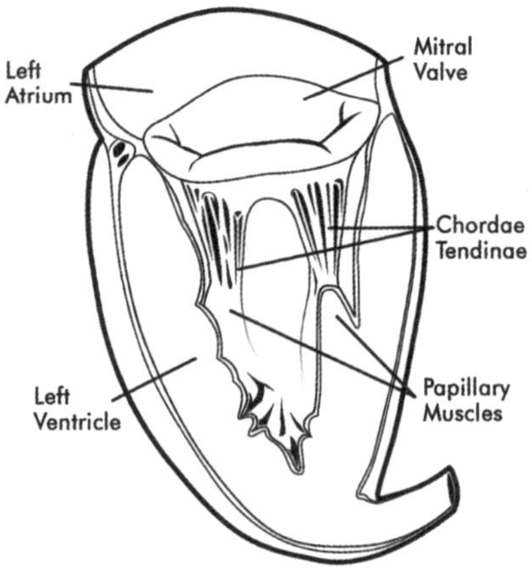

Figure 2.8: The papillary muscles are attached to the heart's valves.

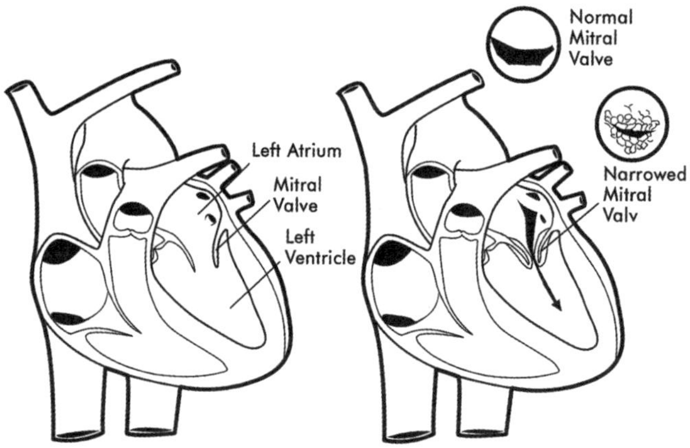

Figure 2.9: Compare the healthy mitral valve on the left to the significantly narrowed one on the right.

Infections such as rheumatic fever, syphilis and bacterial endocarditis also fatally damage heart valves. Myocardial infarctions damage valves just as they do any other tissue in the heart. Longstanding high blood pressure damages valves too. The damaged valve may change shape in a way that prevents the valve's leaflets from closing tightly anymore or narrows the aperture through which blood must flow (see Figure 2.9). As a result, sometimes blood flows backwards through the valve with each beat. Untreated, these valve changes lead to years of congestive heart failure before death results.

Congestive heart failure is not the only way valvular heart disease kills. While most people die over a period of years, others die suddenly when the heart's electrical system produces a fatal arrhythmia. Sometimes turbulence in the blood flow around damaged valves causes clots to develop with fatal results, especially when large ones enter the lungs and block the pulmonary arteries. Clots flowing from the heart into the aorta become fatal by causing strokes.

Higher pressure in the left side of the heart damages the left-side valves faster, which makes aortic stenosis and mitral stenosis the two most common causes of valvular fatality. Nowadays operations have been developed to fix them.

Cardiac Surgery

Cardiac surgery is one area of medicine that has made rapid strides in the past half century. Damaged valves can now be replaced with human, pig, or artificial valves.

Installing a new heart valve is risky surgery, often performed in old, unhealthy people. Though dying is an obvious risk of such surgery, in only about 2% of operations does a patient die on the operating table or shortly afterwards.[6] Coroners may be notified of these deaths, but they usually do not investigate them. Death is a known complication of risky surgery. The review of such a death is more appropriately carried out by the hospital's cardiac surgery department.

Replacement valves do not last forever either. Tissue valves usually only last 10 to 20 years.[7] If not replaced, death can be expected from the grafted valve loosening, clot development causing a fatal stroke or pulmonary embolus, and/or sepsis when infection collects around the graft. Both sepsis and emboli usually cause death in people with artificial valves who stop taking anticoagulant medication to prevent clotting. Coroners won't investigate these deaths any more frequently than they will investigate deaths in valve replacements.

Ruptured Wall

A "broken heart" is a metaphor common to romance novels and grocery checkout-counter celebrity magazines that refer to the end of a romantic relationship. Real hearts actually do break, though a pathologist reporting one describes the heart as "ruptured." That word is chosen because it is a better description of the injury than a "tear" or a "shatter."

The consistency of a heart's wall changes following a myocardial infarction. Through the process of fibrosis, dead muscle fibres turn into scar tissue. Usually the heart wall fibroses uneventfully, but the period right after the heart muscle fibres die is dangerous. Dead muscle fibres are very weak until they turn into scar tissue.

One factor that determines whether these weak muscle fibres will rupture is the heart wall's thickness. Scar tissue forms uneventfully in heart walls of average thickness; the heart returns to normal function and life goes on.

However, when cardiac wall muscle is thin just the pressure of circulating blood may be enough to rip apart dead muscle fibres. Blood will then quickly gush through the tear into the pericardial sac surrounding the heart. Death is sudden because the heart stops pumping.

Two factors are involved in this type of death. First, a large volume of blood collecting in the pericardial sac squeezes the heart. This pressure could become enough to prevent any more pumping action even if the heart's electrical system tries to keep it beating. Second, electrical conduction is usually disrupted too – pumping stops right away, consciousness is lost immediately, and death follows in a few minutes. A large tear in dead heart muscle probably doesn't hurt much. No living nerve fibres would remain to conduct any pain message to the brain. Only if the tear involves living tissue could pain accompany the rupture.

A smaller rent in cardiac muscle that simply allowed blood seepage into the pericardial sac would likely be painful, unless it disabled the heart's electrical conduction system enough to stop it beating. A tiny stab wound to the heart muscle, say with an ice pick or a slightly larger implement, that does not affect the heart's capacity to continue beating has a similar effect. Pain would be felt while the ice pick cut through the skin, muscles, and any bone margin (periosteum) on the way into the heart. Most pain would come from injured tissue around the heart. If the person remained conscious as blood slowly collected in the pericardial sac, he or she would feel an increasing pressure and increasingly sharp pain from the build-up of blood. Even if the person stabbed were not the anxious type, increasing anxiety and a much faster heart rate would accompany the heart's increasing difficulty to pump. Gradually worsening anxiety and discomfort would only end with loss of consciousness.

External Mechanical Obstruction

Pressure build-up from blood entering the space between the pericardial sac and the heart though a slow leak from a small hole in the cardiac muscle is one way that increasing pressure around the heart muscle stops it beating. Large holes cause sudden death.

A virus inflaming the sac, or pericardium, wrapped around the outside of the heart produces a slower death. This sac always has a drop or so of lubricant between the pericardium and cardiac muscle to allow the pericardium to slide smoothly over the cardiac muscle. Only once pericarditis starts do a few drops of lubricating fluid turn into millilitres fluid that can become lethal.

Fluid build-up within the pericardial sac may be rapid, but more often it accumulates slowly, causing a sharp chest pain that worsens with each breath. As time goes on an increasing chest heaviness develops, and the heart starts to beat faster. A volume of fluid so large that it affects the function of the heart is called a cardiac tamponade; see Figure 2.10. This tamponade becomes lethal once the fluid collected around the heart causes the heart to pump so little blood that shock develops. At that point the person, if still alert, collapses and loses consciousness.

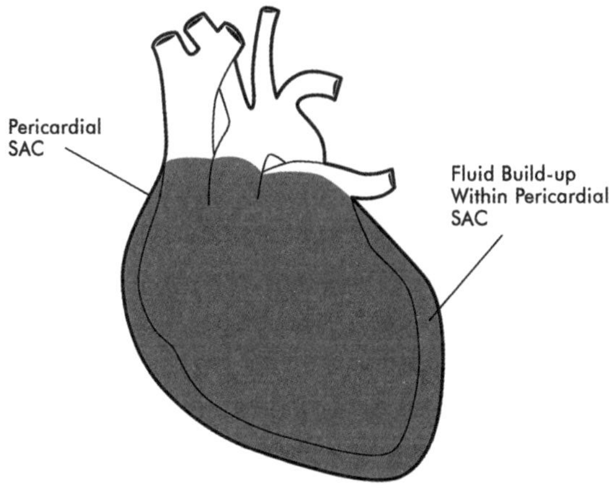

Figure 2.10: Cardiac tamponade

Pericardial fluid accumulation may go on for days. As the heart becomes increasingly dysfunctional, anxiety and even a sense of doom develops. These sensations only end with loss of consciousness. Pain may be less distressing than the anxiety pericarditis creates. People with a terminal pericardial effusion cannot figure out why they are suffering increasing shortness of breath, chest discomfort, and loss of energy and immobility.

Roughly 90% of fatal cardiac tamponades are caused by a ruptured heart resulting from a myocardial infarction or a ruptured ascending aortic aneurysm. The remaining 10% of cases[8] can arise from any one of the following reasons, including:

- metastasized cancer (Cancer that metastasizes to the pericardium can produce a fatal pericardial effusion.)
- severe kidney failure
- a tear or dissection of the aorta just below the aortic valve (This causes sudden death.)
- regular myocardial infarctions
- viruses
- bacteria (In Africa, tuberculosis is a common cause.)
- lupus erythematosis
- severe blunt chest trauma
- complications arising from many cardiac surgeries

Regardless of the specific cause of cardiac tamponade, all people die the same way.

It is hard to get a handle on precisely how many people die from a pericardial tamponade because most of the causes are due to a ruptured heart resulting from a myocardial infarction. Coroners almost never investigate deaths from fatal pericardial tamponade that develop after an operation on the heart, because pericardial tamponade is a known complication in many cardiac surgeries.

Taken as a whole, cardiac deaths are probably the most common cause of death in most developed countries. Percentages vary. In the United Kingdom, United States, Australia, New Zealand and Canada, the rates for cardiac death are between 25% and 30% of all deaths. In Europe the figures are a bit higher at 40% to 50%.[9]

This chapter deals with natural cardiac death. Fatal gunshots and stab wounds through the heart are dealt with in Chapter 21.

Now let us turn from the heart to the lungs.

NOTES

1 Fruitman, D. S. (2000). Hypoplastic left heart syndrome: Progress and management options. *Paediatrics & Child Health, 5*(4) 219–225.

2 Jiang, H., He, B., Guo, X., Wang, X., Guo, M., Wang, Z., … Cui, D. (2020). Brain–heart interactions underlying traditional Tibetan Buddhist meditation. *Cerebral Cortex, 30*(2), 439–450.

3 Smolina, K., Wright, F. L., Rayner, M., & Goldacre, M. J. (2012). Incidence and 30-day case fatality for acute myocardial infarction in England in 2010: National-linked database study. (2012). *European Journal of Public Health, 22*(6), 848–853.

4 Paudel, R., Beridze, N., Aronow, W. S., Ahn, C., Sanaani, A., Agarwal, P., … Panza, J. A. (2016). Association of chest pain versus dyspnea as presenting symptom for coronary angiography with demographics, coronary anatomy, and 2-year mortality. *Achives of Medical Science, 12*(6), 742–746.

5 Virmani, R., Robinowitz, M., Geer, J. C., Breslin, P. P., Beyer, J. C., & McAllister, H. A. (1987). Coronary artery atherosclerosis revisited in Korean war combat casualties. *Archives of Pathology & Laboratory Medicine, 111*(10), 972–976.

6 D'Agostino, R. S., Jacobs, J. P., Badhwar, V., Fernandez, F. G., Paone, G., Wormuth, D. W., & Shahian, D. M. (2018). The Society of Thoracic Surgeons Adult Cardiac Surgery Database: 2018 update of outcomes and quality. *The Annals of Thoracic Surgery, 105*(1), 15–23.

7 Hoffmann, G., Lutter, G., & Cremer, J. (2008). Durability of bioprosthetic cardiac valves. *Deutsches Arzteblatt International, 105*(8), 143–146.

8 Swaminathan, A., Kandaswamy, K., Powari, M., & Mathew, J. (2007). Dying from cardiac tamponade. *World Journal of Emergency Surgery, 22*. doi: N10.1186/1749-7922-2-22

9 Nowbar, A. N., Gitto, M., Howard, J. P., Francis, D. P., & Al-Lamee, R. (2019). Mortality from ischemic heart disease. *Circulation: Cardiovascular Quality and Outcomes, 12*(6). doi: 10.1161/CIRCOUTCOMES.118.005375

3

Respiratory Deaths

All humans need air to stay alive. Should they stop breathing it, death follows in minutes. Air is composed of almost 80% nitrogen and a little more than 20% oxygen. It is the oxygen in air that is the key to life. Whenever they cannot breathe in enough oxygen, people suffocate. While the coroner's definition of *suffocation* follows below, most people use the word colloquially in this fashion. Physicians prefer to say they die of asphyxia, but the words are used synonymously throughout this chapter.

When humans draw a breath, the nose and mouth are the air's entryways into the body. It then flows across the vocal cords, through the trachea (or windpipe) into bronchi of increasingly diminishing size in the lungs. The bronchi finally become microscopic bronchioles leading to alveolar sacs. Once the inhaled air reaches the alveolar sacs, oxygen passes through the wall of an alveolar sac and the tissue between it and the wall of a capillary (the smallest blood vessel). That is where the oxygen in air enters the bloodstream. Oxygen's pathway from air to the blood is set out in Figures 3.1 and 3.2.

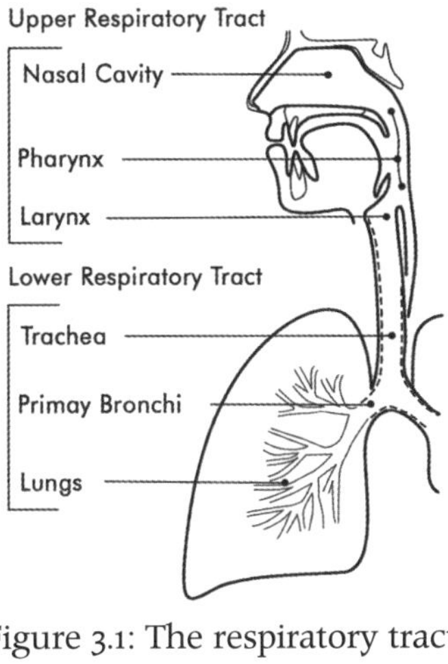

Figure 3.1: The respiratory tract

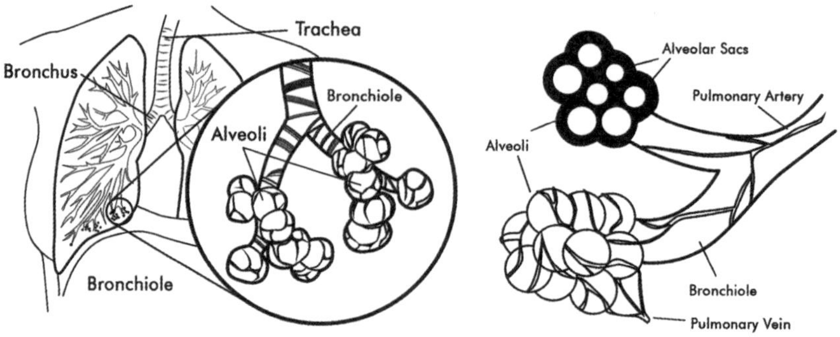

Figure 3.2: Microstructures of the lung
— the bronchioles and alveoli

Humans have an involuntary, or autonomic, nervous system programmed to make adults breathe at least 12 times a minute whether awake or asleep. Children breathe three to five times more rapidly, depending on their age.* The younger the child the faster its breathing. A brain reflex that responds to carbon dioxide levels in the blood controls how fast we breathe. Carbon dioxide is simply a waste product of the body's metabolism, and the higher its level in the blood the more rapidly a person will draw a breath.

As long as breathing keeps oxygen in the blood at a high enough level, life is uneventful. One measure of how much oxygen is in blood is that oxygen's partial pressure. Once its level drops below 25 mm to 30 mm of mercury (which is how partial pressure is measured), a person faints and will stay unconscious. Awakening requires the blood oxygen's partial pressure to rise back up to 25 mm to 30 mm of mercury. When oxygen in the blood continues to decline nerve cells in the brain begin to die. Once new oxygen stops being delivered to the blood death follows. When the brain has been deprived of oxygen for six minutes or more, so many neurons will die that breathing becomes impossible.

There are two reasons for alveoli to contain an inadequate amount of oxygen to support life. In the first scenario, not enough oxygen

* Age 0 to 12 months: 30–60 breaths/minute; age 1 to 2 years: 24–40; age 3 to 5 years: 22–34; age 6 to 12 years: 18–30; age 13 to 17 years: 12–16 breaths per minute.

enters the alveolar sacs. Even if all the oxygen in the sacs is transferred into the blood, there still won't be enough circulating in the blood to keep tissues viable. Death from asphyxia will result from not inhaling enough oxygen. This can occur when (a) the surrounding atmosphere simply does not contain sufficient oxygen to support life, or (b) something blocks the flow of perfectly good air into the lungs.

In the second scenario adequate oxygen is inhaled and enters the alveoli. Fatal asphyxia results because oxygen cannot pass through the tissue between the wall of the alveolar sac and the inner wall of an arteriole. Many diseases cause structural change in the wall of the alveoli, the wall of the arterioles and the tissue between them that will cause this type of asphyxial death.

Both of these fatal scenarios are most often the result of natural causes. The most common one, chronic obstructive lung disease, is discussed later in the chapter. This condition only involves coroners when it leads to death outside a hospital and nobody other than a coroner is available to complete a death certificate. Lots of respiratory deaths are unnatural though. Those are the fatalities coroners usually investigate.

Environmental Asphyxia

The air in some parts of the globe contains too little oxygen for many people's comfort. This is rarely a concern for seaside residents, but the higher one rises above sea level the lower the air's oxygen content. Even the healthiest person probably cannot survive a climb to the top of Mount Everest without the assistance of supplemental oxygen. People with poor lungs would asphyxiate long before they attain the mountain's upper reaches.

Miners have known for centuries that something lethal lurked in mines. Now it is known that odourless gases, like carbon monoxide and methane, have been their killers. In the United Kingdom from 1911 to 1986 miners carried canaries into mines to detect the presence of lethal gases. The birds are small and breathe more rapidly than do humans. As a result, birds die from inhaling noxious gases far faster than a miner. A canary's death warned miners to get out of that shaft quickly or they would suffocate too. The expression "a canary in a coal mine" is now often used in colloquial speech as a warning of danger.

Gases are either lighter or heavier than air. A heavy gas (such as hydrogen sulphide or chlorine) can only kill a person standing erect when it occupies all the space from the floor to the level of the mouth and nose. When the upper level of a noxious gas is lower than that, people will walk through it safely, breathing only air above the gas — as long as they hold their heads high and don't bend down very often.

Noxious gases that are lighter than air, like carbon monoxide, are lethal only when a person enters a space where the gas is trapped, preventing its rise. These gases are fatal if their lowest level reaches below a person's mouth. Gas higher than that will not be inhaled. A person can carry on all normal activity breathing only heavier normal air. The lighter noxious gas will occupy a space somewhere above the person's head.

Oxygen and carbon dioxide react with human tissue, which means that they can be metabolized, but some gases are non-reactive. They are called inert gases. For example, helium is lighter than air, but it is also inert. When inhaled under pressure, helium displaces air from the lungs. This action deprives the blood of oxygen very rapidly because, as an inert gas, helium does not trigger the reflex to take another breath that usually happens when the level of oxygen in the blood becomes too low.

After four to six breaths of helium, the lack of new oxygen entering the circulating blood quickly results in loss of consciousness. Death follows a few minutes later. We believe that a person in this situation feels nothing more than increasing sleepiness on the way to death. For that reason, death societies consider inhaling helium to offer the optimal method of committing suicide because it asphyxiates so painlessly.

Lethal gases that react with body tissues are quite a different story. Some burn and cause pain. All World War I veterans have now died. However, many physicians who treated them in their later years remain alive. These doctors heard that those elderly veterans never forgot the discomfort chlorine gas caused them in the trenches. While those physicians' patients survived, their fallen comrades experienced varying degrees of pain in their eyes, noses, throats and chests before they died. Death usually resulted from lethal lung damage that caused them to cough, feel a burning pain in their chests, develop headaches and nausea, and then vomit until they lost consciousness. Most gassed soldiers did not die that quickly. While 30 minutes' exposure to a high concentration of chlorine could be fatal, many took much longer than that to die.*

Modern-day terrorists have access to similar and even more lethal chemical weapons than were used in the Great War. A coroner in any part of the world may be called upon to investigate a terrorist homicide caused by exposure to a lethal gas. If that gas burns exposed body surfaces (as was the case with chlorine), then skin, eyes, nose, mouth and chest will all hurt. Breathing will become increasingly difficult and distressing until loss of consciousness ends all the pain.

Other gases do not just asphyxiate or burn — they are neurotoxic. An example is sarin, which was used by Japanese terrorists in the 1995 Tokyo subway attack. These neurotoxic gases poison the nervous system and cause death by paralysing the muscles in the chest wall, which prevents further breathing. People collapse, fall into a coma and die. But this takes time. Symptoms of sarin poisoning start with a runny nose, tightness in the chest, nausea and drooling. Increasingly dysfunctional nerves lead to vomiting and loss of both bowel and bladder control. Muscle spasms, especially in the arms and legs, precede or accompany loss of consciousness a short time before death. Sarin and other poisonous gases are discussed in more detail in Chapter 18.

Smothering

A noxious atmosphere is one way to deprive a person's lungs of adequate oxygen. Smothering is another. People smother whenever air cannot enter through the nose or mouth. For smothering to be fatal, both orifices need to be totally blocked. If either nose or mouth remains partially open, a natural reflex keeps breathing going.

One common method of suicide by smothering involves a plastic bag pulled over the head. It becomes airtight when some sort of

---

* Chlorine requires a concentration of 300 parts per million in the air before it will kill in half an hour. In many instances the concentration never reached that level on World War I battlefields. Sometimes chlorine was mixed with phosgene, a much more lethal gas. Phosgene takes 24 hours to do its lethal work, so the soldiers died the day after their exposures.

ligature is tightly secured around the neck. Using duct tape to close both the mouth and nose is usually, but not always, homicide. Adults smother infants by pressing a pillow, towel or soft plastic over the baby's face to prevent air from entering both mouth and nose. The infant becomes unconscious within seconds.

Death from smothering follows quickly when both nose and mouth remain completely blocked. Death takes longer when incomplete blockage of both passages allows some air to be breathed in. Until a person passes out, air hunger during smothering triggers a sense of panic. Some chest pain is felt while the person is still conscious. A dying person struggles against any smothering material. Infants can do very little. Older children and adults flail their arms and legs if not held down. These movements become increasingly less purposeful as the brain receives less oxygen. It only takes a minute or less to lose consciousness. Death follows five minutes or so after smothering starts.

Choking

Choking occurs when a piece of food, or anything else large enough, prevents air from reaching the lungs' alveolar sacs. Inhaled material may not initially completely block air flow. As long as some air gets all the way down to the lungs a person will remain conscious, though anxious and uncomfortable. As less and less air is breathed in restlessness increases and limbs flail more. A partially blocked windpipe's discomfort keeps worsening until the irritated tracheal lining swells so much that it completely blocks all air from reaching the alveoli. Seconds later the person loses consciousness, and death follows a few minutes after that.

Depending on what is inhaled, substances may lodge in the windpipe, large bronchial tubes or even in smaller bronchi. Death from carelessly eating and inhaling French fried potatoes (chips in the United Kingdom), for example, happens this way. In most of these cases, the person has some form of mental impairment. French fries can travel quite far down the bronchial tree before totally blocking airflow through the bronchial tubes. A person who inhales French fries usually lives in distress for several minutes at least. Death comes once the potato chips soften enough to mould themselves to the walls of the bronchial tubes, thus completely blocking all airflow.

Children have died from choking on soothers, balls or other toys they put in their mouths. Adults more often die from inhaling chunks of meat, fruit, pasta or regurgitated stomach contents. Inhaled blood clots, dentures and tumours all have been known to fatally choke older adults.

Strangulation

Choking stops breathing from inside the airway while strangulation stops it with external pressure. Strangulation occurs when hands, arms or a ligature apply force to the neck. A strangulation death does not simply arise from restricting airflow to the lungs.

Pressure on the neck also cuts off the brain's blood flow. Carotid artery compression prevents blood from arriving in the brain. Jugular vein compression prevents blood from leaving the head. Strangulation may also be fatal when it triggers a "carotid body reflex." These different possibilities, though interesting, are of little importance to coroners. Nobody can tell which mechanism came into play in a strangulation death. Relatives seek nothing more than to know that their relative was strangled.

Manual strangulation is also termed "throttling." Most strangulation uses only the hands, but arm "chokeholds" can strangle too. *Choke* is a misnomer for these lethal holds. They strangle people rather than choke them, though when enough pressure is applied to the front of the neck the anterior wall of the trachea can be pressed against its posterior wall to completely block air entry to the lungs.

Occasionally a police baton blocks air from entering the lungs in this way in a similar form of strangulation. In such cases a pathologist may discover a broken hyoid bone or larynx when dissecting the neck. A coroner looking at the dusky face of a strangled adult will see pinpoint spots of blood (conjunctival haemorrhages) speckling the whites of both eyes. Strangulation may visibly bruise the neck too, although this happens infrequently in children.

When the ligature is removed after a strangulation, one side of the neck's skin contains a depression with a size and contour that matches the form of the ligature. Coroners sometimes see cords or shoelaces partially or completely tied around the necks of strangled people. More often the ligature was removed for resuscitation and will be found nearby.

It only takes 10 to 15 seconds (one study says 11 seconds[1]) to lose consciousness once a tight ligature cuts off all blood flow to the brain. Dying takes a few minutes more. But a strangulation death is not always that rapid. Unsuccessful hangings often result in slow strangulation rather than fractured necks. When executions were public, both spectators and journalists frequently described condemned people suspended from the gallows and thrashing about for quite a long time before their bodies finally fell limp.

Restlessness and thrashing about accompany any slow strangulation. The panic of air hunger and neck pain make a person grab the ligature to try to pull it off. When it can't be removed, all limbs wildly flail until the strangled person finally loses consciousness and then dies.

Compression

Any weight that compresses the chest enough to prevent the lungs from filling with air is lethal. This traumatic asphyxia usually occurs accidentally. After seconds, consciousness is lost; death follows a few minutes later. Any object too heavy to easily move can fatally pin a person's chest against any hard surface. Equally lethal chest compression arises when innumerable tiny substances surround a person. Farmers in silos or hoppers who become immobilized by grain pouring around them suffocate when the grain's weight prevents their lungs from expanding. Construction workers suffer the same fate when their chests are buried by soil as earthen walls collapse on them. Even if their heads remain uncovered, these people are doomed. The pressure of the grain or soil against their chests prevents them breathing.

The demented elderly sometimes die wedged between bars in their beds or between their beds and a wall. Their inability to understand the predicament they are in makes it impossible for these people to extricate themselves before their struggling finally suffocates them.

When drunk or drugged, anyone can die in a similar manner. They pass out, collapsing into a position that compresses their chests enough to prevent drawing a breath.

Dead thieves are sometimes discovered tightly wedged after they have been unable to exit a small space they climbed into. Their chests became compressed. Breathing stopped. They suffocated. Heating and ventilation workers die the same way when they become wedged inside metal ventilation ducts. The pathologists' names for these deaths are either positional or postural asphyxias.

Crushing

Traumatic asphyxia can result when any force crushes the chest wall or causes bleeding inside the chest. Fractured ribs on both sides of the chest create a floating plate of chest wall that presses down upon the lungs when the person attempts to breathe in. This is called a flail chest (see Figure 3.3). A flail chest becomes lethal when the floating plate of chest wall is too heavy to allow the lungs to fill with air.

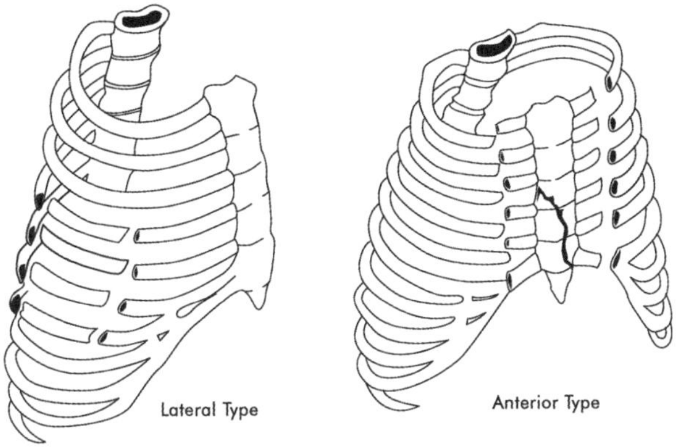

Figure 3.3: Fractured ribs may cause a flail chest.

Sometimes a crushing force ruptures the lungs' arteries enough to fill the pleural spaces between the lungs and chest walls with blood. In these instances, this build-up of blood is called a haemothorax. In cases investigated by coroners, haemothoraces became so large that the lungs could no longer expand and breathing stopped.

Erotic Asphyxia

Any discussion about types of asphyxia would be incomplete if it did not mention erotic asphyxia. When practised alone, autoerotic asphyxia can get mistaken for suicide. Should an investigation conclude that a death resulted from autoerotic asphysxia, it has to be classified as an accident. The practice of erotic asphyxia may have arisen from the observation that, when publicly hanged, males sometimes developed penile erections and then ejaculated.[2] Subsequent practice determined that a lack of oxygen in the brain for a short period of time produces pleasant sensations and hallucinations.

The brain can temporarily be deprived of oxygen by partially cutting one's oxygen supply. This is usually done by tightening a ligature around the neck, placing a bag over the head or duct-taping the mouth and nose. A similar sensation can arise from inhaling volatile solvents or simply compressing the chest. Both sexes can experience these sensations, but the overwhelming majority of participants in erotic asphyxial activity are male. In Ontario and Alberta between 1974 and 1987, there were 117 deaths due to unsafely practiced autoerotic asphyxia. Only one was a female.[3] There are estimated to be between 250 and 1000 autoerotic deaths per year in the United States.[4]

Most of those who die of autoerotic asphyxia are in their twenties, but adolescents also die, as do men in their seventies. Quite often men learn to experience pleasurable autoerotic asphyxia safely through repeated practice. Some even videotape themselves undergoing the experience. Then when something happens, such as a chair slipping leading to a hanging, the death is recorded on fim. Police investigating the death seize the video and use it for training purposes.

A lot of these failed cases end up as hangings. A coroner should be alerted to the possibility of this not being a normal suicide when the man is completely naked or if his fly is undone. It is also suspicious when some item of female clothing is found on the male's body, as fetishistic apparel and even crossdressing are a usual component of autoeroticism.

So is an escape mechanism. People practising partial asphyxiation know they need some way to ensure they begin breathing properly again. If a young man were found dead with tape over his nose and mouth and a pocket watch in his hand, autoerotic asphyxia should immediately come to mind. The fatal episode is not usually the first time the person attempted autoerotic asphyxia. The man learned by experience just how long he could deprive himself of oxygen before he had to rip the duct tape off to prevent loss of consciousness. The coroner becomes involved because one time he made a fatal miscalculation — he lost consciousness before he could remove his gag.

Erotic asphyxia is sometimes enjoyed with a sexual partner who, for example, may apply a ligature around the neck. When on too long or applied too tightly, the person seeking partial asphyxia dies. This often leads to a suspicion that a crime may have been committed. Any investigating police officers need to rule out murder. With a coroner explaining the components of autoerotic deaths, police will come to the conclusion that death arose from a fatal form of sex play.

Fluids

Fluid in the alveolar sacs prevents the air's oxygen from moving into the adjacent capillaries. The resulting asphyxia resembles drowning. Lethal fluids can either be inhaled or ooze out of the lungs' interstitial tissue. Fluid suddenly pouring into lungs causes chest discomfort and air hunger that lasts only a short time before consciousness disappears.

As fluid collects in the lungs (see Figure 3.4), the blood's oxygen level slowly declines. Breathing speeds up in an attempt to inhale more air and the associated chest discomfort increases. "Water on the lungs" makes breathing increasingly rapid and laborious. Once the blood's oxygen level drops too low the person passes out. From then on breaths become totally involuntary, slow down and steadily weaken.

At this point an unconscious dying person feels nothing. Once both lungs have filled with fluid, life ebbs away in a few minutes as in any other respiratory death. The way that person dies is similar to drowning. Drowning is such a common cause of asphyxia that it is discussed separately in Chapter 12, which deals with immersion deaths.

Inflammatory Conditions

Whenever anything inflames the lungs' linings enough to prevent adequate oxygen from entering the blood, death follows. Asthma, an airway disease affecting roughly 10% of people worldwide, inflames the lungs. Most asthma produces only minor, easily manageable breathing problems. Severe asthma can cause death. Lethal asthma was fairly common until the discovery of prednisone in the 1950s. Nowadays asthmatic deaths are rare.

Asthmatic flare-ups cause several changes in the bronchioles, three of which can be used to explain how a person dies from asthma. First, all bronchioles are surrounded by a small circular muscle. When this muscle contracts it narrows the diameter of the bronchiolar tube. Second, cells in the bronchial lining normally produce a small amount of mucus to trap dust particles. As asthma flares, these cells swell and also narrow the diameter of the bronchiole. Third, these swollen cells produce much more mucus. The extra mucus plugs the narrowed bronchial tube to effectively block air entry to the alveoli. This stops delivery of oxygen to the circulating blood.

Death from asthma does not happen rapidly. Worsening asthma shortens each breath. More rapid breathing triggers increasing anxiety

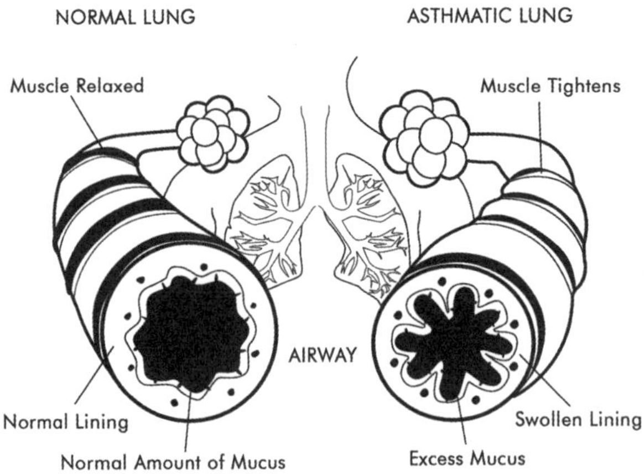

Figure 3.4: Comparison of healthy and asthmatic lungs

that only ends once unconscious. After the person becomes insensible, death from asthma is painless.

Infections inflame the lungs too. While other organisms can cause fatal pulmonary infections, viruses and bacteria are the most common. Both are airborne and cause bronchitis or pneumonia, depending on whether just bronchi or also the lungs are involved. Once bacteria move into the bloodstream they can cause sepsis.

Infection inflames and narrows the diameter of bronchial tubes from the trachea to the bronchioles. In pneumonia (see Figure 3.6), fluids or pus collect in the alveolar sacs blocking oxygen from entering the bloodstream. A sharp chest pain is often felt with each breath; breathing speeds up, becomes more difficult and day by day is more distressing. Eventually the bloodstream receives so little oxygen that consciousness fades, coma develops and death follows.

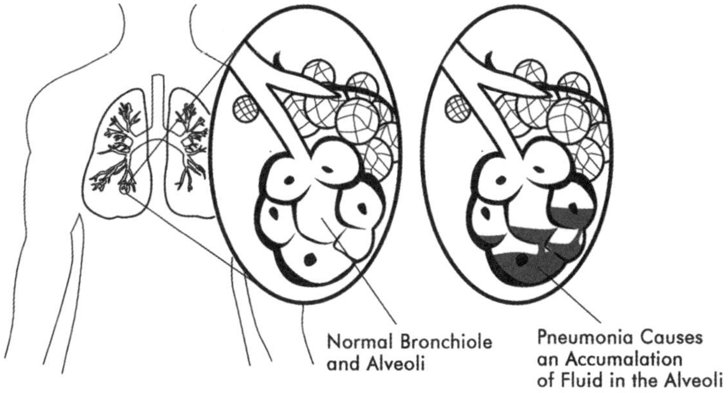

Figure 3.5: The shaded areas represent the fluids or pus that accumulate in the alveoli, causing pneumonia.

Emphysema (see Figure 3.7) is the best known potentially fatal inflammatory lung disease that slowly but steadily worsens. Collectively, all inflammatory lung diseases are called chronic obstructive pulmonary disease (COPD). Up to 40% of deaths caused by COPD are due to too little oxygen entering their blood. The rest die from congestive heart failure, pneumonia, pulmonary emboli, or lung cancer.

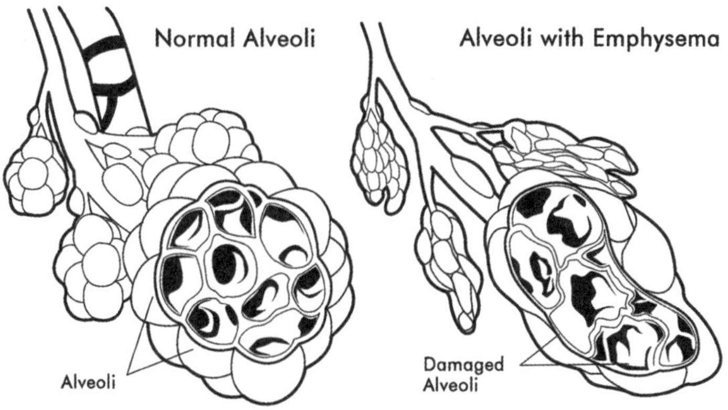

Figure 3.6: Comparison of healthy alveoli and those damaged by emphysema.

Depending on the circumstance, COPD can be the primary cause of death or simply a contributing factor.

Figure 3.7 explains why one dies with emphysema. The recurrent infections and consequent inflammation of chronic bronchitis thickens the walls of the bronchi and bronchioles. Tissue between the wall of the alveolar sacs and the inside wall of the capillaries thickens too. Many alveolar sacs have been totally destroyed by repeated attempts to cough up increasing amounts of mucus.

Lessening the number of healthy alveolar sacs decreases the area for oxygen to pass into the blood. Alterations to walls of those alveoli that remain intact slow oxygen's passage from the air into the circulating blood. These two changes lead to increasingly frequent and lengthening naps that one day turn into a terminal coma. This very common disease has a slow and inexorable progression.

Emphysema often becomes terminal once the heart gets involved. Destruction of more and more alveolar sacs forces the heart to pump harder to deliver oxygen to the lungs. Harder pumping increases pressure in blood vessels and forces fluid out of them and into the alveolar sacs; this becomes congestive heart failure. Fluid in the remaining alveolar sacs makes it even harder to deliver oxygen to the blood, causing a terminal period of coma before death.

Often emphysema is found in smokers. Workers in mining industries (coal and asbestos are well studied) develop the disease too. Death from emphysema is slow and usually takes decades. Activity gradually decreases from normal to a state of being barely being able to get out of bed to sit or walk to the toilet. Families become very familiar with the changes emphysema has wrought. By the time death occurs, it has long been expected.

Fortunate emphysematous people simply die in their sleep. Death while awake starts with a period of confusion, increasing agitation and the restlessness that follows. Breathing speeds up until they slowly lose consciousness. Once unconscious, their breathing steadily slows until ceasing after a few minutes. Families don't usually ask much about how an emphysematous relative died. They tend to talk about smoking, how workplace conditions years before may have caused the emphysema or bounce back and forth between these topics.

Death in severely ill hospital intensive care patients often results from acute respiratory distress syndrome (ARDS). This is a generalized lung inflammation occurring in many of the critically ill, up to half of whom die from it. ARDS is a terminal death event, but coroners attribute its cause to sepsis, pneumonia, pancreatitis, chemical exposure, or the traumatic injury that triggered ARDS in the first place.

Inflammation or trauma don't just produce fluid in the lungs (effusions). They can also cause fluid build-up in the pleural spaces around the lungs. This fluid collection is called a pleural effusion; it looks just like a haemothorax. The only difference is that this pleural effusion consists of clear serous fluid rather than blood. Since an intact rigid ribcage cannot expand, the pleural fluid compresses the lungs. As the lungs gradually expand less and less, the person gradually asphyxiates, lapses into a coma and finally dies.

Lung diseases are not the only ones that collect fluid in the pleural cavity. Congestive heart failure at the end of many cases of heart disease, cirrhosis of the liver and terminal kidney disease can do the same thing. Both primary and metastatic tumours in the lung or pleura (often a mesothelioma in asbestos workers) also trigger lethal pulmonary effusions.

While a pleural effusion may end life, the coroner attributes the cause of death to whatever underlying disease caused the fluid to develop. That disease should be the prime focus of any discussions with inquiring relatives.

Cancer

Malignant tumours in the lungs are very often lethal. Since all blood passes through the lungs, lots of cancer cells float into the lungs where they reproduce and become metastatic lesions. Whether cancer originates in the lungs or metastasized there from elsewhere, dying follows a similar course. Fatal lung cancer is discussed in more detail in Chapter 7.

Anaphylaxis

Television ads for autoinjectors constantly remind viewers of the possibility of an anaphylactic death from exposure to a substance to which a person is very allergic. While a risk exists, those advertisements need to be considered in context. In the United States, almost 60% of anaphylactic fatalities result from medical treatment (such as anaesthesia, antibiotics, and radiocontrast media). Food consumption triggers just over 5% of all anaphylactic deaths, while insect and other venomous stings are responsible for three times that number. For roughly 20% of fatal anaphylactic cases the cause is unspecified or undetermined.[5] These deaths are very uncommon. Only 500 to 1000 people are likely to die from anaphylaxis in the United States in a year, 20 in the United Kingdom and 15 in Australia.[6]

The most common way people die from anaphylaxis is asphyxia. Anaphylaxis usually consists of bronchospasm developing in the lungs, but it can also result from changes in the mouth. The tongue, lining of the mouth, and the lips can swell so much that it becomes impossible to draw air into the lungs. Sudden anaphylactic deaths commonly involve oral airway swelling. Anaphylaxis is mentioned in this chapter because, when fatal, it usually causes death by asphyxia.

However, asphyxia is not the only anaphylactic route to death. A lesser number die a cardiac death, particularly when having bad coronary artery disease. Anaphylaxis drops the blood pressure. This slows delivery of oxygen to all parts of the body. In the coronary arteries inadequate oxygen leads to a fatal myocardial infarction.

I suspect that families will be satisfied by simply being told that death was due to an anaphylactic reaction rather than exactly how it took place. In any case, this is an unlikely conversation since coroners are rarely asked to investigate such a death.

Now that we have looked at how the brain, heart and lungs can cause death, it is time to consider how other parts of the body — called endocrine organs — can become equally lethal.

NOTES

1 Sauvageau, A., Ambrosi, C., & Kelly, S. (2012). Three nonlethal ligature strangulations filmed by an autoerotic practitioner: comparison of early agonal responses in strangulation by ligature, hanging and manual strangulation. *American Journal of Forensic Medicine and Pathology, 33*(4), 339–340.

2 Erotic asphyxiation. (1997). *Lust* Magazine.

3 Blanchard R., & Hucker, S. J. (1991). Age, transvestism, bondage and concurrent paraphilic activities in 117 cases of autoerotic asphyxia. *British Journal of Psychiatry, 159*(3), 371–377.

4 Uva J. L. (1995). Review: Autoerotic asphyxiation in the United States. *Journal of Forensic Sciences, 40*(4), 574–581.

5 Jerschow, E., Lin, R. Y., Scaperotti, M. M., & McGinn, A. P. (2014). Fatal anaphylaxis in the United States, 1999–2010: Temporal patterns and demographic associations. *Journal of Allergy and Clinical Immunology, 13*(4), 1318–1328.

6 Lee, J.K. & Vadas, P. (2011). Anaphylaxis: Mechanisms and management. *Clinical and Experimental Allergy, 41*(7), 923–938.

4

Endocrine Deaths

All endocrine organs secrete hormones, along with other products, into the body. This makes them glands. The words *organs* and *glands* are used interchangeably throughout this chapter. A few organs do more than just secrete, but once their essential functions cease, they "fail." Injuries, diseases and simply ageing may end in fatal endocrine organ failure. Most of these deaths occur naturally and don't involve a coroner. Among the deaths that do are injuries and cases where the person never sought medical treatment. The following sections outline what people feel when their endocrine organs die. The glands are presented in alphabetical order.

Adrenal Gland

The adrenal gland sits atop the kidneys. This vital organ secretes "stress" hormones, sex hormones, minerals and glucocorticoids, including hormones that help the kidneys control the concentrations of salt and water in the body.

Failure of the adrenal glands is first diagnosed as Addison's disease. It worsens slowly, and initially doctors manage it by simply monitoring symptoms and adjusting medications. These symptoms start with increasing fatigue and irritability, loss of both appetite and weight, and salt cravings. Nausea, vomiting, abdominal pain, diarrhoea, muscle pain and joint pain also occur. As failure worsens people faint, develop darker skin, lose hair from their bodies, and become increasingly depressed.

Past experience tells people these symptoms usually have other causes. They are frequently ignored until unbearable, at which point the adrenal failure has probably become terminal. In many cases it takes years before feeling the need to visit a doctor.

In some other cases, untreated adrenal gland failure becomes lethal quite rapidly. Without knowing what actually happened a coroner can only speculate about the symptoms felt while dying. Adrenal glands fail when severe bacterial infections cause septic shock or when the glands are badly damaged by tuberculosis, mumps or AIDS. Any trauma that results in bleeding in the gland can be lethal; more rarely, autoimmune processes in the gland can cause death. In fatal autoimmune disease, the body's immune system fails to recognize its own tissue and destroys it. Don't try to explain this at all. Refer all inquiries to a knowledgeable physician, Wikipedia, or other reliable web sources.

Coroners rarely investigate hospital deaths from terminal adrenal failure. In the cases in which the coroner does get involved, the glands' malfunction usually has a natural cause. Hospitals sometimes record terminal symptoms on the charts in the emergency department. Additional notes made by the treating nurses and physicians may be found covering the period after the patient was admitted to a ward. Family members usually have some idea of what their deceased relative went through and tend not to ask questions.

Adrenal gland deaths that coroners do investigate usually involve recluses. Typically, neighbours know nothing about their state of health. By the time the person is discovered, their body is at least partially decomposed. Adrenal failure is often secondary to some other cause, like cancer or trauma. Relatives tend to be "out of the loop", and most have little if any idea about the decedent's state of health. They don't usually ask any questions about these deaths either.

Kidney

Kidneys are the start of the urinary tract, which is shown in Figure 4.1. Kidney failure arising from disease or injury becomes fatal when the kidneys excrete such a small amount of the products of the body's metabolism in the urine that a lethal quantity of urea collects in the blood. Urea collected in the blood creates a condition called uraemia. When severe and untreated by dialysis, uraemia causes death.

Uraemia — an elevated level of urea in the blood — usually develops gradually in one of three ways:

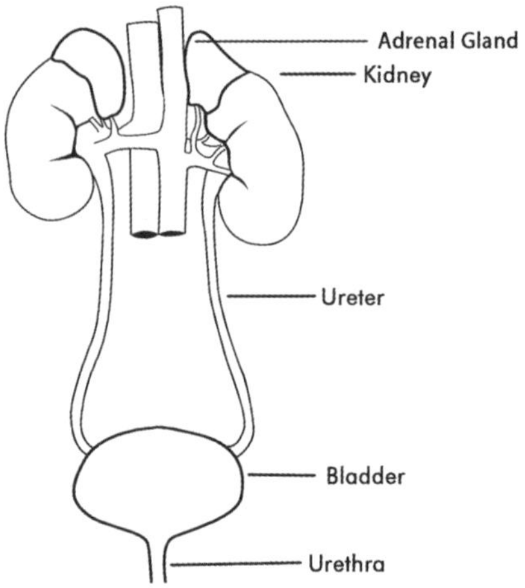

Figure 4.1: The urinary tract

1. Too little blood flows into the kidneys to produce enough urine to get rid of the products of the body's metabolism.
2. Diseases or injured kidneys lose the ability to produce urine.
3. Some sort of blockage of the urinary tract beyond the kidneys prevents urine from leaving the body.

Both severe congestive heart failure and any type of shock can become lethal when they drop a person's blood pressure so low that the kidneys don't receive enough blood to filter. Terminal kidney failure also results whenever the liver produces more urea than the kidneys can excrete.

Advanced diabetes, atherosclerosis and glomerulonephritis (inflammation of the tiny filters in the kidneys) eventually impair kidney filtration enough that a lethal uraemia develops. Uraemia can also arise when urine flow is blocked after leaving the kidneys by kidney stones, tumours or a large prostate.

Most people die slowly from uraemia over a period of years. The sole time death occurs rapidly is when a person receiving haemodialysis decides to stop treatment. Even in that case death will not be immediate. Urea builds up in the blood day by day until it reaches a lethal level. After treatment ceases, death nearly always follows in two to four weeks.

A uraemic death is generally considered to be quite pleasant. In their final months uraemics usually lack energy to do much more than sit around. Most become drowsy and nap a lot. They lose their appetite, eat less and defecate less frequently.

Uraemia eventually leads to shortness of breath as fluid collects in the lungs and builds up everywhere else in the body. Half the people dying of uraemia develop nausea. Some become distressed about their impending death, experience muscle twitching or become delirious. Others feel no distress at all. All have itchy skins long before they die from kidney failure.

Although uraemia itself can be fatal, most uraemics die from other causes. Most of these are cardiovascular; some are respiratory; and at other times people die from uraemic encephalopathy, which may be accompanied by bleeding in the brain and stomach.

Liver

Coroners sometimes find that liver disease is the cause of death in people who die at home. The liver plays many roles in the body's metabolism, one of which is detoxification. When liver function fails, ammonia, bilirubin and many other substances build up in the blood. Eyes and skin turn yellow. The whole body becomes quite itchy. In most cases seen by coroners, arms, legs and abdomen have swollen. Bleeding may have occurred spontaneously somewhere in the body.

Increasing metabolic toxic waste build-up in the blood makes people forgetful and confused. Many make up stories to cover their inability to remember facts. Near the end of life their brains swell. People lose consciousness and become comatose until finally expiring. This lengthy pathway from liver disease to death is called hepatic encephalopathy.

Hepatic encephalopathy causes a lot of trying times — the whole household has, with varying degrees of success, tried to cope with the difficulties their dying relative experienced. After an autopsy, all a coroner can do is explain that the brain was damaged and suggest that the death was painless in the end. The only time that won't be true is when liver encephalopathy is accompanied by a damaged gag reflex, which often leads to death from choking on food.

The death of a terminally ill relative with liver failure is often a relief for caregivers who have long laboured hard to look after them. Fluid retention may have caused their relative's body to swell; the resulting weight gain and increasing immobility would make lifting or moving the person much harder. It is back-breaking work looking after a near-comatose relative in liver failure.

Often, caregivers also come to their wits' end dealing with their relative's erratic, untrustworthy behaviour that worsened as the brain function deteriorated. Often they know that Wernicke's encephalopathy or Korsakoff's syndrome was the explanation. Many family members read about these conditions to try to cope with their relative's unpredictable actions.

Many people with these conditions have indulged themselves in a lifetime of excessive alcohol consumption. But coroners should know that, besides alcohol abuse, viral infections and other diseases cause cirrhosis or scarring of the liver. Regardless of the cause of a cirrhosis, the pathway to death from liver failure is the same.

While death can occur from cerebral oedema (brain swelling), liver failure can also trigger lethal bleeding when the body stops making enough clotting factors. Fatal haemorrhages may arise from any blood vessel in the body.

Cirrhosis dilates veins around the umbilicus (belly button), the vulva, the scrotum and the rectum (where they become haemorrhoids). Since these veins are small, death from their rupture would require bleeding to continue for hours. Should this happen, the end is painless while the person is intoxicated and unconscious. Those awake and conscious weaken and tire before lapsing into a comatose state that precedes death.

Veins in the oesophagus of cirrhotic people also dilate and bleed, usually in small amounts. However, in the cases coroners investigate oesophageal bleeding would have been very heavy (see Figure 4.2). The death scene is usually coloured by massive amounts of blood that poured out of the dying person's mouth or into the stomach or lungs. Out of control bleeding from a large oesophageal vein rupture induces panic. The bleeding itself may be painless, but blood pouring out of the oesophagus gets aspirated, making breathing difficult and causing chest pain. Increasing blood loss worsens weakness and fatigue

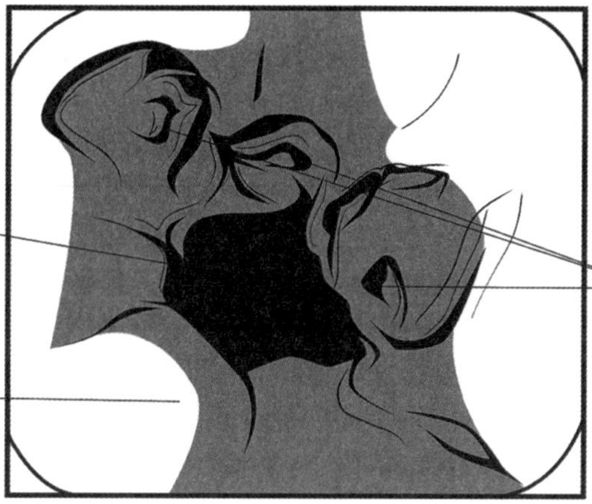

Figure 4.2: The large black area in the centre is the oesophageal lumen (tube). The ruptures around it are also shown in black.

and eventually causes the person to lose consciousness and lapse into a terminal coma. Death results from either haemorrhagic shock or asphyxia. Dying takes only minutes when bleeding is heavy.

Most deaths from liver failure end a longstanding chronic disease process. Occasionally they come more quickly. Chemicals, such as an overdose of Tylenol (acetaminophen or paracetamol), or a meal of poisonous toadstools can rapidly destroy enough liver cells to trigger sudden and severe liver failure. These people experience a steadily worsening pain in their damaged livers (under the lower right ribs), severe vomiting and finally a coma for some period preceding death. But even in these cases, death from liver failure is not immediate. For example, dying from an overdose of Tylenol may take four to seven days.

Pancreas

The pancreas is the organ that most people know produces insulin. It also produces enzymes to assist digestion. Without a functioning pancreas life becomes impossible. Pancreatic deaths usually arise from cancer, pancreatitis, or the complications of diabetes mellitus. Since death from cancer of the pancreas is fully discussed in Chapter 7 it need only be mentioned here.

Pancreatitis

Death from pancreatitis occasionally comes to the attention of a coroner. The families of people with chronic pancreatitis watch them suffer for years. Severe chronic pancreatitis leads to numerous hospital admissions, often in the intensive care unit, where death frequently occurs. Even in acute pancreatitis, death occurs during the first hospital admission less than 10% of the time.

Pancreatitis pain, felt across the upper half of or even the whole abdomen, is dull and radiates to the back. When severe in cases of acute pancreatitis, parts of the pancreas die. This produces a pain as intense as any a human can experience. Abscesses then develop in the dead parts of the pancreas.

Pain may be the worst misery pancreatitis causes, but the nausea and vomiting that frequently accompany pancreatic inflammation are miserable too. A coroner can assume these symptoms probably occurred at some time when investigating the death of a person who died alone at home without medical care.

Pancreatitis causes a variable amount of suffering before death. Chronic pancreatitis pain can sometimes be tolerated without using medication. More often, it hurts enough to require some sort of analgesia to make it bearable.

When a person with chronic pancreatitis dies it usually comes from a complication of the disease rather than the pancreatitis itself. Acute pancreatitis is different. It may be mild, but when severe it is fatal in more than 20%* of cases.[1] Severe acute pancreatitis stops the pancreas from working properly. As mentioned above, parts of it die or become infected; cysts and abscesses develop. Shock results from the body directing more fluid and nutrients to the pancreas in an effort to repair its damage.

Many relatives are aware that their family member's pancreatitis was very painful. They probably will not want to discuss it. When a coroner needs to talk about pain in the case of a death from chronic pancreatitis, try to avoid any detailed discussion. Just observe that the surviving family members can be thankful that the pain of chronic pancreatitis is much less than that when the condition is acute.

---

* The death rate ranges from 2.2% when the acute pancreatitis is mild to 45.1% when the acute pancreatitis is severe; 21.1% is the average overall.

If that intended deflection does not end the conversation, observe that fatty diarrhoea probably developed. Point out that this type of stool always floats on water in the toilet. Most people find this topic so revolting they stop asking questions or at least switch to a different line of questioning. When a relative has died of acute pancreatitis, agree that the pain was probably severe but stop at that. Don't catastrophize.

If a knowledgeable questioner still wants more explanation, try to guide the conversation toward the mechanism of death. Explain that when the body diverts fluids to the pancreas in an attempt to repair its damage, blood volume elsewhere in the body drops, leading to shock. Ask them to imagine their relative becoming clammy and feeling weak, anxious and confused while starting to breathe rapidly. There is nothing too distressing in that picture. When nobody knows what actually happened, suggest that loss of consciousness, coma and death likely followed in rapid succession. That is a best-case scenario. Reiterate that once the person became unconscious, their death was painless.

"Why does pancreatitis happen?" may be asked by relatives who are not close to the decedent, but who have, through happenstance, become the next of kin. Roughly 80% of cases of pancreatitis are caused by either gallstones that block the flow of the pancreatic enzymes out of the pancreas or by alcohol abuse.[2] Since most of these cases are discovered at autopsy, the pathologist may be able to help define the cause.

Should relatives attribute death to excessive alcohol use, agree it may have been the case. Many relatives know just how much their deceased relative drank. Many will also recount a lifelong habit of heavy smoking and ask, "Did it play a role in the pancreatitis?" The answer is "Perhaps not, but maybe." Many medical papers have been written discussing whether the connection is significant. A coroner can safely observe that smoking certainly did nothing to prevent pancreatitis developing.

A coroner may investigate the death of a person who appears to have suffered a fatal haemorrhage, infection, kidney failure or lung collapse. After more investigation it may become clear that this terminal mechanism of dying arose from an underlying pancreatitis. The coroner should consider that the death arose from a complication of pancreatitis.

Diabetes Mellitus

Diabetes arises when the body simply lacks enough insulin or cannot properly use it to metabolize sugar. As a result, blood sugar levels go out of control. Diabetes develops when pancreatitis destroys too many insulin-producing islets of Langerhans cells, which are located throughout the pancreas. Diabetes is a complication of pancreatitis, but pancreatitis may not be the cause of death.

In fact, most people who die from diabetes don't have pancreatitis. How the diabetes arose is irrelevant to how one dies from it — regardless of the cause, dying follows the same path. When blood sugar levels drop too low (hypoglycaemia) or rise too high (hyperglycaemia) to sustain life, people lose consciousness.

People with hypoglycaemia may pass out very quickly. People infrequently die from hypoglycaemia, but when they do, it is often the result of an accidental, (or occasionally deliberate) injection of an excessive amount of insulin. Hypoglycaemia causes lethal brain damage when blood sugar remains low long enough. In people with heart disease, a common condition in middle age, it may trigger a fatal cardiac arrhythmia.

Death from hyperglycaemia is more common than from hypoglycaemia. To understand dying in diabetics a little biochemistry follows. The living human body requires many continual biochemical reactions that cease only with death. The levels of hydrogen ions (atoms missing an electron) in a biochemical reaction make the body's fluid acid, alkaline or neutral.

Acidity is a state most people understand. Very acid substances burn human skin.

The opposite of acidity is alkalinity. Extremely alkaline liquids or substances burn skin too. The burns look similar but result from a different biochemical reaction. Neutral compounds do not burn skin at all.

More than a century ago, scientists developed pH as a method of measuring acidity. A pH of 7.0 is neutral. In humans, pH is measured in the blood or urine. A drop in pH (for example, from 6.8 to 6.6) indicates increasing acidity. A rise in pH (for example, from 7.5 to 7.7) means increasing alkalinity. The pH scale is the tool used to measure all the body's biochemical reactions.

Human body tissue is designed to be a bit alkaline, though the pH is not uniform throughout the body at all times. A healthy person's pH ranges from 7.35 to 7.45. A pH outside these parameters makes people start to feel sick. Any extreme pH movement in either direction beyond these parameters that lasts for too long becomes fatal.

The body's pH is commonly measured in the blood. It changes slightly moment by moment. Every organ in the body works hard to keep the body's pH within its desirable range. Once the pH moves outside the body's comfort zone, compensatory mechanisms kick in to try to bring it back within its desirable range.*

When the body produces too much acid, or the kidneys don't excrete enough, a state called metabolic acidosis occurs — blood acidity and pH move above or below the body's range of tolerability. Metabolic acidosis, caused by diabetes allowing glucose in the blood to get too high, is called diabetic ketoacidosis when organic products called ketones develop as well. Ketones have a fruity smell, a bit like nail polish. Untreated diabetic ketoacidosis leads to death. Most diabetics and their families know this. Coroners may smell ketones if an investigation starts soon after a death from hyperglycaemia.

Death from metabolic acidosis often comes slowly. It starts with symptoms of weakness and nausea, sometimes accompanied by vomiting and abdominal pain. These people become anxious, develops palpitations, experience chest pain and get headaches.

Their vision may become blurry, and their breathing speeds up and deepens. While these hyperglycaemics commonly feel thirsty and urinate frequently, up to a third of the people who die from diabetic ketoacidosis don't even know they have diabetes. That shows how insidious and hard to diagnose the condition is. Sometimes coroners find no evidence that the person knew they had diabetes. That's always unfortunate. Diagnosis and proper treatment of diabetic ketoacidosis

* The body's hydrogen ion levels can make a difference between life and death. Too low a hydrogen ion level is acidity, a state that makes it hard for the blood's haemoglobin to pick up oxygen. When the body remains acidic for too long, inadequate oxygen kills more and more of the brain's neurons until the brain stops working. When the blood gains too many hydrogen ions the pH rise makes blood alkaline for too long a period. That causes blood vessels bringing oxygen to the brain to constrict and fatally deprives the brain's nerve cells of oxygen. In both states the loss of brain neurons causes death, but the mechanism differs between alkalinity and acidity.

reduces its mortality rate to less than 1.9% in those aged between 12 and 69 years.[3]

Thyroid Gland

While thyroid gland problems are generally not fatal, the gland's overactivity, called hyperthyroidism, is statistically associated with an increase in many types of deaths. Fatal hyperthyroidism's highest correlation is to cardiac deaths and strokes. When faced with both conditions, most investigating coroners attribute death to the cardiovascular or cerebrovascular cause and call hyperthyroidism simply a contributing factor.

Longstanding hypothyroidism (not producing enough thyroid hormone) makes people feel quite tired and cold, even in warm weather. This is common in the elderly, especially females. A younger hypothyroid woman may find her menstrual period becomes irregular. At any age, hypothyroidism can cause melancholia, dry skin, headaches and constipation. Some hypothyroid people find their voices hoarsen. Many accumulate fluid throughout their bodies in a condition called myxoedema.

Hypothyroid people usually die from other causes — an infection, a stroke, heart failure or some sort of injury. Only in significant myxoedema will death ensue, starting with confusion, frequent napping and weight gain when fluid collects throughout the body. Congestive heart failure begins. Pneumothoraces (fluid between the outer walls of the lung and the lining of the chest wall) may develop. Breathing becomes very difficult, coma starts, and breathing slows. Death follows.

A coroner is highly unlikely to investigate a case of a death arising from a myxoedema coma. In the event of that happening, it is safe to assure the family that death was painless.

There are several other endocrine glands, including the parathyroids, prostate, pituitary, pineal, hypothalamus, testes and ovaries among them. Coroners will run across people who die from cancer of the prostate and cancer of the ovary, and how they die is discussed in the cancer chapter. Few die from disorders of the other glands in situations requiring a coroner's investigation. Should a coroner be called upon to investigate a death due to one of these other organs, read up on the subject before talking to the relatives, whenever possible.

NOTES

1 Popa, C. C., Badiu, D. C., Rusu, O. C., Grigorean, V. T., Neagu, S. I., & Strugaru, C. R. (2016). Mortality prognostic factors in acute pancreatitis. *Journal of Medicine and Life, 9*(4), 413–418.

2 National Institute of Diabetes and Digestive and Kidney Diseases (NIDDK). (n.d.). *Pancreatitis.* U.S. Department of Health and Human Services. Retrieved February 7, 2021, from https://www.niddk.nih.gov/health-information/digestive-diseases/pancreatitis

3 Hardern, R., & Quinn, N. (2003). Emergency management of diabetic ketoacidosis in adults. *Emergency Medicine Journal, 20*(3), 210–213.

5

Deaths Related to Blood Vessels

Blood can be involved in two ways of dying — some people bleed to death, and at other times it is blood clots that kill. We begin with bleeding.

Bleeding to Death

Coroners sometimes arrive at extremely bloody death scenes. Several police officers will have arrived quite a bit earlier. One may be responsible for taking many photographs for use in any future legal process. Some pictures will be quite gory, and police usually won't show them to relatives. Quite often, juries at inquests or trials won't see them either. A dead body lying in a pool of blood makes many people feel squeamish. Defence lawyers often successfully argue these pictures bias juries against their clients. That may be true, though any impression these images make on a juror pales in comparison to their effect on relatives.

Regardless of how it begins, dying from exsanguination always follows the same course. The injury that starts the bleeding may be very uncomfortable, but the path to death that follows usually involves steadily decreasing pain. Just saying that may not satisfy upset relatives though. A little physiology is useful to explain why.

Average, healthy adult human bodies contain about five litres (10 pints) of blood. A woman has a blood volume that is slightly less than a man's. That difference can be attributed to (generally) smaller female bodies needing less blood to function properly than (generally) larger male ones.[1] The bigger a person of either sex, the greater the blood volume needed to keep them functioning properly.

The human body uses blood to transport oxygen to and carbon dioxide from all its tissues. Though blood's physiology is complex, most of it is irrelevant to understanding blood's role in death. To explain a blood-related death simply, consider blood as having only three components — plasma, blood cells and platelets. One or more of these usually plays a major role in blood-induced deaths that coroners investigate.

Plasma is the fluid suspending blood cells and platelets while they travel around the circulatory system. Blood cells come in two types — white and red. Red blood cells deliver oxygen to all the body's tissues and carry away to the lungs the carbon dioxide that is produced by the body's metabolism. White blood cells fight infection. Platelets are integral to clot formation that stops bleeding.

For bleeding to be fatal it must be heavy. As past blood donors can attest, the human body easily tolerates siphoning off 450 mL (a pint) of blood. In fact, blood losses up to 750 mL don't affect a person's well-being very much at all. Losing a pint of blood may cause momentary light-headedness when first getting up from a chair. Not much else happens. Only once about a third of the body's blood is lost will the process of dying likely start. After the circulatory system is depleted of two or more litres (four pints) of blood, death become probable.

It takes about four months for the body to replace any lost blood. Millions of blood donors feel perfectly fit throughout the 120 days it takes for their red cell numbers to return to normal.[2] This lack of unpleasant side effects encourages some donors to regularly donate blood multiple times year after year.

Fatal haemorrhages have many causes. Injuries, gun shots, blood thinners, cancer, bleeding uteri, peptic ulcers and inflamed blood vessels can all end with bleeding to death. A body's genetic inability to produce blood clotting factors, a blood vessel that leaks or a ruptured organ all can produce an equally lethal loss of blood.

Bleeding to death on the operating table is always painless; anaesthesia sees to that. Operating room deaths almost always follow an extensive period of resuscitation. Neither surgeon nor anaesthetist wants an operation to end as a death "on the table." The whole surgical team resuscitates a patient dying in the operating room for a long time before finally giving up.

The time it takes to bleed to death depends on the rate blood flows out of the body. That, in turn, partly varies with the size of the damaged blood vessels. The aorta is the biggest artery in the body. Blood flows from the heart into the aorta at a rate of roughly five litres per minute. If the aorta is completed severed (transected), all blood could flow out of the circulatory system in less than 60 seconds. Loss of consciousness would be almost immediate, and a rapid, painless death would follow. Automobile accidents and falls from great heights are two common types of trauma that lethally lacerate aortas.

On the other hand, blood from completely severed smaller arteries flows out of the body more slowly. Blood from a transected radial artery at the wrist spurts out at a maximum rate of 80 mL per minute. That means that to lose enough blood to cause death will take at least half an hour. With an only partially lacerated artery, blood is lost less quickly and death will take even longer.

A severed brachial artery has a flow rate of just under 240 mL per minute, making death is possible within 10 minutes. The femoral artery is bigger still. Depending on how severely atherosclerosis has narrowed a lacerated femoral artery, blood can flow from it at a rate of 200 mL to 500 mL per minute. That means death from exsanguination should occur from as few as four minutes to slightly more than 10.

The common carotid artery branches into the internal and external carotid arteries. Depending on which one is completely severed, blood flows from the body at a rate varying from over 100 mL per minute to well over 500 mL per minute. Death can occur in anywhere from three or four to minutes to as many as 20.

The external jugular vein is more often severed than an artery. That leads to a much slower death, since blood flows much more slowly from a lacerated vein. Twenty minutes or more must elapse before enough blood flows out of a large transected vein to make a person lose consciousness. Death will take another 40 minutes or more. When a vein is only partially lacerated, the blood flows more slowly and death will take even longer.

It would be unethical to discover the time it takes a person to bleed to death experimentally. These figures arise from mathematical calculations using the speed blood flows through an individual artery. Death is more rapid the faster blood flows out of a damaged blood vessel. If an estimate of the length of time it took to bleed to death becomes unavoidable, suggest the shortest time possible. The wisest course is to decline to reply on the basis that any guess would be too speculative.

Exsanguination is not uncomfortable. Bleeding tires and weakens people. They lose motivation. Skin pales; hands and feet cool. As more blood is lost, people become aware their breathing speeds up. Usually only very anxious people or those exercising a lot notice their hearts beating. But anyone who is haemorrhaging to death will notice their heart beating at some point. As more and more blood flows out of the body, tissue demands for oxygen make a heart beat faster in a desperate effort to meet the need. As long as blood vessels can continue to constrict enough to provide a minimally adequate blood flow to the brain, consciousness will continue, though alertness drops. The person also notices their skin becoming clammy.

Confusion begins once about 30% of a body's blood is lost[3] and arterial constriction trying to keep the blood flowing starts to fail. A terminal coma begins, and internal organs sequentially shut down. Breathing ceases, the heart stops beating, and brain death follows.

While anxiety provoking, none of this process is very uncomfortable. Most sensations felt while dying from exsanguination are quite tolerable. Pain while dying always concerns relatives. A coroner can safely say that very little discomfort arises from bleeding to death. (However, pain from any injury that caused the haemorrhage will continue to some degree as long as any degree of alertness remains).

Source of Fatal Bleeding

Every blood vessel in the body has the potential for lethal haemorrhage. A cut to any part of the skin produces some bleeding. Most lacerations clot easily, but not all do. Death from exsanguination is the fate that some people born with a bleeding disorder or taking a blood thinner experience when they cut themselves and their blood won't clot.

Gastrointestinal Tract

People sometimes do bleed to death from their mouths. In unusual circumstances any oral laceration, even a self-inflicted bite, can prove fatal. Dental regulators usually severely punish any dentist whose patient dies from a bleeding socket following a tooth extraction.[4] The fatal haemorrhage usually results from a "blood thinning medicine" that the dentist didn't know about or ignored. Dentists expect no patient should die as the result of a properly performed tooth extraction. Though coroners also investigate along with the dentist's regulatory body, few will ever be involved with a fatal dental haemorrhage, since these deaths occur very rarely.

Ear, nose and throat surgeons always worry about heavy bleeding during the first two weeks following a tonsillectomy. It doesn't happen very often, but between 1 in 12,000 and 1 in 16,000 people bleed to death this way after their tonsils have been removed.[5] Not all post-tonsillectomy bleeding deaths require a coroner's investigation. This haemorrhage it is a known complication of tonsillectomies.

Surgeons try very hard to stop this bleeding. When death follows what may have been the failure of quite heroic surgery to try to stop a lethal post-tonsillectomy bleed it is quite appropriate for the death to be reviewed by the hospital's department of otorhinolaryngology. A coroner's investigation is likely to find only that the death was an unavoidable known complication of the tonsillectomy.

Tongue lacerations are rarely fatal. The tongue's lingual artery is capable of pumping out a fatal volume of blood if the bleeding continues steadily for two to three hours. People with oral cancer occasionally bleed to death when the tumour ruptures that artery, but rarely. More often people with oral cancer die of starvation. Coroners frequently view bodies where massive quantities of blood have poured out of their mouths. Few coroners' investigations will conclude a haemorrhage started in the mouth.

Bleeding to death from the oesophagus is a different story. Every coroner will investigate many of these cases. Varicose veins, called varices (just one is called a varix), in the oesophagus (see Chapter 4, Figure 4.2) frequently rupture. Something swallowed, like a chicken bone, can lacerate a varix. The speed that blood flows out of the mouth varies with the size of the hole in the bulging vein.

Most fatal varices develop as a complication of liver cirrhosis. These bulging, thin-walled veins burst spontaneously and tear easily. Half of all people with cirrhosis have them, and 30%–50% of these varices leak blood. Almost half of people with a ruptured oesophageal varix die within six weeks, even when hospitalized.[6]

Ruptured oesophageal varices may leak slightly, or in the cases coroners investigate, bleed massively. As oesophageal varices start to haemorrhage, people can initially spit all the blood out of their mouths. Continued bleeding leads to weakness, collapse, and loss of consciousness. Should the haemorrhaging be too heavy, or a person too confused or weak to spit any longer, the blood may start to be swallowed or simply run down the oesophagus into the stomach.

Though a stomach full of blood may trigger vomiting, not all blood necessarily leaves the mouth. Breathing while vomiting draws blood down the windpipe into the lungs in a process called aspiration. Only coughing can blow this aspirated blood out of the lungs. When people become too weak to cough the blood just collects there. Chest discomfort is felt while the person is alert and still able to cough. That state does not last very long before coma ends all discomfort. Death follows a few minutes later.

Most people with ruptured oesophageal veins make it to hospital to receive at least some treatment. Their deaths in hospital rarely involve a coroner at all. Coroners investigate deaths at home of people who, for some reason, did not seek medical care for their terminal oesophageal haemorrhage.

At the death scene in the case of a variceal haemorrhage, usually the body is lying at the end of a trail of blood that may start anywhere in the residence. Its path usually runs through the kitchen or bathroom and involves a sink or toilet at some point along the way. Many trails end at one of those locations, or a bedroom.

How a head ends up after collapsing determines the direction of any blood flow during the final minutes of consciousness. Blood flows out of the mouth when the head is turned sideways or the body lands face down. When the person fell after passing out, some blood will have collected in the stomach and perhaps the lungs if the head remained upright.

Lung cancer rupturing a pulmonary artery leads to an equally bloody scene. This type of terminal bleed doesn't last very long because of the speed with which blood flows out of the pulmonary artery. An emaciated body will raise a coroner's suspicion of lung cancer when contemplating the cause of so much bleeding.

When oesophageal veins rupture, people also often have lots of fluid, called ascites, that greatly distends their abdomen. Viewing a body with a big belly makes ruptured oesophageal varices the likely reason for the fatal haemorrhage. A roomful of empty beer cans, wine bottles or spirit bottles tilts the odds further in favour of that being the cause of the bloody death. Certainty in either case requires confirmation by autopsy.

The stomach, the small intestine, and the alimentary canal starting at the mouth are all considered the upper gastrointestinal tract. More haemorrhages arise from the stomach and small intestine than from that tract's upper parts. Bleeding commonly arises when a tumour ruptures a blood vessel, when a peptic ulcer develops and erodes the wall of a blood vessel, and perhaps even when an ulcer perforates the stomach or duodenum. Commonly, especially in the elderly, gastrointestinal erosions that arise from taking non-steroidal anti-inflammatory medications like aspirin, Motrin, or naproxen cause lethal haemorrhage. The frequency of upper gastrointestinal haemorrhages becoming fatal varies with available care. One study in 2014 cited a range of 5%–10% dying from upper gastrointestinal haemorrhages in the United Kingdom and the United States,[7] so coroners in developed countries could quote those percentages, if asked. Lower gastrointestinal haemorrhage is less often fatal and rarely investigated by a coroner.*

* Bleeding to death from ulcerative colitis or Crohn's disease occurs too. More commonly an ulcerative colitis death arises from some a complication – toxic megacolon, cancer or an infection. Diverticulitis can cause arterial bleeding. Haemorrhoids sometimes produce heavy venous haemorrhage. So can angiodysplasia, a large intestine vascular malformation. All five of these conditions theoretically can make a person bleed to death, but fatal haemorrhage occurs rarely. Cancer can also rupture any artery in some part of the abdomen and thereby cause fatal internal bleeding. These causes of death are only discovered by autopsy.

Abdominal pain of varying intensity flares recurrently with gastrointestinal bleeds. Unless death follows a first attack, family members will understand their relative's suffering during a flare-up. Most relatives assume any terminal pain resembled what they have already witnessed. Unless asked, don't raise the prospect of discomfort having been worse when the pathologist discovered peritonitis. Family members aware of the discomfort produced by past attacks rarely ask coroners about what happened in the final one.

However, coroners usually only investigate the deaths of people who received little or no medical treatment. Many of these people avoided doctors. Some were reclusive, others mentally ill, and a third group chose to shun conventional medical care. Almost all will have had little contact with family members. Next-of-kin informed of the death of an estranged or distant relative rarely delve deeply. They tend to accept any explanation a coroner offers and don't inquire about the process of dying.

Blood Vessels

Any arterial damage is potentially fatal. All arteries rapidly pump blood out of the circulatory system the moment an opening in one of their walls develops. Speed of blood loss varies. Death takes but a few minutes when the laceration's size and the bore of the damaged artery are large enough. The body's largest artery is the aorta. The quickest death from exsanguination results from aortic transection and can take less than five minutes.

Aortas tear either spontaneously or as a result of trauma. People die from tears in abdominal and thoracic aortas differently. Trauma sometimes quickly kills young people by damaging healthy aortas. More frequently, lethal aortic tears arise when an older vessel has been weakened by atherosclerosis.

Like all blood vessels, the aorta has three layers beyond its basement membrane, as illustrated in Figure 5.1. Its innermost layer, the tunica intima, helps provide a smooth surface to allow blood flow without creating any turbulence. The middle layer, the tunica media, is a muscle surrounding the intima that, whenever necessary, constricts the artery's diameter. The outermost layer, the externa, is tough connective tissue encapsulating the two inner tunicas.

Atherosclerosis gradually hardens arteries by depositing cholesterol in their walls; this is shown in Figure 5.2. They also weaken and bulge to form aneurysms; this is shown in Figure 5.3 In most cases seen by coroners, the intimal lining of an aortic aneurysm tear at the edge of a cholesterol deposit has extended through the media and the externa so that blood has poured out.

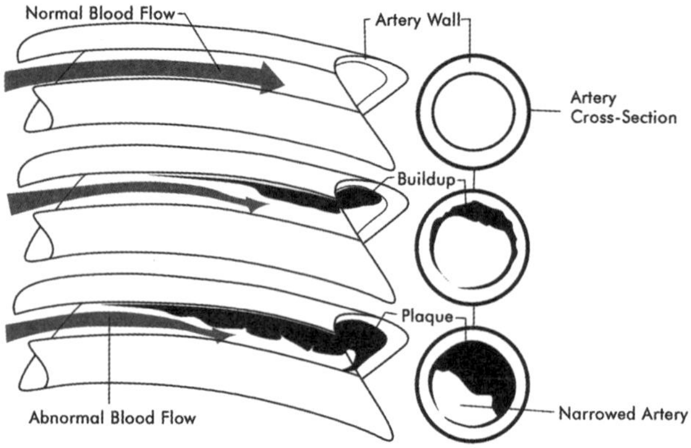

Figure 5.2: The build-up of plaque inside the arteries is caused by deposits of atherosclerotic cholesterol.

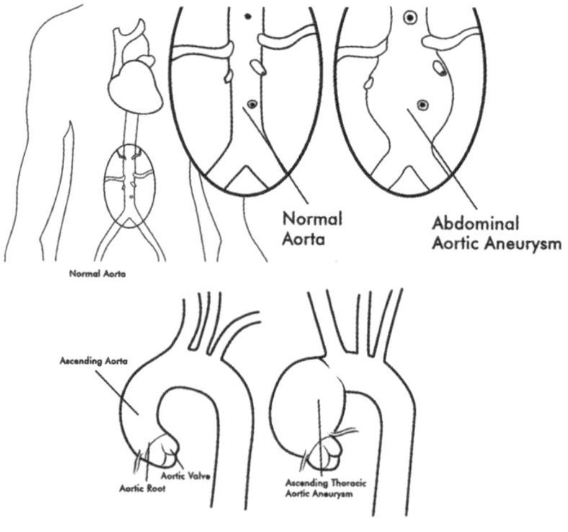

Figure 5.3: Aortic Aneurysm

Most aortic aneurysms rupture in the abdomen. The pain experienced when an aneurysm ruptures varies with the part of the aorta that tears. A rupture of the anterior wall of an aortic aneurysm produces momentary excruciating pain before the person lapses into a terminal comatose state. Blood flows into the surrounding peritoneal cavity so rapidly that loss of consciousness takes only seconds and death follows in minutes.

An abdominal aortic aneurysm that ruptures posteriorly has different consequences. Blood is pumped into a steadily enlarging space between the aorta and tissues behind it. Bleeding is relentless because it is so forceful. The rate of blood flow out of the aorta varies with the tear's size. Minutes, hours and occasionally even days may pass before the volume of blood lost from the circulatory system becomes lethal.

Thoracic aortic aneurysms occur less commonly than abdominal ones. Should the thoracic aorta dissect and rupture into the pericardial sac around the heart, the sac will fill up with blood. Death is sudden, because the heart stops beating almost immediately. Surgical repair, though rarely successful, can be attempted in some cases when an aneurysm's rupture is recognized early enough. Repair of ruptured abdominal aneurysms is frequently attempted.

The prognosis for survival in either case (abdominal or thoracic aortic aneurysms) is poor. Thoracic aneurysm ruptures are almost uniformly fatal, and coroners can say that almost every attempt to surgically repair a ruptured thoracic aortic aneurysm fails. The survival rate of people whose haemorrhage is caused by an abdominal aortas rupture is 10%–50%.[8]

When an aortic wall tears, pain continues until the tearing stops. Some aortic tears, called *dissections* (see Figure 5.4), extend only into the middle of the aorta's wall. In those cases, pain varies with the dissection's location. Dissections don't usually result from accidents, and they aren't only found in people with atherosclerosis. Coroners investigate sudden deaths of unfortunate young people who suffer from diseases that weaken muscle fibres in their arterial tunica media, which often first dissects and then fatally ruptures.*

* These conditions are called connective tissue disorders. The two most commonly resulting in deaths coroners investigate, Marfan syndrome and Ehlers-Danlos syndrome, are often known to families who are usually aware of the possibility of fatal arterial ruptures.

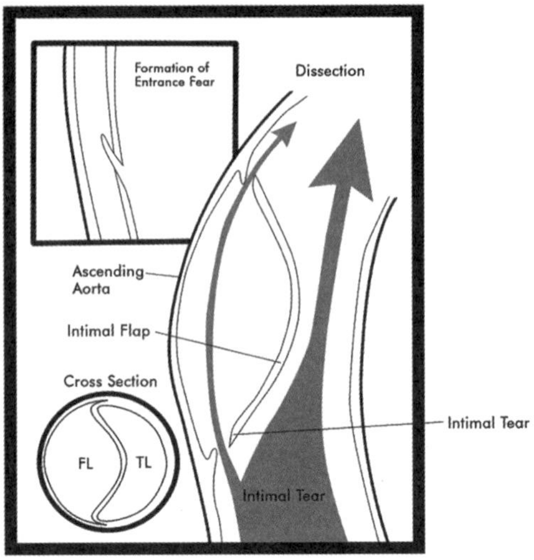

Figure 5.4: Aortic Dissection

A dissecting thoracic aorta will cause upper back pain that is occasionally intermittent, sometimes continuous and occasionally occurs just once. Though uncomfortable, the pain of a dissection is not always totally disabling. Aortic wall dissections vary in length from a centimetre or two to perhaps 20 centimetres before rupturing.

Any blood vessel in the body can potentially dissect or rupture. The method of dying when an artery within the skull tears is discussed in Chapter 1. A coronary artery dissection stops that artery's blood flow and causes sudden death. Coroners never expect a coronary artery dissection to be the cause of death. These dissections are only discovered by a pathologist. Most deaths from any ruptured aneurysm investigated by a coroner occurred suddenly where there was no possibility of getting to a hospital.

Respiratory Tract

A nosebleed (epistaxis) is rarely fatal. Only four Americans among the 2.4 million who expired in a recent year died from a nosebleed.[9] Absent unusual circumstances, any death from a nosebleed usually follows heroic surgical efforts to try to stop the bleeding and is unlikely to involve a coroner. Coroners are only likely to investigate fatal nosebleeds that occurred in people who were never taken to hospital.

Any nosebleed death scene is likely to be bloody. Without someone to explain that a nosebleed was fatal, the cause might not be apparent at the death scene. The origin of a lethal nasal haemorrhage can only be identified at autopsy. Dying from a nosebleed undoubtedly provokes a lot of anxiety, but little pain accompanies it until weakness finally prevents spitting or swallowing. At that point, aspirating blood might be uncomfortable for a short time before loss of consciousness. Only if an autopsy reveals a lot of blood collected in the lungs should a coroner consider that the death was painful.

Fatal bleeding from the trachea (windpipe) is uncommon too. Tracheostomies are holes surgeons create in the windpipe to ease breathing when something obstructs normal respiration. The windpipe hole into which a tracheostomy tube is inserted is called a stoma. That stoma can become infected and start to haemorrhage. The bleeding could become fatal when using blood thinners, but this type of fatal bleed is uncommon. When it does happen the death is a foreseeable complication of the condition for which the tracheostomy was created. Coroners are unlikely to ever investigate such a death.

Tracheal trauma that compresses the windpipe's anterior wall against the back of the tube suffocates when it completely blocks all air flow to and from the lungs. Bleeding that may accompany tracheal compression is often simply one of many potentially fatal injuries. Death is more properly attributed to multiple injuries rather than just the tracheal injury alone.

The same is true of bleeding into the lungs. An asphyxial death follows any injury to the lungs' arterioles or capillaries that fills the lungs with blood. In many circumstances this process takes some time. With bleeding from a pulmonary artery, often caused by stabbing or shooting, dying is much more rapid. Any sudden force that compresses the chest can tear enough of the lungs' blood vessels to be fatal. This too is often one of several injuries that are each potentially fatal.

Pulmonary arteries are large. Blood flows through them at almost four litres per minute. Once severed, consciousness can continue only for 20 seconds or so. Death follows minutes later. Trauma is not the only reason for fatal pulmonary haemorrhages. Anticoagulants (medications used to stop blood from clotting) and congenital bleeding disorders can also cause lethal bleeding in the lungs.

When death is caused by a fatal haemorrhage from a natural disease (like cancer) anywhere along the respiratory tract in a hospitalized patient, a coroner will almost never investigate the death. Those occurring unexpectedly at home or out of doors fall within the coroner's purview. Coroners always investigate fatal traumatic haemorrhages.

Head and Neck

In a "closed" head injury the skin and skull remain intact. Bleeding becomes fatal when elevated intracranial pressure pushes the brainstem downward through the foramen magnum and breathing stops. In open head injuries the skull is fractured, and lacerated scalp above the fracture exposes both the brain and torn cranial arteries to the air.

The fatal head injuries coroners investigate are so severe that in most cases consciousness was lost immediately. Even though the volume of blood lost might not have been enough to cause death, combined with the brain injury it will turn out to be lethal. A coroner need not choose between these physiological processes that lead to death. The term "open head injury" covers both possibilities.

Fatal head injuries are quite common. One study looked at what it called traumatic brain injury (TBI) deaths in Europe. The rates of TBI deaths (which almost always involve bleeding) varied from 9 per 100,000 and 28.1 per 100,000 deaths, depending on the country.[10] Rates in that range would probably be found in North America and Australasia as well.

Urinary Tract

Bleeding commonly arises throughout the urinary tract — in the kidneys, ureters, bladder or urethra. Haemorrhage only becomes lethal once an artery is lacerated or ruptures. The renal artery, with a rate of blood flow of 1.2 litres per minute, is the usual source of fatal haemorrhages. Coroners rarely investigate these deaths unless they were caused by an injury. In most trauma cases death arises from multiple injuries; bleeding kidneys are simply two of many lethal haemorrhages.

Bones

Bones bleed whenever broken. Death is more likely when a piece of broken bone tears an adjacent artery. Both the fracture and the pressure caused by blood collecting around the site of the break cause pain. A fracture may become lethal when broken bone pierces the skin, allowing high-pressured arterial blood to rapidly spurt out of the body.

Though using an anticoagulant may lead to bleeding within the bone itself, the haemorrhage is rarely fatal because a bone's rigidity limits the amount of bleeding possible. However, a lot of pain accompanies bleeding inside a bone. Dying as a result of fracturing a bone is very common, particularly when frail elderly people break a hip. In most of these cases, death arises from complications of the fracture other than bleeding.

The consequences of skull fractures and anticoagulant bleeds into the brain are discussed in Chapter 1.

Bleeding Disorders

Several congenital bleeding conditions, collectively called haemophilia, make injured people bleed excessively. Humans have 13 clotting factors involved in the cascade of actions that lead to the formation of blood clots. How those clots develop is learned by every medical student and remembered by every haematologist. Fortunately for coroners, they don't need to understand how clotting factors work.

Genes that deprive people of any clotting factor make even the slightest bump a potential cause of a lethal haemorrhage. Haemophilia, a medical condition in which the ability of blood to clot is severely reduced, is a natural occurrence. Coroners will only investigate the death of a haemophiliac when it was accidental or when death occurred unexpectedly somewhere outside a hospital.

Bleeding into either a joint or muscle can be very painful. Autopsies may reveal such haemorrhages that are not obvious to a coroner. Any pains a dying haemophiliac experienced will likely resemble previous discomfort. Inquiring family members generally make that assumption. They are unlikely to discuss the pain of dying at all.

Besides bleeding factors, platelets are needed for blood to clot. Anything that decreases the number of platelets increases the chance of a fatal haemorrhage. Alcoholism, infections like HIV, and conditions that lessen the spleen's ability to function all may cause a lethal decrease in platelets.

Talking about the pain of haemorrhage is simple. Bleeding into body tissue hurts. Bleeding that leaves the body is painless. Nobody ever asks a coroner about platelets. Nevertheless, coroners should be aware that lethal bleeding may occur when a person lacks them. While relatives of alcoholics seem to accept the fact that chronic alcohol abusers commonly bleed to death, some inquire about the source of the terminal bleed.

Clotting

Sometimes a fatal blood clot develops in either an artery or a vein. The medical term for a clot is a thrombus (plural thrombi). A clot big enough to stop all blood flow through an artery kills all the tissues that the vessel supplies. When that tissue is in a vital organ like the heart, lungs or brain, the clot becomes lethal.

Blood flowing around either an intact or ruptured cholesterol plaque of an arterial wall becomes turbulent. Consequent clot development is discussed in the chapters on brain and cardiac deaths (Chapters 1 and 2). Atherosclerosis, the common factor in both situations, can also lead to lethal clotting in both pulmonary arteries and the aorta. These thrombotic deaths are relatively uncommon and almost never investigated by coroners.

Most people know that smoking, obesity, lack of exercise, and high blood fats are factors that make blood clots likely to develop. Coroners frequently hear from relatives that they repeatedly tried to get the person to change some behaviour that the relatives were sure would eventually cause premature death. It is important not to let relatives believe that the death resulted from any failure on their part. Emphasize that people can only be responsible for their own health, not for that of anybody else.

Many medical conditions encourage blood to clot. Some families have several members affected by a clotting disorder like polycythaemia rubra vera, protein C deficiency, or an antiphospholipid syndrome. When speaking to knowledgeable relatives a coroner should listen more than talk. Knowledgeable relatives can teach an investigator a lot about the fatal disease while going through their grieving process.

It is rather complicated to explain why red blood cells stick together to form a clot. If asked, talk about electrostatic charges sticking red blood cells together in the same way that paper sticks to a sweater. A coroner can usually safely add that dehydration and conditions producing too many circulating red blood cells make clotting more likely without requiring further explanation. For more information, direct questioners to Wikipedia or other reputable online sources.

Thrombi form in veins too. Venous clots rarely cause death at their time of creation. Death results from part of the clot breaking off and travelling through the bloodstream to a blood vessel far away, where its arrival blocks blood flow and fatally deprives some vital body part of oxygen. A mobile clot is called an embolus (plural emboli).

Immobile patients lying in bed after an operation tend to develop large clots in veins in their legs. Congestive heart failure and cancer are two other medical conditions in which venous thrombi commonly develop and then fatally embolize. Some people's genes promote such clot development more. Sitting in aeroplanes on long-haul flights for such people may be hazardous.

In cases that coroners see, the fatal clots typically break loose from leg or pelvic veins before travelling toward the lungs. These emboli pass through increasingly larger veins to enter the right atrium of the heart. From there, the clots pass through the tricuspid valve into the right ventricle, which then pumps them through the pulmonary valve into the pulmonary arteries.

Small emboli travelling this route simply produce a sharp chest pain with each breath. Larger ones, called saddle pulmonary emboli (see Figure 5.5), prevent blood from entering the lungs, which causes immediate loss of consciousness and a sudden, painless death. Less commonly, people die following a sharp chest pain, coughing up bloody sputum, or perhaps experiencing symptoms mimicking a myocardial infarction.

Fatal clots also form within the heart itself when an atrium fibrillates. In fibrillation, an atrial chamber weakly flaps rather than squeezes. The fibrillation creates blood turbulence that forms thrombi. Death follows different paths, depending on which atrium contains the clot.

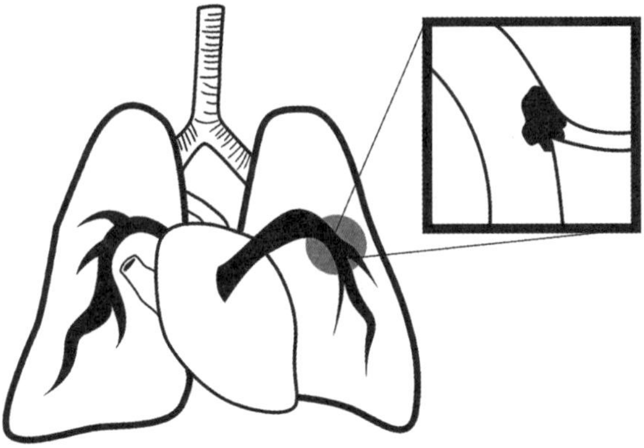

Figure 5.5: A large blood clot that prevents blood from entering both lungs is called a saddle pulmonary embolus. This pictured clot affects only one lung.

A clot arising in the right atrium passes through the tricuspid valve, into the right ventricle, and ends up in the right pulmonary artery. Once lodged there, it has the same effect as any embolus that might have arrived from a faraway vein.

There is one situation in which a clot can travel to the opposite side of the heart. Should the person happen to have a large hole in the wall (septum) dividing the right from the left atrium or ventricle, the clot may pass through that hole into the left side of the heart. Once there, that embolus follows the same fatal course as would a thrombus generated in the left atrium.

In cases coroners investigate, the left ventricle pumps the clot into the aorta and upward toward the brain to lodge in an artery causing a fatal stroke. How this happens is described in the chapter on brain death (Chapter 1).

Disseminated Intravascular Coagulation

Disseminated intravascular coagulation (DIC) is a widespread, and often fatal, clotting syndrome. DIC arises from shock and affects both veins and arteries. DIC deaths differ from other clotting deaths. In some DIC cases, the body's clotting cascade has been set in motion to form thrombi at different sites in the body. In other DIC cases, bleeding occurs in different places in the body. Most DIC haemorrhages arise at surgical sites or in the mouth or nose, but virtually anywhere in the body is a possible site of bleeding.

DIC starts for many reasons, with an underlying bacterial infection somewhere in the body being the most common. Once the germ spreads into the bloodstream, septic shock develops and triggers DIC. While DIC usually arises from bacterial infections, viral, fungal and protozoan infections are occasional causes.

DIC is also associated with obstetrics. In the twenty-first century birth still poses dangers for women. DIC sometimes starts after the placenta tears away from a woman's uterine wall, and the lifeless foetus remains in the mother's womb. Pre-eclampsia and eclampsia are shock-like states that sometimes precede DIC.

Bits of placenta or other foetal products that remain in the uterus after birth are also sometimes associated with fatal DIC. Septic abortions and post-partum haemorrhage are other DIC causes. Coroners investigate every DIC death of a pregnant woman.

Severe trauma causing massive body tissue injury, including severe head injuries, commonly leads to a fatal DIC. Life following deep extensive burns into muscle sometimes ends with DIC. Lethal DIC also arises when other sorts of massive muscle destruction, called rhabdomyolysis, result from electrocution, extensive surgery, or even occasionally a protracted high body temperature.

Transfusing the wrong type of blood also may result in a lethal DIC. The syndrome can be the fatal end to severe allergic reactions or venomous snake bites. People with giant haemangiomas (clusters of blood vessels) or large aortic aneurysms sometimes develop DIC. Promyelocytic leukaemia and some other cancers are known to terminate in DIC.

Nowadays most people who experience DIC die in hospital. In the bulk of these deaths DIC is the terminal fatal complication of some natural disease. Unless the disease resulted from an accident or the family has concerns about medical care, coroners won't be involved.

If a coroner has to investigate a DIC death, when evaluating the hospital care, remember that up to half of people developing this condition can be expected to die. This is particularly true when DIC arises from bacterial sepsis; in those cases, death rates are over 80%.

When fatal cases of DIC result from septic shock, the person went through a period of alternately feeling hot and shivering, then confusion, and finally loss of consciousness. Those may be the only symptoms felt while dying of DIC. There is no pain at all in its final comatose stage. Most symptoms experienced by people dying from DIC arise primarily from the condition that triggered DIC's development. Some pain may be felt when a large volume of blood collects in any tissue or joint space. People with DIC also could feel pain if they were awake while their blood-deprived organs shut down. However, at that point most are in a coma, making the terminal process of dying from DIC relatively painless.

NOTES

1 Wadsworth, G. R. (1954). The blood volume of normal women. *Blood, 9*(12), 1205–1207.

2 Fernandez Arias, C., & Fernandez Arias, C. (2017, April 5). *How do red blood cells know when to die?* Royal Society Open Science. https://royalsocietypublishing.org/doi/10.1098/rsos.160850 Retrieved February 1, 2021.

3 Tintinelli, J. E. (2010). *Emergency medicine: A comprehensive study guide.* McGraw Hill Companies.

4 Lowe, Y. (2019, October 23). Dentist suspended due to Patient Bleeding to Death after he Extracted Ten of Her Teeth. *The Telegraph.*

5 Cohen, D. (2008). Morbidity and mortality of post tonsillectomy bleeding: Analysis of cases. *Journal of Laryngology & Otology, 122*(1), 88–92.

6 Graham, D. Y., & Smith, J. L. (1981). The course of patients after variceal hemorrhage. *Gastroenterology, 80*(4), 800–809.

7 Kim, B. S. M., Li, R. T., Engel, A., Samra, J. S., Clarke, S., Norton, I. D., & Li, A. E. (2014). Diagnosis of gastrointestinal bleeding: A practical guide for clinicians. *World Journal of Gastrointestinal Pathophysiology, 5*(4), 467–468.

8 Shiraev, T., & Condous, M. G. (2013). Incidence and outcomes of ruptured abdominal aortic aneurysms in rural and urban Australia. *ANZ Journal of Surgery, 83*, 834–843.

9 Tabassom, A., & Cho, J. J. (2020, August 8). *Epistaxis.* In NCBI Stat Pearls. https://pubmed.ncbi.nlm.nih.gov/28613768/

10 Majdan, M., Plancikova, D., Brazinova, A., Rusnak, M., Nieboer, D., Feigin, V., & Maas, A. (2016). Epidemiology of traumatic brain injuries in Europe: A cross-sectional analysis. *The Lancet Public Health, 1*(2), e76–e83.

6

Deaths from Infection

Infection has always been a great, but mysterious, killer of mankind. Until a couple of hundred years ago nobody on Earth knew what infections were, or how they killed people. Our ancestors thought those dying of an infection simply succumbed to a "fever." "Fevers" were thought to have been brought about by humours or flux. Even though van Leeuwenhoek first saw bacteria in his microscope around 1674, it took centuries more for people to learn how these germs caused illness or death when transmitted from insects, other people or food.

In the not very distant past, children and a lesser number of adults commonly died of diphtheria, measles, polio and many other infections now prevented by immunization. Infected wounds frequently led to a septic death until Sir Alexander Fleming discovered penicillin during Second World War. Death from tuberculosis (TB) was once so common that special hospitals, called sanitariums, had to be built for tubercular patients to languish in for years before many died. Sanitariums only disappeared in the 1950s after the discovery that three antibiotics in combination could kill the bacillus (germ) that caused TB.

In previous centuries, infections were so common and basically untreatable that society considered deaths from infection unavoidable and possibly divinely inspired. A coroner would only investigate such a fatality if someone in the community suspected that the infectious death had been maliciously inflicted by a curse or some other sort of magic spell.

Nowadays a country's number of deaths from infections varies with that state's ability to provide adequate medical services. In many countries, especially in parts of Asia and Africa, health care is rudimentary and sanitation is poor. Many people on those continents die once an easily transmitted infectious disease becomes widespread. Fatal infections are common. Coroners in underdeveloped countries rarely investigate deaths caused by infections.

Even though the situation is better in countries with excellent public health services, coroners still rarely investigate infectious deaths. Comprehensive childhood immunization prevents almost all death from measles, tetanus, polio, diphtheria, meningococcal meningitis, hepatitis — in fact, any disease against which a vaccine has been developed. The usual investigation of a death caused by a preventable infectious disease becomes the province of the medical officer of health.

Nowadays, everyone knows the ease with which infectious disease is transmitted between people who live in squalor. Every year or two a new disease is discovered to have spread from an animal to a human, causing widespread illness — even a pandemic in the case of the novel coronavirus, Covid-19. Cat bites are notorious for causing bacterial infection of the fat (cellulitis) caused by the germ, *Pasturella multocida*, that resides in their mouths. Fortunately, cat bites are rarely fatal. Bat bites that spread rabies are a different matter. Without immediate antibody administration a bite by a rabid bat will always be lethal. Some *Anopheles mosquitos* transmit malaria by their bites. Malaria can be fatal. Again, such deaths are considered natural events that are of concern primarily to public health officials.

Institutional Deaths

Hospital Deaths

Most members of the public know that germs abound in hospitals. Emergency departments were reminded of this truism when the Covid-19 outbreak stopped people coming during the first few months of the pandemic. In fact, hospital-acquired infections are so common that a term has been coined to describe them — nosocomial. Nosocomial infections have many sources — patients, staff, any surface in a room, dirty linen, used bandages or a surgical operation. Almost anything in a hospital is a potential source of an infection. Fortunately, these infections are usually not lethal.

Most nosocomial deaths are unfortunate, but foreseeable, complications of the problem that brought the patient to hospital in the first place. Infections often follow surgery. In fact, infection is one of the two most frequent types of post-operative complication. (The other is bleeding.) Before being administered an anaesthetic, patients are warned to expect either problem during their period of recovery and are told that nosocomial infections can sometimes be fatal.

The number of fatal hospital-acquired infections is higher than one would think. The United States estimates it has 98,000 such deaths annually.[1] One Norwegian study found almost 5% of people who developed nosocomial infections died within 30 days.[2] Since infection is a risk of hospitalization, only if malpractice is suspected does a coroner investigate a nosocomial death. More commonly, hospital staff involved in the patient's care review the case to see whether there is any action they could take to prevent a future similar death. A couple of situations where nosocomial infections are regularly reviewed involve the use of urinary and central venous catheters.

Urinary Catheters

The first common source of lethal nosocomial infections is the urinary catheter (shown in Figure 6.1). Hospital patients require urethral catherization for many reasons and for different lengths of time. Once inserted, a urinary catheter may stay in place for anywhere from a few minutes to many hours. Sometimes the catheter becomes "indwelling" when it has to stay in place for a day or two. More unfortunate patients require an indwelling urinary catheter for the rest of their lives.

The longer the catheter remains in situ the greater the chance of a nosocomial infection. Every day a catheter remains in a urethra the chance of infection increases by 5%. Infection develops first in the

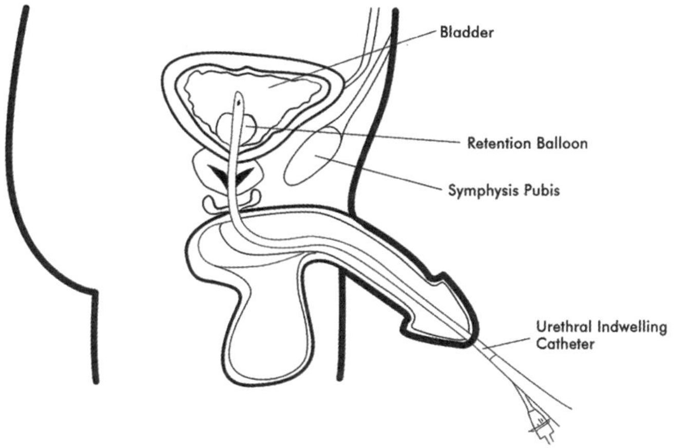

Figure 6.1: Urinary catheter inserted in a male.

urine but easily crosses into the bloodstream; once it does so, it is called bacteraemia. Bacteraemia can lead to sepsis and potentially fatal septic shock.

In one United Kingdom report, 40% of catheterized people who developed bacteraemia from a urinary infection developed septic shock and died within a month. Three quarters of those deaths occurred within the first week.[3] Men and women are equally susceptible to urinary catheter infections, but men tend to develop sepsis — and die from it — more often than women.[4] Regardless of sex, over half who develop septic shock (called urosepsis) are over 70 years of age. Deaths from catheter infections are considered a foreseeable complication of catheter use.

Central Venous Catheters

In hospital, very ill patients who need a large volume of fluid often get it delivered through a plastic tube called a central venous catheter (see Figure 6.2). The central venous catheter is inserted into a large vein using a sterile procedure that usually takes place in an emergency room, operating room or intensive care unit. Most catheterization is uneventful, but even the best sterile procedure cannot always prevent infections. When infection does occur, the position of the catheter's tip in the bloodstream allows bacteria to immediately circulate around the body and cause sepsis.

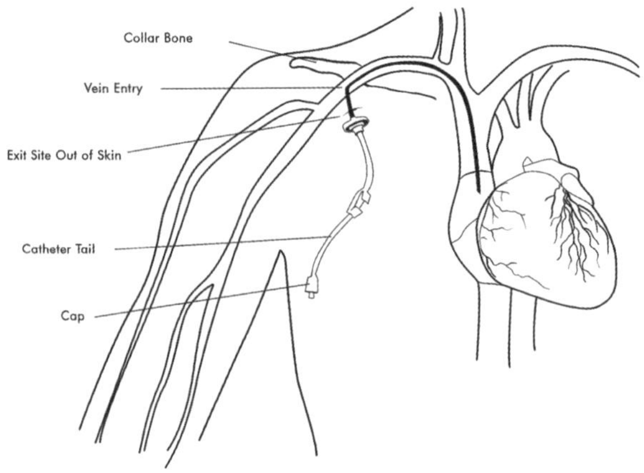

Figure 6.2: A central venous catheter inserted into a major vein in the chest.

Fatality rates from sepsis caused by a central venous catheter vary from country to country and institution to institution. In the United States central venous catheter mortality rates probably vary from 12%–25%.[5]

In 1998 one American surgical intensive care unit cultured 232 central venous catheters. Only 114 were found to be germ free. Of the total, 17% were colonized with bacteria, but with too few germs to cause an infection while 34% were considered infected.[6] Roughly 20% of those infected died. Fifteen of these patients died from infection-related causes within two weeks, two of them within three days. All of the central lines studied were put into very ill post-operative patients. Many people with central lines may be less ill than those included in this study. It is hard to get accurate figures for how many Americans actually die from central venous catheter–caused sepsis. Fatality estimates range between 500 to 4000 annually throughout the United States.

Septicaemia develops from a central venous line 64 times more often than from the usual intravenous plastic tube inserted into a peripheral vein in an arm or leg.[7] The tunnel produced by the catheter permits bacteria to pass from the skin through the space between the outer wall of the catheter and the adjacent tissue, right into the vein's blood. Some germs continue to grow on the catheter tube afterwards too. Bacteria carried by the blood from elsewhere in the body also tend to collect on a catheter tip.

A fatal septicaemia announces itself with chills and fever. Temperature and many other biologic parameters are usually carefully monitored in all patients who have a central venous line. A nurse wants to be sure that their blood pressures do not start to drop. The septicaemic patient starts to feel generally unwell, becomes nauseated and then vomits. Muscles hurt as they go into spasm. Collections of bacteria stuck together on the catheter tip break off and travel to other places their venous blood flows. These bacterial clumps might lodge in the heart, joints, bones or spinal cord. Wherever these clusters of bacteria end up, a collection of pus develops.

The bottom line is that infection from a central venous catheter or a urinary catheter is a common complication that cannot be completely eradicated even with the best sterile practices. For that reason, resulting deaths are considered natural, and they are rarely investigated by a coroner. Instead, these deaths are reviewed by the hospital to see whether some slightly different practice might decrease future fatalities. Coroners usually only investigate deaths caused by catheterization when a family believes malpractice is involved.

Surgery

Post-operative infection rates in the United States are roughly 2%–5%.[8] Most of these infections are not fatal. Nevertheless, any wound infection makes death more likely. Post-operative death is twice as common with an infected wound as one that remains "clean." In 2002, just over 8,200 Americans died of infections at surgical wound sites.[9] Undoubtedly, most of those deaths were not investigated by a coroner. In less developed countries the figures for surgical site infections and fatalities may be much higher.[10]

The bacteria that cause these fatal nosocomial infections come from many places. The patient's own body, the operating room table, surgical instruments, surrounding air or attending surgical staff are all possible sources. Predisposing factors in some patients make their death from a post-operative infection more likely. Age is one of them — the very old and the very young are most prone to death from surgical infections. Diabetics, smokers, people taking steroids or immune suppressing drugs, or anyone who cannot fight infections very well because of an inadequate immune system is also more likely to die of a post-operative infection than someone in good health.

The longer a person remains in hospital the greater the chance of a nosocomial infection. Preoperatively, any part of the body is a potential infection site. Post-operatively a wound adds a new and common nosocomial infection site. People die more frequently when undergoing surgery while an active infection is present in some part of their body far away from the location of the operation. Having an abscess or pneumonia makes a person more likely to die from a knee replacement than if the patient were perfectly healthy. Weight matters too. The obese and the malnourished are more prone to wound site infections. Surgical post-operative deaths occur more commonly when the incision has to be made through an area of the body that is already infected.

Both surgeons and anaesthetists classify the infection risk of any proposed surgery. But a high risk does not preclude an operation taking place; it just makes surgery more dangerous. Some patients believe they have no choice but to opt for an operation even though post-operative survival is improbable. All operating room staff and surgeons follow a mandated system to minimize chances of a post-operative infection. All hospitals use variants of a regime requiring preoperative antibiotics, lengthy surgical scrubbing of hands, antiseptic treatment of skin in the operative area, good operating theatre ventilation, sterile instruments and techniques to shorten operative times as much as possible.

An elective patient's preoperative instructions to minimize infections could include not smoking for a month before surgery, showering before elective surgery and using a disinfectant like chlorhexidine as a cleanser. Diabetic patients are asked to control their blood sugar perfectly right up to the date of surgery.

Only when someone believes a fatal surgical infection death might have arisen from some form of malpractice is a coroner asked to undertake its investigation. The coroner's investigation should include a review of the need for hospitalization, treatment, central line insertion for catheterization, surgery, and the hospital processes associated with care throughout the admission. It is impossible to know how long people scrubbed their hands, of course.

Usually the coroner will conclude that required precautions, preoperatively, intraoperatively and post-operatively were taken. Nevertheless, the patient died from an infection. The verdict will be a natural death due to sepsis, a common complication of surgery. Family members who are angry about the loss of their loved one are often unhappy to hear that conclusion. A coroner must understand their unhappiness, show empathy, but also clearly explain that the death is not an unnatural one. The coroner must remain resolute in the opinion that there is no evidence of malpractice when that is the finding.

The Military

Senior military officers have long been concerned about infectious diseases killing their troops. During the American Revolution eight times more soldiers in the British army died from disease than died from fighting. In the American Civil War, more than half a century later, two thirds of the estimated 600,000 soldiers' fatalities were attributed to infections.[11] Malaria, typhoid fever, dysentery and pneumonia accounted for most of the deaths. As recently as the First World War, infections still killed enormous numbers of both combatants and civilians in all theatres of that conflict.

Nowadays, the military in most developed countries endeavours to provide serving members with comprehensive protection against infection, partly through immunization. Conditions, even in combat areas, are kept as sanitary as possible. Onsite medics administer preventive medications to infected soldiers. Wounded combatants are moved speedily from their place of injury to cleaner areas. Water is clean and food uncontaminated. Infections rarely kill modern-day warriors from wealthy countries.

Troops are still deployed to areas of the world where deadly infectious diseases afflict both armed forces and the civilian population. In areas where tropical diseases are endemic and where no current prevention exists, troops might become ill and die, but this is uncommon. When deaths from infections occur on duty overseas the military will review them, but no coroner will be involved. Coroners may investigate deaths in the home country.

Jails and Prisons

Coroners investigate the deaths of most people who die in jail. Infection happens commonly during a sojourn in prison. Injection of drugs, tattooing and anal intercourse commonly spread potentially fatal bloodborne viral infections like HIV, hepatitis B and hepatitis C throughout the inmate population. By one American calculation, in recent years 18 of every 100,000 prisoners died of the complications of AIDS.[12] The disease was usually not caught in jail. Ninety percent of these inmates entered prison already infected.

Many prisoners also start their incarceration afflicted with hepatitis B and C acquired from intravenous drug use while "on the outside." These diseases take a long time to become fatal, so prisoners with lengthy terms of imprisonment are those most likely to die in jail. Should an inmate begin serving a sentence late in the course of one of these diseases, death can occur even during a short period of incarceration.

Older prisoners also die of pneumonia and urosepsis. The penitentiary is their retirement home. The ways in which aged inmates die resemble those found in any long-term care facility for the elderly. In any jurisdiction where legislation requires investigating any death in prison, coroners frequently find that these conditions were lethal, causing natural deaths of elderly convicts who spent their last days in penitentiaries.

Nursing and Retirement Homes

Both nursing- and retirement-home residents regularly die from infections. Weakened immune systems of ageing people eventually become unable to stop a fatal multiplication of germs somewhere in their bodies. Lethal infections in the elderly occur most commonly in the lungs and the urinary tract. Pneumonia that ends life in the demented elderly has long been termed "the old man's friend."

In these natural deaths, an institutional physician usually pronounces death and signs the death certificate. Coroners only enter the picture when someone expresses concern about the care provided or when that physician is unavailable. The cause of death is usually obvious. The coroner's investigation considers whether different care would prevent a future similar death and may make recommendations whenever that is the case. The coroner does not offer any judgemental opinion on whether the care is adequate or substandard, however.

Nursing-home and retirement-home deaths are on the increase as more elderly people throughout the developed world spend their last years in one of these institutions. At one time Ontario coroners investigated all nursing-home deaths. The provincial government eventually removed that requirement once it decided that nursing homes had improved through regulation, and the province's ministries were satisfied that both nursing-home medical care and management had become generally satisfactory.

Common Infectious Diseases

Lung Infection

The genesis of a pulmonary death is a germ inhaled into the trachea. Its numbers multiply as it travels through the bronchial tubes to become a full-blown pneumonia upon its arrival and reproduction in alveolar sacs. The lethal germ need not be a bacterium. Viruses, mycoplasma and fungi are other organisms that cause pneumonia. A worsening

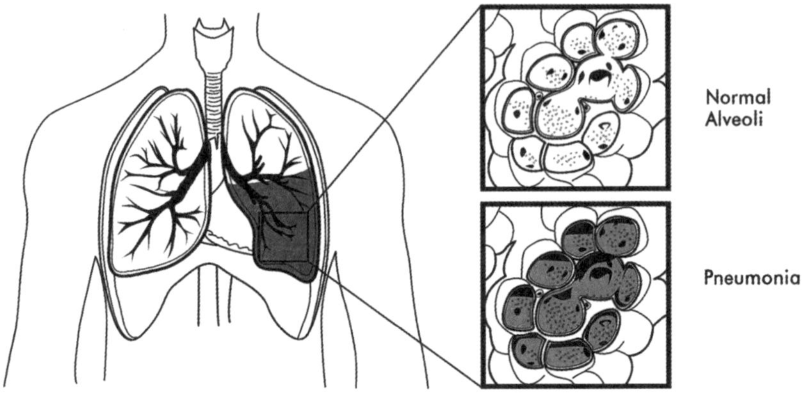

Figure 6.3: Pneumonia occurs when pus, mucus, blood or clear serous fluid clog the alveoli in the lung.

infection fills the lungs with a mixture of pus, mucus, blood or clear serous fluid, as shown in Figure 6.3. These substances make it hard for oxygen to pass from the lung's alveolar sacs into the adjacent capillaries.

As the amount of oxygen passing from the lungs into the bloodstream decreases, respirations speed up. Breathing becomes laboured. Younger people and healthy older people on this downward course initially gasp while trying to catch their breath. They make strenuous efforts to get more air into their lungs and become very restless.

Eventually the oxygen in a dying person's blood drops below the level required to maintain consciousness. Coma may happen quickly, but in other cases consciousness slowly fades. In their final days these oxygen-deprived people sleep for increasing periods of time. Their waking intervals shorten between naps. Finally, they become comatose until death stops all breathing.

It is sometimes very hard to appreciate severe respiratory distress in a frail, demented elderly person. Quite often the diagnosis of a fatal chest infection is made retrospectively after a caregiver, on a routine visit, has discovered a dead body.

Respiratory infections also become fatal when bacteria spread into the bloodstream causing bacteraemia, sepsis, septic shock and ultimately death. A more detailed explanation of how lung infections become fatal is found in Chapter 3. Lung infections usually kill people via asphyxia or septic shock.

Urinary Tract Infection

Urinary infection is commonly fatal in unhealthy elderly people. (Younger people can certainly die of urinary tract infections too, but their deaths are much less common). Death results from bacteria passing from the urine into the bloodstream; this causes urosepsis that ends in a fatal septic shock.

Infections occur, particularly in women, when bacteria gain access to the urinary tract. This is a common occurrence and usually far from lethal. However, fatal cases commonly involve catheterization. Each day a catheter remains lodged in a person's urinary tract there's another 5% (actually 3%–7%),[13] but we'll use 5% for convenience) chance of a urinary tract infection. Consequently, the longer a urinary catheter remains in a person's bladder the more likely an infection will develop, turn into bacteraemia and end as fatal septic shock.

In 2008, over a period of a year, British researchers studied 437 hospitalized patients who developed bacteraemia (bacteria in the blood) as a result of having urinary catheters. Twenty percent of the patients were dead within a week, and 35% of them died within a month.[14] The risk of death from urosepsis varies between institutions, but this type of death is common in all of them. Coroners usually only investigate such deaths when the family is concerned about some aspect of their relative's care.

Sepsis

Sepsis is the body's chemical immune response to a blood-borne bacterial infection. The most common sources are the lungs (pneumonia), the urinary tract, the abdomen and the bloodstream itself (for example by injecting drugs using a dirty needle). Sepsis accounts for at least 25%–30% of hospital deaths in developed countries, perhaps even 35%,[15] and probably 50% or more of hospital deaths in underdeveloped countries.

Sepsis starts with fever, chills and rapid breathing. The pulse races and breathing becomes difficult. Urination is scanty because the kidneys produce less than a normal volume of urine. Thinking becomes muddled. Nausea, vomiting and diarrhoea sometimes follow. Generalized weakness turns into coma. Since all these symptoms are common in many conditions, sepsis is often not recognized until the person is comatose, by which time it is too late to do anything about it.

As sepsis worsens blood pressure drops. The drop may be imperceptible at first, but eventually shock develops. Septic shock brings with it clot formation in the arteries. These clots cause gangrene to develop in the part of the body supplied by a blocked artery. The gangrene may be painful, but nature is sometimes kind about this. Quite often gangrene only develops from septic shock after the person becomes unconscious. It is unusual for a coroner to ever investigate a case of fatal urinary sepsis.

Meningitis and Encephalitis

Coroners also rarely deal with deaths caused by either meningitis or encephalitis. Most of these deaths that they do investigate are among recluses who avoided doctors. The coroner only learns of either cause of death from a pathologist who discovered it at autopsy.

The most common causes of encephalitis and meningitis are viruses and bacteria – more commonly viruses. In both cases death arises when the brain or the meninges (the coverings around the brain) swell so much that they drive part of the brainstem through the foramen magnum. Half of people with untreated meningitis die. Some types of encephalitis are more lethal than others. For example, even with the best treatment, 30% of people with herpes simplex encephalitis still will not survive. The fatality rate for untreated encephalitis reaches 70%–80%.[16]

Cerebral infections often start with vague symptoms like those felt when a cold is coming on. Symptoms become more worrisome when severe headaches and a very painful, board-like stiff neck appear as the encephalitis or meningitis worsens. In fatal cases seizures often precede the period of coma that ends with death. Dying may take no more than a few hours from the first symptoms' appearance. However, time frames need to be elastic when talking about encephalitis and meningitis. While symptoms may start from three to seven days following exposure to the source, death may not occur for days or even months afterwards.

Many viruses and a couple of bacteria cause meningitis and encephalitis. Deaths are infrequent in developed countries, and most occur in hospitals. For that reason, coroners are usually not involved at all, since these are natural deaths.

Rarely Investigated Infectious Diseases

Malaria

Many malarial parasites cause fatal disease. Around the world malaria killed about 409,000 people in 2019, primarily young children and mostly in Africa.[17] Of the four types of malarial parasite the *Plasmodium falciparum* is the most lethal. Falciparum malarial parasites cause death when they plug up cranial arteries, reducing blood flow to the brain cells they supply. When a critical number of the brain's neurons die the whole brain stops working.

Malaria used to be found all over the world. Nowadays the disease is rare in temperate zones. Humans become infected when bitten by an infected *Anopheles* mosquito, an insect eradicated from most temperate-zone countries. Malaria still ravages people who live around the equator, though. In developed countries, people who acquired the disease in an infected area can still die from it after coming home, usually in a hospital's intensive care unit.

Malarial deaths always interest the local medical officer of health. A coroner does not become involved unless the family questions some aspect of terminal hospital care. Tropical-zone coroners see death from malaria as a foreseeable consequence of life in their country — as does the population in general. Tropical-zone coroners are only likely to investigate a malarial death when its cause was initially unsuspected. Temperate-zone coroners will likely never investigate a malarial death at all.

Other Fatal Parasitic Diseases

There are lots of parasites in the world, and at least five others besides malarial ones can kill people. The average coroner almost certainly will never investigate a case, so there is no need to discuss them. In the unlikely event that an investigation reveals that one of these other parasites was the cause, read about it in Wikipedia or other reliable web resources.

Other Viral Infections

Over 200 viruses are known to infect human beings. Most do not kill the people they settle into, but some do. One of the deadliest, smallpox, has now been eradicated. Polio has almost vanished as well. However, local outbreaks of Lassa, Marburg, and Ebola infections still cause many fatalities in parts of Africa. All three diseases have very high death rates, cause significant bleeding before death occurs, and are almost never seen by a coroner. Anyone with one of these diseases should have been quarantined by the local medical officer of health. Their discovery is a public health emergency.

Hantavirus inhabits rats in the American southwest and kills people in two ways. One path to death is acute renal failure that is fatal in 5%–10% of the cases in which it occurs.[18] Hantavirus also causes pulmonary oedema that is lethal 35% of the times it develops.[19]

Dengue is a tropical virus carried by mosquitoes; it usually resolves without treatment. Most people just complain about sore joints a lot until they get better, but sometimes a severe form follows three or four days of fever. Gums begin to bleed and blood is vomited. Blood appears in the urine and bloody spots called petechiae start to appear all over the body. With treatment 5% of people with severe dengue die; among the untreated 50% do. Roughly 22,000 people around the world die from severe dengue each year.[20] Again, this is more a matter of public health interest than a coroner's concern.

Influenza is actually a huge killer. The Spanish flu, back in the days of the First World War, killed 50 million people, most of whom were young and healthy before becoming infected. The type of influenza virus that strikes change each year. The Spanish flu was probably the most virulent pandemic in recent history.

Influenza still kills many people today, but usually only the frail elderly or people whose medical condition made the virus especially lethal. Children die too, but half of all those who die from influenza are perfectly healthy before becoming infected. In the United States in the 2017–2018 season, about 61,000 people died from that year's influenza virus.[21]

Australia and Canada both estimate about 3,500 of their residents die from flu per year. Britain calculates deaths differently. It reports that only about 600 people die from the disease itself annually. However, when you take into account influenza's aggravating effects on pre-existing conditions, the number rose to 7,500 in the 2019–2020 season.[22]

Influenza's appearance in a human body triggers a vigorous immune response. About one third of flu deaths arise when the virus simply overwhelms the immune system. Another third of deaths are actually caused by secondary bacterial infections, usually pneumonia. The last third of influenza's deaths arise when organs shut down after the virus inflames the heart, brain, muscles or spinal cord.[23]

The recent Covid-19 pandemic caused by a coronavirus caused deaths in a similar manner to ordinary influenza. It was also similar in that most who died were elderly inhabitants of long-term care homes. Covid-19 differed a bit in that almost no children died.

A number of childhood diseases that have killed people in centuries past today are prevented from so doing through immunization. Childhood diseases that occasionally cause a fatal encephalitis or meningitis like measles, German measles, chicken pox or mumps no longer do this in areas where most people are vaccinated. Nowadays the herpes simplex virus found in cold sores is the most common cause of fatal encephalitis — but only two per million annually.

Fungal Infections

Fatal fungal diseases only incidentally interest coroners. It is estimated that about 1.5 million people a year die from fungi.[24] The most common human fungal infections are blastomycosis, aspergillosis, cryptococcus, pneumocystis, candidiasis and coccidiomycosis. Today, most fungal deaths in developed countries occur in people with AIDS or who have otherwise compromised immune systems.

Fungi can cause sepsis. Sometimes a fatal encephalitis or meningitis develops. More often the fungi are aspirated, sometimes developing into a fatal pneumonia. This is probably the most common cause of fungal deaths. All these fungal deaths are natural diseases, usually treated in hospital, that are almost never investigated by a coroner.

Infections from Intravenous Drug Use

Coroners always investigate illicit drug use deaths that happen shortly after the person used the abused substance. Those deaths are considered accidental. Coroners rarely investigate a death from an infection brought on by using dirty needles to inject street drugs into the veins. That is because these deaths happen years later in hospital, where dying is considered a natural terminal consequence of the viral infection. The three most common fatal diseases spread this way are hepatitis B, hepatitis C and AIDS (acquired immune deficiency syndrome) caused by the human immunodeficiency virus (HIV).

Hepatitis B and hepatitis C cause death in the same way: people die either as a result of complications from cirrhosis or liver cancer. Many people around the world die of these diseases. The WHO estimates of 880,000 die of hepatitis B each year and about 400,000 people around the world die from hepatitis C annually. In 2015 a total of 1.34 million people were estimated to die of all types of hepatitis combined.[25] How they die is described in Chapter 4 (Endocrine Deaths) and Chapter 7 (Deaths from Cancer).

In 2018, 15,820 adults and adolescents diagnosed with HIV died in the United States and its six dependent areas.[26] Most died from some sort of overwhelming fatal infection caused by the body's immune system being suppressed by the disease. Though there are many other possibilities, pneumocystis pneumonia, toxoplasmosis and tuberculosis are three common infections that often prove fatal for people with AIDS. Cancer of many sorts can also be the lethal agent. One tumour particularly associated with the disease is Kaposi's sarcoma. Nowadays death usually follows many years of successful treatment. Coroners who investigate a death caused by AIDS can usually expect the family to not ask questions about how the disease progressed. They will already know.

Infections are always a natural occurrence. It is only when nothing was known about how a person died, or when there is some suspicion of malpractice in the terminal management of an infectious death that a coroner's investigation is sought. Fatal infections are of professional interest but are only occasionally within the coroner's ambit.

NOTES

1 Haque, M., Sartelli, M., McKimm, J., & Abu Bakar, M. (2018). Health care-associated infections — An overview. *Infect Drug Resist, 11*, 2321–2333.

2 Koch, A. M., Nilsen, R. M., Eriksen, H. M., Cox, R. J., & Harthug, S. (2015). Mortality related to hospital-associated infections in a tertiary hospital: Repeated cross-sectional studies between 2004-2011. *Antimicrobial Resistance & Infection Control* 4, 57.

3 Meltzer, M., & Welch, C. (2013). Outcomes in UK patients with hospital-acquired bacteraemia and the risk of catheter-associated urinary tract infections. *Postgraduate Medical Journal, 89*, 329–334.

4 Nasir, N. Jamil, B., Siddiqui, S., Talat, N., Khan, F. A., & Hussain, R. (2015). Mortality in sepsis and its relationship with gender. *Pakistan Journal of Medical Sciences, 31*(5), 1201–1206.

5 Srinivasan, A., Wise, M., Bell, M., Cardo, D., Edwards, J., Fridkin, S.,...Pollock, D. (2011, March 4). Vital signs: Central line–associated blood stream infections: United States, 2001, 2008, and 2009. *Morbidity and Mortality Weekly Report, 60*(8), 243–248.

6 Charalambos, C., Swoboda, S. M., Dick, J., Perl, T., & Lipsett, P. A. (1998). Risk factors and clinical impact of central line infections in the surgical intensive care unit. *Arch Surg, 133*, 1241–1246.

7 Gahlot, R., Nigam, C., Kumar, V., Yadav, G., & Anapurba, S. (2014). Catheter-related bloodstream infections. *International Journal of Critical Illness & Injury Science, 4*(2), 162–167.

8 Loyola University Health System. (2017, January 19). Surgical site infections are the most common and costly of hospital infections. *Science Daily*. https://www.sciencedaily.com/releases/2017/01/170119161551.htm#

9 Klevens, R. M., Edwards, J. R., Richards, C. L., Jr., Horan, T. C., Gaynes, R. P., Pollock, D. A., & Cardo, D. M. (2007). Estimating health care-associated infections and deaths in US hospitals, 2002. *Public Health Reports, 122*(2), 160–166.

10 Sattar, F., Sattar, Z., Zaman, M., & Akbar, S. (2019). Frequency of post-operative surgical site infections in a tertiary care hospital in Abbottabad, Pakistan. *Cureus, 11*(3), e4243.

11 Hamidullah, I. K. (2002). *The impact of disease on the Civil War*. https://teachers.yale.edu/curriculum/viewer/initiative_10.06.02_u

12 Maruschak, L. M., & Bronson, J. (2017). *HIV in prisons, 2015—Statistical tables*. Washington, DC: US Department of Justice, Bureau of Justice Statistics. https://www.bjs.gov/index.cfm?ty=pbdetail&iid=6026

13 Nicolle, L. E. (2014). Catheter associated urinary tract infections. *Antimicrobial Resistance & Infection Control, 3*(23). https://doi.org/10.1186/2047-2994-3-23

14 See note 3 above.

15 Brigham and Women's Hospital. (2019, March 11). Sepsis a leading cause of death in US hospitals but many deaths may not be preventable. *Science Daily*. https://www.sciencedaily.com/releases/2019/03/190311125242.htm

16 Easton, A. (2019). *Death from encephalitis*. https://www.encephalitis.info/death-from-encephalitis

17 World Health Organization. (2020, November 30). *Malaria fact sheet*. https://www.who.int/news-room/fact-sheets/detail/malaria

18 Jiang, H., Du, H., Wang, L. M., Wang, P. Z., & Bai, X. F. (2016). Hemorrhagic fever with renal syndrome: Pathogenesis and clinical picture. *Frontiers in Cellular and Infection Microbiology*. https://doi.org/10.3389/fcimb.2016.00001

19 MacNeil, A., Ksiazek, T. G., & Rollin, P. E. (2011). Hantavirus pulmonary syndrome, United States, 1993–2009. *Emerging Infectious Diseases, 17*(7): 1195–1201.

20 Centers For Disease Control and Prevention. (2019, May 3). *About dengue: What you need to know.* https://www.cdc.gov/dengue/about/

21 Centers for Disease Control and Prevention. (n.d.) *2017–2018 estimated influenza illnesses, medical visits, hospitalizations, and deaths and estimated influenza illnesses, medical visits, hospitalizations and death averted by vaccination in the United States.* https://www.cdc.gov/flu/about/burden-averted/2017-2018.htm

22 Public Health England. (2020, June 25). *Flu annual reports winter 2019–2020.* Retrieved February 8, 2021, from https://www.gov.uk/government/statistics/annual-flu-reports

23 Jabr, F. (2017, December 18). How does flu actually kill people? *Scientific American.* Retrieved February 8, 2021, from https://www.scientificamerican.com/article/how-does-the-flu-actually-kill-people/

24 Bongomin, F., Gago, S., Oladele, R. O., & Denning, D. W. (2017). Global and multi-national prevalence of Fungal diseases — Estimate precision. *Journal of Fungi, 3*(4), 57.

25 World Health Organization. (2017, April). Global hepatitis report, 2017. https://www.who.int/hepatitis/publications/global-hepatitis-report2017/en/

26 HIV.gov. (n.d.). *US statistics: Fast facts.* https://www.hiv.gov/hiv-basics/overview/data-and-trends/statistics

7

Deaths from Cancer

Cancer accounts for about a quarter of deaths in developed countries but a much smaller proportion of coroners' investigations. That's because coroners consider them natural occurrences, regardless of any possible trigger. Mesothelioma is an example of a lethal cancer found in people who inhale asbestos. Coroners consider mesothelioma development years after asbestos exposure an expected complication of contact with particles of that substance and don't investigate those deaths.

One goal of coroners' investigations is to try to prevent similar future fatalities. A death that occurs years after exposure makes it impossible to make useful recommendations about dealing with a substance. Coroners never assign responsibility. Mesothelioma deaths set many people on a quest to blame somebody for the tumour's development. Coroners cannot help these endeavours. Only judges or other types of adjudicators determine responsibility for cancer deaths.

Coroners usually only learn about cancer after autopsy. Its discovery is common enough that coroners need to know how to talk to relatives about various types of malignancies. Whenever possible, the conversation should generalize about dying from cancer. It is best to avoid the pathophysiology of any specific tumour. Most families know coroners are not oncologists, but there are relatives who want some explanation about how their relative might have died. Any explanation should be general and brief. People wanting to know more detail than a coroner can offer should be directed to a knowledgeable physician, such as a specialist dealing with a specific type of cancer. Better still, refer them to a reputable cancer website such as one of those produced by the American Cancer Society.

Coroners often get asked the unanswerable question "How long did dying take?" The correct response is that the coroner does not know and, further, that no physician can accurately tell either. Physicians who are asked the variant "How long will it take for me to die?" reply to the question with a statistic. That statistic is the "five-year survival rate" – the percentage of people with the disease who are still alive five years after they were diagnosed.

Cause

What causes most cancers remains a mystery. Clinical observation and statistical analysis have identified the origins of some malignant tumours. As early as 1775, Sir Percivall Pott realized that soot caused chimney sweeps to develop scrotal tumours. During the twentieth century epidemiologists (medical statisticians) definitively tied smoking tobacco to lung cancer. Carbon particles can be quite carcinogenic in other parts of the body besides the lungs. Smoked or charred food is associated with gastrointestinal tumours. Icelanders, who usually smoke their fish before eating it, develop a lot of stomach cancer as a result.

Viruses like hepatitis B or the human papilloma virus can cause cancer. Ionizing radiation is carcinogenic too. Since 1945, large numbers of survivors of the hydrogen bombs dropped on Hiroshima and Nagasaki that ended the Second World War have died of cancers, especially leukaemia. Radiation from too many X-rays, radon gas in the basement, and even excessive sun exposure will cause malignant cancer. Deaths from malignant melanomas from too much sun exposure are a particular problem in Australia.

Gene variations can make people prone to one sort of cancer or another. Two of the best known are the BRCA1 and BRCA2 genetic mutations associated with breast cancer. Many other gene variations, for which no tests are yet available, have been associated with other sorts of cancer. Future research will undoubtedly discover that there are many more.

Statisticians have tied other factors to malignant tumours. Cancer is more likely to be found in those who drink too much alcohol, who are obese, or who have excessively high blood levels of some hormones. Bacteria, like the *Heliobacter pylori*, commonly found in the stomach, parasites, liver flukes, and tissue inflammation all are statistically associated with an increased risk of cancer. Some tumours are hereditary. Yet all these factors taken together cause only a minority of cancers.

Most malignancies arise from random spontaneous gene mutations (changes) that transform normal cells into cancer cells. Though researchers around the world study cancer's origins at the molecular level, a coroner need know little about cancer's origins. Relatives virtually never ask.

Development

Once a cancer arises, its progression differs with its type. There are too many malignant tumours to remember how each develops. Coroners should stick to generalities when entering into a conversation about the subject.

Cells double their numbers through a process of repeated division called mitosis. Both healthy cells and cancer cells do this. Healthy cells have a control mechanism that stops cellular division once the body has produced enough of those cells. Cancer cells lack that control. Cancer cells don't divide any faster than healthy cells; they just won't stop increasing their number.

A human body consists of billions of different cells, every one specialized to perform a particular function. Each cell dies after replacing itself in a continuous cycle ending only with death. Cancer cells, on the other hand, are undifferentiated. The body's inability to stop these cells from multiplying results in cancer spreading into the surrounding tissue.

Cancer cells also break loose, enter the blood stream, or travel along lymphatics to end up in some distant part of the body. The lymphatic system, unfamiliar to many, is very important in spreading cancer. Lymphatics are channels linking glands that fight infection. Most people become aware of these glands only when they swell in the neck to fight a "strep throat" or bouts of tonsillitis. Cancer cells use the lymphatic channels between groups of glands to travel around the body.

The spread of cancer cells to some distant body part is called metastasizing. Once a cancer cell finally stops moving and begins to divide and multiply in one place, it becomes a metastasis and starts to steal nutrients from its surrounding tissue. Under the right conditions, a metastasis can grow larger than the original tumour. Cells from any metastasis are also able to break loose and float around the body, spreading the cancer even further. Cancers that spread either locally or by metastasis are considered to be malignant.

Cancer can develop anywhere in the body. Symptoms from a malignancy vary depending on the speed with which a cancer grows, its location, and its eventual size. Small, slow-growing tumours, which are often only incidentally discovered on autopsy, may be totally asymptomatic. Larger, faster-growing cancers produce symptoms by invading surrounding tissues or by damaging an organ's function.

The site of a metastasis is all-important to understanding the symptoms a malignant growth produces. No matter their place of origin, all cancer metastases that are located in the same tissue have similar symptoms. A boney metastasis from breast cancer hurts just as much as a boney metastasis from thyroid cancer. However, the symptoms of a tumour's metastasis into a bone differ greatly from those into a lung.

In some cases, the cancer victim's poor immune system may have offered little resistance to the cancer's spread. People with HIV-AIDS have especially poor immune systems. The same is true for people who take high doses of immune suppressant drugs, which are being increasingly prescribed to treat people with autoimmune diseases like ulcerative colitis and rheumatoid arthritis. Immune systems in the elderly are weaker than those in the young. Ineffectual immune systems shorten the dying period, minimizing the length of time the person experiences cancer symptoms.

Cancer Deaths Coroners Investigate

Almost everyone has thought about getting cancer at some time. People who actually become afflicted with the disease are unhappy about their initial diagnosis, but they all eventually come to terms with it, to a greater or lesser degree. Even the best cancer treatment cannot prevent everyone from being killed by a malignant tumour. Therefore, as a rule, coroners don't investigate fatal cancers that have been treated. Cancer deaths that involve coroners typically occur in lonely folk who live by themselves, many of whom are mentally ill, have no relatives nearby, and lack contact with their neighbours. The smell of death emanating from a residence is a common clue that leads to the discovery that they have died.

Recluses constitute part of a larger group of deaths coroners investigate — those who choose not to seek medical attention. People ignore doctors for a number of reasons. Some simply live in fear of a nasty diagnosis. Others dislike authority. A suspicious few think organized medicine is conspiring against them. Frequently, past bad personal or family experiences have put them off doctors for good. Some lived with a spouse who noticed their physical decline but were unable to convince them to seek medical attention.

Coroners often investigate cancer deaths in the mentally ill, who tend to fall into one of three groups: those who were unable to appreciate the significance of their cancer symptoms, those who mistakenly attributed any problems they noticed to a harmless cause, and those who were incapable of giving an accurate enough history to alert their physicians to the need to investigate the possibility of cancer.

Coroners also are involved with cancer deaths in the growing number of people whose unconventional medical beliefs preclude the use of standard medical therapies. To cure their cancers, these people will have selected homeopathy, therapeutic touch, naturopathy, diet, or some other form of complementary medicine that failed them. Such therapies are usually expensive and, to the regret of the surviving family members, never cure cancer.

Adults in democratic countries are free to choose any therapy for themselves no matter how unconventional it may be. A coroner who learns of a cancer death in a person treated solely with complementary medicine should still investigate it thoroughly. The coroner needs to inquire whether the therapy's value and limitations were accurately represented to the decedent. If not, the coroner needs to consider the need to publicize that type of complementary medicine's inability to cure cancer. The reason: to try to prevent future deaths where more conventional therapies might offer a chance for survival.

Children who die after undergoing such a treatment are investigated by both the coroner and the police. Coroners always investigate a child's cancer death when parents chose "quack medicine" over conventional therapy to treat a malignant tumour. The investigation's outcome should ensure that the public understands such treatment does not work in an effort to prevent its use in treating a future similar problem. Police will also conclude that such therapy is inappropriate for children. Criminal charges against the parents usually follow.

Symptoms Common to All Cancers

Some cancer symptoms vary with the cancer's type and location while others are common to all malignancies. Pain experienced can range from nothing at all to a discomfort that is quite intolerable. Keeping this in mind avoids catastrophizing when talking to upset relatives. They listen carefully. Assume every word you say will be remembered! Minimizing all cancer symptoms, especially pain, provides a small degree of comfort.

Most early symptoms of cancer are found in many minor ailments. Cancer tires people, but a lack of sleep, overwork, too much exercise, etc. are more common causes for fatigue. Nothing about feeling tired normally makes anyone rush off to see a doctor. Cancer's fatigue is not initially ignored — just misconstrued.

In the same vein, the weight loss accompanying cancer is commonly welcomed until its cause becomes known. This is especially true for dieters who may give self-discipline undue credit for such weight being shed. Even a rapid 20 kg (44 lbs) weight loss may not be enough to alarm people bent on slimming. Many rejoice at their significant decrease in weight.

Only when a symptom impairs some regular activity do people tend seek medical attention. Stoics take longer than others to visit a physician. The length of time taken to visit a doctor results from a combination of personality traits and philosophy. In a conversation with a relative who is overly critical about the length of time the decedent took to seek medical help, it is quite all right to point this out. When obvious symptoms seem to have been ignored, a description of the deceased person as "probably very tough" is often both accepted and appreciated.

Only when cancer weight loss leads to weakness does the need to discover its cause always arise. The young become alarmed more quickly. Initially, elderly people may attribute weight loss and weakening to their ageing. Once muscle wasting becomes apparent, patients usually decide its cause is something more than age. Withering will have been visible to others who are often the first to suspect its cause.

People with malignant tumours become anaemic. With fewer red cells circulating, brains receive less oxygen. Dizziness results. Lightheadedness and poor balance cause falls. These are common symptoms before any person dies from cancer. When a fall results in a broken bone a hospital visit usually ensues.

All malignancies weaken the immune system, resulting in both more frequent infections and a diminished ability to resist them. Pneumonia commonly kills elderly people with malignant cancer by asphyxiating them. Often the bacteria that cause pneumonia enter the bloodstream and cause a fatal sepsis to develop. Cellulitis (infected skin and fat), urinary tract infections and, in fact, bacteria located anywhere within the body, can produce a fatal septic shock.

Pain is not felt by everyone dying with cancer, but when it does arise most people seek medical help to discover its cause. Since pains (and other symptoms) vary with the site of a malignant growth, it is necessary to look at some specific cancers to understand them.

Specific Cancer Site Symptoms

Local symptoms are the same whether the tumour arose in or metastasized to the site. Most autopsies can accurately describe the type of cancer, but when discussing symptoms the cancer type is less important than the tumour's size and location. For informed remarks beyond general cancer symptoms, either an autopsy or imaging studies are needed to define the size and location of both the original tumour and its metastases. Cancer originates in and spreads to many sites in the body. Basic information for coroners about some of the more common cancers, in alphabetical order, follows.

Adrenal Gland

The adrenal gland lies just above each kidney. A malignant adrenal cancer increases the production of a hormone called cortisone. Cortisone is responsible for many of this cancer's unique symptoms, including weight gain and pink or purple stretch markings on the skin. Women dying of adrenal cancer develop facial hair but go bald and develop irregular periods. Men find their breast tissue enlarges and their testicles shrink.

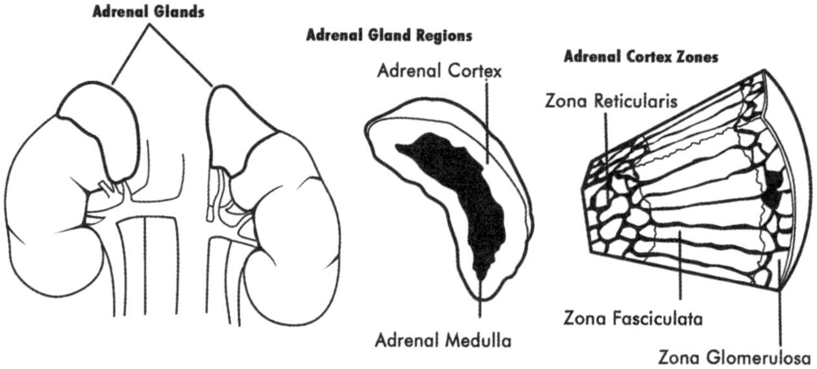

Figure 7.1: The adrenal gland

Nausea, vomiting, loss of appetite, bloated abdomen, back pain, and fevers accompany growth of a malignant adrenal tumour. Once advanced, the dying process caused by an adrenal cancer resembles that caused by any other malignancy. Weight is steadily lost, weakness increases, and cachexia (wasting) may develop terminally.

Many relatives of people treated for adrenal cancer understand the suffering involved. For those unaware, or when no medical treatment preceded discovery of an adrenal malignancy at autopsy, a coroner can suggest these symptoms might have occurred while dying. This adrenal carcinoma, found in only 1 or 2 per million population, is the least common type of cancer mentioned. Its overall five-year survival rate is 51%.[1]

Bladder

Bladder cancer is initially asymptomatic. When a bladder tumour is incidentally discovered on autopsy and is not the cause of death, the cancer likely caused no symptoms. If anything were felt before death, the person might have urinated a lot, felt some burning or frequently experienced an urgent need to void. Starting to urinate might have been difficult; the stream of urine might have been weak with only a scanty amount of urine produced each time.

For bladder cancer to cause death it must be quite advanced. This will have led most people to receive medical attention that might have even included bladder removal and its reconstruction using intestinal tissue at some point. Knowing that all that therapy took place, most relatives understand their deceased relative's suffering and don't ask questions. Coroners rarely investigate these cases.

When an autopsy reveals that a person who received no medical care died from bladder cancer, a coroner can assume that all the usual symptoms common to cancer generally occurred, along with some of those specific to bladder cancer.

Malignant bladder tumours that metastasize to nearby lymph nodes may cause feet to swell. Bladder cancer that spreads to the liver, lung, peritoneum or bones causes symptoms. Once a pathologist identifies metastasis sites, a coroner can deduce what symptoms are likely to have been felt.

Bladder cancer is less lethal than many other malignancies. The general five-year survival rate for people with bladder cancer is 77%. The overall 10-year survival rate is 70% and the overall 15-year survival rate is 65%. In metastasized bladder cancer cases that coroners investigate, the expected five-year survival rate is only 5%.[2]

Blood

Blood cell tumours come in three types — leukaemias, lymphomas and myelomas. Pathologists, not coroners, make the distinction since microscopic examination is needed to define the type. In developed countries most people with these diseases receive continuous treatment until it becomes no longer useful. The cancer's course is well known by any family members keeping in touch. In all three tumour types, fatigue and unexplained weight loss appear at some point. Leukaemias and lymphomas impair the immune system, causing recurrent, finally fatal infections.

Bone marrow manufactures blood cells. Leukaemias, and lymphomas especially, increase the number of cells within bone marrow so much that increasing pressure within the bone may lead to bone pain virtually anywhere. Multiple myeloma usually causes spinal and chest pain. Leukaemia is often discovered after bruises develop or bleeding starts somewhere. Nosebleeds and night sweats are common. Fluctuating fevers are part of the process of dying in both leukaemias and lymphomas.

Lymph nodes commonly swell in the neck, armpits and groin in both leukaemias and lymphomas. Lymphomas in the lung cause coughing. All three types of blood tumours (although myelomas least frequently) enlarge the spleen and make it hurt. Myeloma causes the least distress. At first people with myeloma don't feel a thing. Any symptoms myeloma subsequently causes are commonplace — constipation, thirst or confusion — and unlikely to elicit suspicion of a malignancy.

Most family members who keep in touch with a relative suffering from a blood tumour are well aware of their dying relative's symptoms. They don't ask coroners to talk about them. Kinfolk only want to talk about dying when the relative's prior state of health was unknown or when the condition had never been treated. Since a coroner doesn't know what was felt either, it is kindest and perfectly honest to suggest the possibility that symptoms while dying might have been quite manageable, in which case the decedent would have suffered little.

The five year survival rates for people diagnosed with leukaemia in the United States between 2007 and 2013 varied by type. Among people who had chronic myeloid leukaemia, 68.7% lived for five years after diagnosis. The five-year survival rate was 86.8% for those diagnosed with chronic lymphocytic leukaemia, while 71.6% of those with acute lymphocytic leukaemia continued to live for five years. The most lethal form was acute myeloid leukaemia. It's rate of survival after five years was only 28.1%.

The five-year survival rates for lymphomas varied by type as well. During the period 2007 to 2013, 88.4% of Americans diagnosed with

Hodgkins lymphoma lived five years following diagnosis. During that same period 74.1% of those diagnosed with non-Hodgkins lymphoma survived for five years post-discovery. The overall five-year survival rate for people with myeloma during those six years was 52.4%, but it increased to 75.7% for people who were first diagnosed when they were under the age of 45.[3]

Bone

Most tumours found in bones did not originate there but metastasized from somewhere else. Whichever the cause, a dull, deep, constant pain, often worse at night, announces cancer's arrival. Cancer that grows in an arm bone limits its use. Tumours that grow in a leg bone make walking painful. Metastatic cancer in the ribs is tender to touch and leads to pain with each breath.

Cancer weakens a bone's structure, often resulting in a pathological fracture (one caused by disease rather than injury) through the tumour site. That type of fracture is a natural process and not of interest to a coroner. Coroners might infrequently investigate a death arising from a pathological fracture when an operation to repair it fails. More often a coroner learns only about a pathological fracture when a pathologist discovers it at autopsy. Family members understand that many of their deceased relative's day-to-day activities would have been painful before the bone fractured through the metastasis.

The five-year survival rate differs a lot between metastases and tumours that originate in the bone. Survival rates for metastases are low and vary with the cancer's origin from virtually zero to over 20%. When the cancer originates in the bone the overall five-year survival rate varies by cancer type from 60% to over 80%.[4]

Brain and Spinal Cord

Cancer in the brain and spinal cord arising from its own nervous tissue is called primary. However, most lethal cancer in the brain is metastatic or secondary. Whether primary or secondary, the symptoms of fatal brain tumours are similar. Medical students are taught the two most common symptoms are headaches and nausea. Dizziness occurs commonly too. Frequently a seizure will be the first sign of cerebral malignancy. When cancer affects the brain's visual pathways, vision blurs. Some will see double while others lose bits of their vision.

Speaking can become difficult. People with some brain tumours have trouble finding words, often don't make sense and tend to repeat words over and over again. They become confused. Simple tasks become difficult to perform. Moods switch back and forth between happiness and melancholy. Easygoing people become unreasonable, irritable or even aggressive. Increased anxiety caused by an undiagnosed brain tumour is often attributed to simply being overstressed.

Others with brain cancer are apathetic. Some find planning ahead and organizing even simple tasks often beyond their capability. Normal social constraints often disappear. Visitors may discover that a host with brain cancer comes to the door naked or partially clad. Inappropriate sexual behaviour results from brain tumours too.

The type of symptom brain cancer produces varies with the tumour's location in the brain. A growing cancer destroys adjacent brain tissue and increasingly disrupts cerebral function. Frontal lobe malignancies cause personality changes because the frontal lobes are the control panel for mood, knowledge and understanding. Spinal cord tumours can cause complete or partial paralysis that will end only with death. Close relatives know everything that happened to a family member dying from brain cancer. Only those for whom the brain tumour is an unexpected surprise will ask any questions. Respond in generalities about symptoms caused by brain tumours. If pressed to be more specific, simply say that you cannot be.

The length of time brain and spinal cord tumours take to cause symptoms varies by type and location. Some slow-growing (though lethal) brain cancers take years to cause death. More malignant tumours prove fatal within weeks after being diagnosed. Tell anyone who asks that without a witness, it is impossible to estimate how long symptoms, if any, might have existed. The way brain tumours kill is fully described in the chapter on brain death.

The five-year survival rate differs only slightly between men and women. Considering all malignant primary brain tumours, only 35% of people live at least five years. That figure is derived from a 33.8% male and a 36.4% female five-year survival rate. The type of cancer in the brain has a lot to do with the speed of death. Glioblastoma multiforme leads to the speediest death. Only 5.6% of those with a glioblastoma live five years after diagnosis.[5]

The survival rate in metastatic brain cancer varies a lot with its origin. One American study in 2000 found the overall survival rate was 8.1% at two years post diagnosis, 4.8% at three years, and 2.4% after five years. Consider the following for comparison: at two years post diagnosis, patients with brain metastases from ovarian carcinoma had the highest survival rate (23.9%), and patients with small-cell lung cancer brain metastases had the lowest survival rate (1.7%). However, regardless of the type of brain metastases, few lived for five years. In comparison, consider that after five years, survival rates were just 7.8% for ovarian cancer metastases and 2.3% for both melanoma and renal cell cancer metastases.

Breast

Though it only occasionally occurs in men, breast cancer develops in over 10% of all women. Its ubiquity makes many women well-informed about the disease. Breast cancer is usually discovered as a painless breast lump. Surgery along with other treatment follows shortly after discovery. Most women now survive.

Coroners will only become involved with very malignant tumours that have spread to tissues surrounding the breast where they originated or have metastasized, usually to the bone, liver, lungs or brain. A woman dying of metastatic breast cancer has the same experience while dying as anyone dying with similar metastases from any other cancer. Since a lot of breast tissue or even the whole breast may have been surgically removed, most of the discomfort when dying from breast cancer occurs in other parts of the body.

Nowadays about 90% of American women who get breast cancer live at least five years after its diagnosis. Metastases drop the five-year survival rate to 22%. The high overall survival rate reflects how successful treatment is when the cancer is caught in its earlier phases. Coroners are only likely to investigate breast cancer in women with some sort of serious mental disability.

Female Genitalia

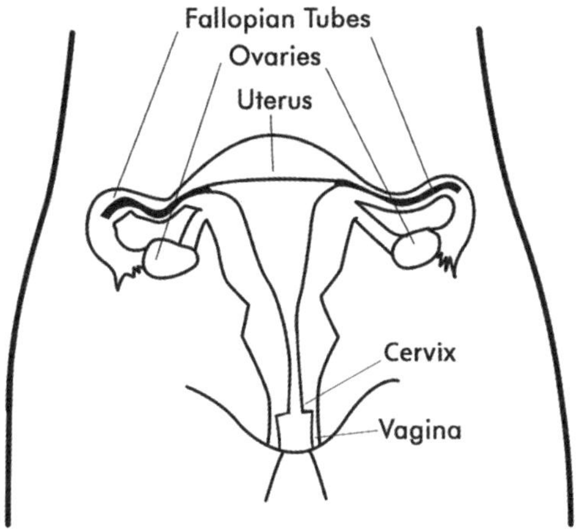

Figure 7.2: The ovaries, fallopian tubes, uterus and cervix

Female genitalia include the ovaries, fallopian tubes, uterus and its cervix. Most cases of cervical cancer are diagnosed by a pathologist looking at a Pap test. Those cervical cancer deaths that coroners investigate are those that have been undiagnosed, untreated or found in a woman who stopped treatment for some reason. Cancer of the cervix or the uterus often causes unexpected painless vaginal bleeding or bleeding following sexual intercourse. Menopausal women are usually alarmed by this, but untimely vaginal bleeding may simply puzzle women during their fertile years.

Some women who die from uterine cancer notice only foul-smelling or pus-like vaginal discharge rather than bleeding. Uterine cancer can be painful or cause a pressure sensation in the pelvis, lower abdomen, back or legs that worsens when urinating or when having a bowel movement. Blood in the toilet bowl following urination or defecation means that uterine cancer has spread into the bladder or the rectum. Swelling of the abdomen and legs follows.

A cancerous tumour in the ovary or fallopian tubes frequently enlarges for quite a while before causing any symptoms at all. Any felt are initially nonspecific – poor appetite, feeling full quickly when eating, vague abdominal discomfort, a bloating sensation and often urinating more frequently than usual. Abdominal discomfort and fullness can be quite marked when the malignant tumour forms a huge cyst. Malignant ovarian cysts weighing as much as 62.5 kg (138 lbs) have been removed from a woman's abdomen.[6]

A cyst even half that large would make a woman urinate frequently and make opening her bowels very difficult. Sexual intercourse would be painful, and her menstrual flow would change. Dull pains in the pelvis, lower back or thighs are common. She would find it hard to even walk around.

The five-year survival rate for cervical cancer is 92%. When it spreads to the body of the uterus, this rate drops to 57%. Once the tumour metastasizes to other areas of the body the five-year survival declines further to only 17%.

Uterine cancer's figures are not much different. There is some variation with the type of tumour, but overall, when localized, 95% of those affected live five years or more. That number drops to 69% with spread to adjacent tissues and drops again to 17% once the cancer has metastasized.

Ovarian and fallopian tube cancers have similar survival rates. Overall, when the cancer stays local 95% live five years. When the spread is only to adjacent tissues and organs the five-year survival rate is still 75%. But once it has metastasized to distant parts, only 29% survive five years. Unfortunately for more than 75% of women, metastasis usually precedes the cancer diagnosis.[7]

Kidney

Because people with kidney (renal cell) cancer frequently have metastases by the time of its discovery, this cancer is often fatal. Dying from a renal cell carcinoma is accompanied by bloody urine, weight loss, fever, night sweats and pain in one flank. Most feel generally unwell, particularly once metastases have spread to the lymph nodes, lungs, liver, adrenal glands, brain or bones.

Coroners will only be involved with a renal cell cancer death when there has been a family concern about care provided or when a person died without receiving medical care at all. This happens infrequently.

American statistics from 2008 to 2014 show people with a localized kidney cancer diagnosis survive for sedat least another five years 93% of the time. Once the tumour spreads regionally that number dropped to 69% and with metastases it drops to only 12%. Unfortunately, 25%–30% of people are only diagnosed at this late stage.[8]

Liver

Primary liver cancer is relatively uncommon in North America and Europe, but since many tumours metastasize into the liver, secondary liver cancer occurs frequently. All liver tumours cause jaundice that turns both skin and eyes yellow and makes the skin itchy. Unless a body is very decomposed when discovered, a coroner can see this yellow colour at the time of death.

Cancer growth enlarges the liver, causing a dull abdominal pain that is felt just below the right ribs and sometimes radiates to the right shoulder. The edge of a very enlarged liver may be felt, or even seen, just below the right ribcage, on the upper right side of the abdomen.

A person's liver continues to function well during most of the time that cancer grows within it. Only once the liver finally begins to fail do litres of fluid, called ascites, start to collect in the abdominal cavity. This large volume of liquid makes the abdomen protrude. The tight skin it causes is uncomfortable, and the fluid pressing on the diaphragm muscles makes breathing difficult.

The American Cancer Society's overall five-year survival rate for all primary liver cancers is 15%, but that number varies with distance spread. When confined to the liver, 28% of patients survive five years after diagnosis. Once spread into nearby organs the rate drops to 7%. Nobody lives five years once the cancer has spread to distant tissues or organs. The usual survival time once liver cancer has metastasized is only about two years. The life expectancy is also two years when the liver tumour is a metastasis from somewhere else.[9]

Lung

A tumour that has started in or spread to the lungs (a common site of metastasis) is discovered in different ways. Shortness of breath would have been one likely clue in cases where an autopsy disclosed fluid in the lungs or in the pleural cavity between the lungs and the chest wall. Hoarseness, which is sometimes produced by an enlarging lung tumour, would be another.

Lung cancer is usually associated with coughing, which is sometimes bloody. It can occur at any time during a tumour's development. While some pulmonary malignancies may be painless, others cause both sharp and dull pains of varying intensity. Pains may be triggered or worsened by simply taking a breath, laughing or coughing.

Lung cancer causes massive terminal haemorrhage when the tumour erodes a pulmonary artery. The blood will be both aspirated and vomited, leaving a trail from the site of the rupture to the place the body was found. This picture needs to be disclosed in a gentle fashion to any unaware family members who will need to clear up the mess after investigators have departed. Dying will have been painless — starting with bleeding, followed by weakness, loss of consciousness, and death in a fairly rapid sequence. Most family members don't even want to know that much.

The five-year survival rate for lung cancer depends on how far it has spread at the time of discovery. With a tumour confined to the lung itself, 61% of people can expect to live for five years or more. Once the nearby lymph nodes are infiltrated the percentage drops to 35%. Metastases farther afield decrease it further to only 6%. Considering all stages of lung cancers together, the five-year survival rate is 24%.

Pancreas

Cancer of the pancreas is almost uniformly fatal. Its discovery immediately raises the question of how long a person is going to live. When pancreatic cancer has not spread to nearby lymph nodes outside the pancreas, the five-year survival rate is 12%. When it has spread to other organs outside the pancreas, usually the liver or lung, only 3% live for five years. Overall, the five-year survival rate is considered to be 9%.[10]

Initially pancreatic cancer is quite painless. Once signs and symptoms develop, as is usually the case when first diagnosed, the tumour has already reached an advanced, incurable stage. Those dying of pancreatic cancer lose both their appetite and quite a bit of weight.

Their skins terminally yellow from jaundice, their stool colour lightens, and their urine turns dark. The most difficult part of dying from cancer of the pancreas is usually a very severe deep, dull abdominal or back pain.

Peritoneum

The peritoneum can be imagined as a large empty balloon separating the abdominal wall from the organs and the rest of the body behind it. Figure 7.3 shows the cavity in cross section. Cancer rarely starts in the peritoneum, but many malignant tumours metastasize there. Cancers from any part of the gastrointestinal tract, such as the oesophagus, stomach, appendix, colon or rectum, commonly spread to the peritoneum.

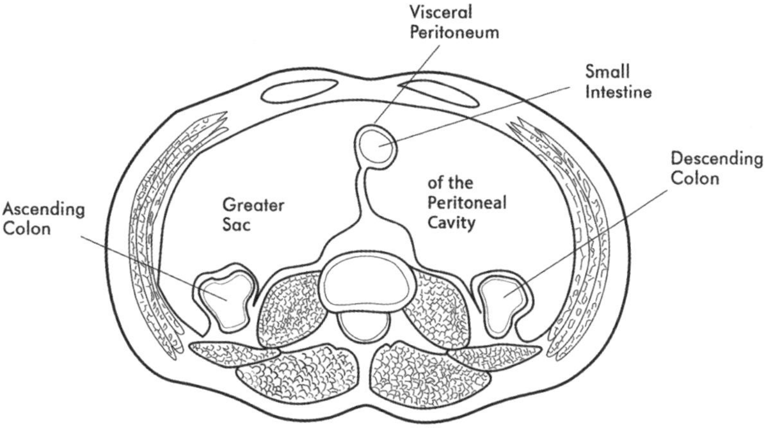

Figure 7.3: The peritoneal cavity

So do many cancers of the gall bladder, pancreas, ovary, liver, breast, and lung, as well as malignant melanomas. Other cancers metastasize to the peritoneum less often. Pathologists can often tell a coroner where a primary cancer arose when death resulted from a metastatic peritoneal tumour, but not always.

Regardless of origin, all types of peritoneal cancers produce the same symptoms. Apart from symptoms common to all cancers, peritoneal malignancies produce litres of a clear liquid that collects within the peritoneal cavity, in a condition called ascites. This fluid distends the abdomen, causing first a bloating sensation and then discomfort when the abdominal wall becomes quite tightly stretched.

Nausea increases as the malignancy grows, but it really worsens once vomiting starts; this occurs when the spreading cancer completely blocks fluid flow through the intestines (a bowel obstruction).

The source of the metastasis is useful for determining which five-year survival rate applies. When the cancer arose elsewhere but spreads to the peritoneum, the rate attributed to a metastasis of that distant cancer is the correct one. In the unlikely event that the cancer arose in the peritoneum, its survival is the same as cancer of the ovary, that is, a 29% five-year survival rate.

Prostate

Prostate cancer the most common malignancy in men, but usually it is not fatal. Men's five-year survival rate with local or regional prostate cancer is nearly 100%. After 10 years, 98% still remain alive. However, once the cancer metastasizes, its five-year survival rate drops to 30%.

Men have few symptoms when prostate cancer remains localized. Early on, it may be difficult to urinate or achieve an erection. Urine streams weaken, and blood may be seen in semen. Generally, prostate cancer is diagnosed by a physician feeling a lump on a prostate gland during a rectal examination.

Local spread of prostate cancer causes pelvic pain. Pain elsewhere starts once the tumour metastasizes, commonly to the bone, brain, liver or lungs. Symptoms produced by metastatic prostate cancer are identical to those of any other malignant tumour's metastases. Any death from prostate cancer a coroner might be called upon to investigate will almost certainly be metastatic, but the likelihood of such an investigation is very low.

Skin

There are three common types of skin cancer, two of which — squamous cell carcinomas and melanomas — are commonly fatal. Malignant melanomas account for about 75% of all skin cancer deaths.

Though people die from skin cancer throughout the world, Australia, New Zealand and South Africa have the highest rates. Death usually results from metastases to the liver, lungs, bone or brain. Symptoms felt while dying of metastatic melanoma are identical to those produced by similar metastases from any other cancer.

Most melanomas in the United States are discovered before there is any spread. That makes the overall five-year survival rate exceed 90% because, with treatment, 97.6% of patients with localized melanomas survive for five years. Survival drops to just over 60% once the tumour spreads to nearby tissues, and the five-year survival rate is only 16.2% when the malignancy has metastasized.

Stomach and Intestines

Cancer developing in the stomach may produce a sense of fullness or even periodic abdominal pains for months before death. Stool often turns black; this symptom often leads to investigations. Heartburn, especially following a meal, and vomiting can both occur while the tumour grows. Stomach and intestinal hyperactivity alone may be enough to trigger vomiting that becomes continuous once the growing cancer blocks either the large or small intestines. Cancer in the small intestine causes a total obstruction much more quickly than does colon cancer. Initially, most people consider something they ate

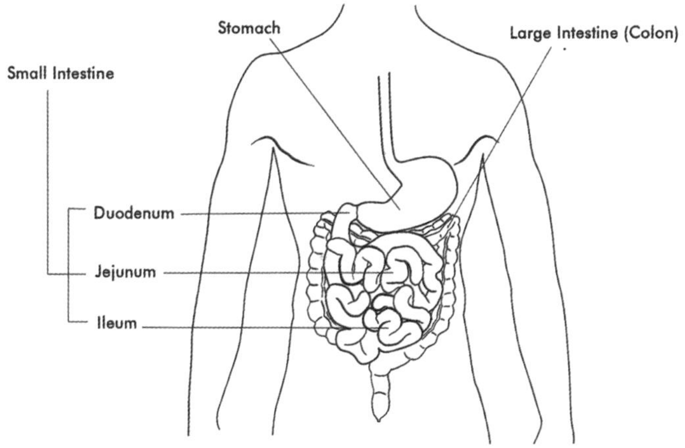

Figure 7.4: The stomach and small intestine

to be the reason for their stomach upset. Once vomiting won't stop, investigation leads to the tumour being discovered.

Malignancies in the large intestine distend the abdomen and cause constipation. Some families will have noticed this and remarked upon a "big belly" developing while their relative was still alive. A coroner can assume the person who died of colon cancer suffered from constipation and abdominal pain if told by a pathologist that the tumour almost completely blocked the colon. Rectal bleeding prior to death would also have been likely. Though hard to miss, this bleeding is sometimes mistakenly attributed to haemorrhoids.

Five-year rates of survival for stomach cancer vary according to its spread. In England and Wales, when the tumour remains localized to the stomach (called stage 1), 65% live for at least five years. Once the cancer enlarges and spreads to adjacent lymph nodes (stages 2 and 3), the five-year survival rate drops to only 35% and 25%, respectively. Nobody lives five years once metastases spread to other parts of the body (stage 4.)[11]

In the United States, the most common small intestine tumour is an adenocarcinoma with a five-year survival rate, if localized to the bowel, of 86%. Among patients who have a regional spread of this cancer, 76% remain alive five years after diagnosis. Distant metastases decrease the five-year survival rate to 46%.

U.S. statistics for colorectal cancer include all large intestine malignant tumours from the caecum to the anus. Considering all stages of

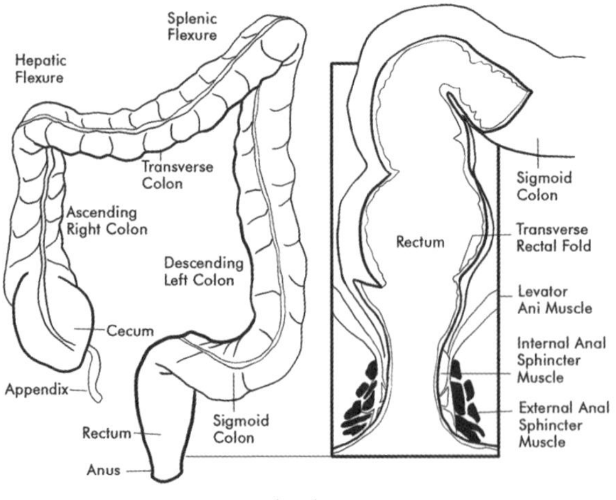

Figure 7.5: The large intestine

these cancers, their overall five year survival rate is 63%. However, when the tumour is confined to the bowel, 90% survive five years from the time of diagnosis. Spread to the regional lymph nodes drops that percentage to 71%. If it has metastasized to distal organs, the five-year survival rate becomes only 14%.[12]

Thyroid

Thyroid cancer typically does not cause any signs or symptoms until a lump can be seen or felt through the skin at the front of the neck. Voice changes or hoarseness, difficulty swallowing, pain in the neck and throat, and swollen lymph nodes in the neck follow. Thyroid cancer most commonly metastasizes to the lungs, bone or liver, and less often to the brain. Again, symptoms in these cases are the same as any metastases from any other type of malignancy.

Survival rates differ with the type of thyroid cancer. The five-year survival rate is almost 100% for localized papillary, follicular, and medullary thyroid cancers. For localized anaplastic (fast-growing cancer cells) thyroid cancer, the five-year survival rate is 31%.

Thyroid cancer spread to nearby tissues or organs or the regional lymph nodes is considered "regional." The five-year regional survival rate for papillary thyroid cancer is 99%. For regional follicular cancer, the rate is 96%, and for regional medullary cancer it is 90%. However, for regional anaplastic thyroid cancer, the rate is only 12%.

Medullary and anaplastic thyroid cancers, which together make up 5% of all thyroid cancers, spread most frequently. The five-year survival rate for metastatic papillary thyroid cancer is 78%; for metastatic follicular thyroid cancer the rate is 63%. But only 39% of metastatic medullary thyroid cancer cases survive at least five years. Metastatic anaplastic thyroid cancer's five-year survival rate is worse still, at just 4%.

While about 25% of deaths in developed countries are caused by cancer nowadays, coroners don't investigate many of them. When they do, coroners should only tell relatives a little bit about the fatal malignancy. It is wiser to refer their inquiries to a reputable cancer organization's website. Its information will be more comprehensive and accurate than anything most physicians could provide.[13]

NOTES

1 This overall figure provided by the American Cancer Society is based on cases from 2009 to 2015. It reflects a spread between 37% and 74% depending on whether it is localized or metastasized. Coroners usually deal with cancer that has spread.

2 American Cancer Society based on 2009–2015

3 American Cancer Society

4 The American Cancer Society's webpages give up-to-date figures for all different types of bone tumours.

5 There is quite a bit of variation between survival based on types of cancer and age. For more detail look at the American or Canadian Cancer Societies' web pages, or that of your own country if one exists.

6 Even larger benign tumours have been removed. The largest recorded was in Texas (where else) in 1905. Dr. Spohn removed a 328 pound (149.1 kg) simple cyst.

7 All these figures are American. The death rates are quite a bit worse in countries with unavailable medical care.

8 American Cancer Society

9 As with all the figures in this chapter, statistics vary year by year and when grouped in collections of different sequences of years.

10 The American Cancer Society is now using a 7% five-year survival figure.

11 More information can be found on the Cancer Research UK Cancer Statistics website.

12 American Cancer Society based on 2009–2015.

13 American Cancer Society based on 2009–2015.

8

Deaths from Neurological Diseases

While everyone with a neurological disease dies, frequently it is not the disease that kills them. A chronic neurological malady often makes people more susceptible to some other illness that turns out to be lethal. Sometimes the neurological disease causes death. That can happen with epilepsy.

Epilepsy

Epilepsy is the term given to a collection of different neurological conditions associated with abnormal cerebral electrical activity. An electrical discharge in the brain triggers body movements described as either seizures or convulsions. Pathological changes to the brain caused by infectious diseases, brain tumours, strokes or a brain injury may all lead to seizures. However, most people who convulse have no abnormal brain tissue at all. The seizure is just a consequence of the brain's electronic malfunction, not a disease in itself.

Before a convulsion starts, some epileptics experience an aura, a moment of awareness that a seizure is about to begin. The aura lasts briefly before a loss of consciousness precedes the seizure's onset. Most seizures don't last very long. Upon reawakening, the person cannot remember anything about the convulsion itself, though wet underwear and a bite mark on the tongue may provide clues that one occurred. Occasionally seizures go on and on in a state called status epilepticus. Most periods of status epilepticus dissipate naturally just like a brief seizure does. They end in a return to normal too — it just takes longer to get there.

Lots of people with conditions causing seizures die as a consequence of having the disease. Most of the time, death results from either the underlying brain condition that caused the seizures or a fatal accident that occurred during the seizure. However, in two to three cases out of 1000 convulsions, when the seizure suddenly stops the person dies.[1]

Since it is not known exactly how a seizure causes death, a fatal seizure is called a sudden unexplained death in epilepsy (SUDEP).*

A seizure may be associated with a blood pressure low enough to deprive the brain of adequate oxygenated blood. Older people who convulse often have coronary atherosclerosis. An excessively slow heart rate during a seizure may trigger a fatal cardiac arrhythmia too. Whatever the mechanism of dying, the convulsing person is unconscious and experiences nothing.

SUDEP happens at different times. Some deaths occur during a seizure. Some people die right afterwards. Others have recovered completely from a seizure only to drop dead a short time later. Epileptics have been found dead in bed with no signs of a seizure and no apparent cause of death on autopsy. Relatives can be told that SUDEP causes death in 8%–17% of epileptics.[2]

Since SUDEP is currently a mystery, inquiring relatives should be told that epileptics sometimes just suddenly die. Most will accept the fact that, right now, nobody has an explanation why. An epileptic's sudden death is always a great shock because it is so unexpected. The only helpful message for grieving relatives about SUDEP is that death was painless; it simply came out of the blue.

Of course, deaths in most convulsing people do not arise from SUDEP. Frequently, the underlying disease somehow causes the death. In many other cases fatal injuries result from the seizure. Convulsing epileptics may fall under the wheels of a bus, off the edge of a cliff or into a lake. In the first two cases epileptics die of traumatic injuries. Those falling into water drown.

Convulsing epileptics also die choking on food while eating. They may fall into a stove or into some form of hot liquid that fatally burns

---

* Some theories relate SUDEP to the autonomic nervous system. That's the part of the body's nervous system over which there is no conscious control. The fatal fault causing SUDEP may be an excessive delay in sending messages to the lungs to take a breath. The autonomic system also controls the heart beating, so SUDEP may also arise from a fatal cardiac arrhythmia. Perhaps there are two physiological pathways to SUDEP.

them. Sometimes death occurs from the medication used to treat the seizures. A number of studies set out the percentages of different types of death experienced by groups of epileptics. These percentages vary in different societies. The information is of little interest to relatives of an epileptic who has just died. They just want to know what happened in the one death that interests them.

Degenerative Neurological Diseases

Many neurological diseases are degenerative. They start to slowly destroy the nervous system cell by cell. This process of neurons dying can go on for decades, but the person's death is the result of malfunction in some other system in the body.

There are a great many neurological degenerative diseases. Since most people suffering with them usually die from a non-neurological cause, six types — some occurring frequently and others of interest to coroners — will be used as examples. Dementia, in its several forms, is the most common. Amyotrophic lateral sclerosis, Parkinson's Disease, Huntington's disease, Creutzfeldt-Jakob disease and multiple sclerosis are five others that people may ask coroners questions about.

Dementia

Right now, an estimated 50 million people around the world suffer from dementia. About 10 million new cases are diagnosed every year. Roughly 60%–70% of all dementia cases are the Alzheimer type, so that name is often used interchangeably when people talk about dementia.[3] Regardless of the type of dementia people die in more or less the same way. All types of dementia worsen as more and more individual brain neurons die.

Death usually arises from complications that result from dementia rather than brain death itself. The inexorable decline dementia causes has usually been witnessed daily by relatives or caregivers for quite a long time. The demented person becomes frail and weakens steadily. The resultant feeble state leads to loss of balance, falls and fractured bones. Death often follows surgery to repair the fracture (typically a broken hip).

Most demented people are elderly. With increasing age immune systems decline and infections develop. Frequently demented people die from pneumonia. Sometimes a germ inhaled simply multiplies enough to eventually kill them. However, that's not the only reason demented people die of pneumonia. Many develop swallowing difficulties with the result that a bit of food finds its way into the lungs instead of the stomach. Breathing in food is called aspiration. Germs collect around the food particles, and aspirated food turns into a fatal pneumonia.

Many demented people die from sepsis when bacteria from (usually) either lung or urinary tract infections spread into the bloodstream. Another common cause of sepsis comes from the pressure from lying in bed in one position for too long. First the skin reddens, and then ulcers are created when continual pressure beaks the skin down. An infected ulcer is another route to fatal sepsis.

Infection and injury are not the only ways life ends when demented. Severely demented people stop opening their mouths when offered food and drink. This behaviour can only go on for a few days before death ends it. Dementia is written as the cause on the death certificate. Its terminal event will have been either dehydration or starvation. Even when the person dies of an infection, dementia is its underlying cause.

Dementia alters many senses and cognitive functions, but not all. One thing people often notice in a demented relative's final days is a continuing ability to feel pain. While dying, a person with dementia can let caregivers know that movement hurts an arthritic joint or a fractured rib. While dementia itself is painless, some of its consequences are not, such as a fractured hip.

Amyotrophic Lateral Sclerosis (ALS)

At one time, the colloquial name for amyotrophic lateral sclerosis (ALS) was Lou Gehrig's disease (Gehrig was a professional baseball player). The fact that Stephen Hawking lived so long with ALS has probably done more than anything since Gehrig's death to make people aware of the disease. ALS is caused by serial deaths of neurons in the motor region of the brain, the spinal cord and the rest of the body. The deaths of these neurons cause a gradual weakening of muscle function.

As motor neurons degenerate and die, fewer activity messages are transmitted to muscle fibres. People notice their muscles gradually weaken, stiffen, cramp, twitch and waste. Twitches commonly start in an arm, leg, shoulder or tongue. As muscles in the mouth and oesophagus weaken, chewing and swallowing become difficult. Speech becomes slurred or nasal. Eventually, a person loses the ability to initiate or control any voluntary movements, including speaking, eating, moving, and finally breathing.

In many people the first signs of ALS may be difficulty buttoning a shirt, writing, or turning a key in a lock. Others first find walking or running awkward. They trip or stumble. Things worsen over the ensuing months.

Most people with ALS die from respiratory failure, when the muscles between the ribs become too weak to move the chest well enough to deliver enough oxygen to the blood. People quite often die in their sleep from respiratory failure. In those cases, death is quite painless. Sometimes people with ALS die with pneumonia, but more often death simply results from muscular paralysis.

Unfortunately, most people with ALS are quite aware of their gradual decline, that nothing can be done about it, and that death is inevitable. Consequently, while ALS may not cause much pain at the time of death, the gradual weakening from amyotrophic lateral sclerosis causes significant anxiety, depression and much suffering. Death usually occurs within three to five years after the symptoms first appear. About 10% of people with ALS survive for 10 or more years.[4]

Parkinson's Disease

Parkinson's disease (PD) is the world's second most common neurodegenerative disorder, after Alzheimer's disease.[5] In North America it affects 572 out of 100,000 people over 45 years of age.[6] The disease is caused by the death of neurons in the area of the brain that controls movement. Once 50%–70% of those neurons die, the symptoms of PD become very evident.[7] A Parkinsonian's hands may begin to tremble; their thumbs start to rub against their index fingers in what is described as a pill rolling movement. Muscles stiffen, movements slow, steps become shorter. The person then starts to shuffle. They become stooped and find it hard to maintain their balance.

This is an understandingly upsetting state of affairs. Fear, anxiety and even quite severe depression can occur at any time. Dementia occurs in the later stages of PD. Swallowing becomes harder as the disease progresses. Some people drool. Others find chewing difficult, resulting in both choking and weight loss. Parkinsonians have trouble sleeping, waking up frequently throughout the night or early in the morning. Often, they fall asleep during the day. Sometimes they lose control of their urine and soak their underwear. Some have difficulty urinating at all.

But none of these impairments kills them. Most people with PD live a normal length of time and die of other natural causes. The complications of PD that kill are swallowing problems that cause people to aspirate food into their lungs. The aspiration leads to pneumonia, the leading cause of death in PD.

The second most common fatal complication of PD starts with loss of balance, falling and breaking a bone. The fracture alone, or complications resulting from its treatment, often lead to death. Finally, when people with Parkinson's disease become demented, death arises from one of the consequences of dementia (see discussion above).

Huntington's Disease

Huntington's disease (HD) is well known and feared by some, but it's not that common. In people of European descent, there are roughly 10 to 17 cases of HD per 100,000 population.[8] In the rest of the world's population HD is rare. Huntington's arises when a person's own genes trigger destruction of motor neurons in various parts of the brain. Their deaths are accompanied by difficulty concentrating, memory lapses and symptoms of depression. Besides becoming melancholy, they lack interest in things, become easily irritability and feel hopeless. These mental changes occur in tandem with starting to stumble and becoming increasingly clumsy and aggressive.

Eventually HD causes involuntary jerks or fidgety movements of the limbs and body. Speaking clearly becomes difficult. Communication may actually become impossible. Many people with HD choke on food, aspirate and develop pneumonia. Physical movements become increasingly slow or rigid. Their personality changes to the point that people often don't seem like their former selves. Breathing becomes harder; moving around becomes more difficult. HD sufferers eventually can lose the ability to walk or sit up by themselves. In the later stages, people with Huntington's disease find all daily activities increasingly difficult. They need full-time nursing care.

Huntington's is uniformly fatal. Death usually is attributed to pneumonia in anywhere from 33%–85% of cases. Terminal pneumonia probably arises from food being aspirated due to swallowing difficulties in about 90% of cases.[9]

Creutzfeldt–Jakob Disease

Coroners rarely investigate deaths caused by Creutzfeldt–Jakob disease (CJD), but they are frequently involved with funeral directors who are very aware of this disease. Undertakers have been taught that CJD is a uniformly fatal degenerative brain condition caused by an odd form of protein called a prion. Like so many other neurological diseases, CJD causes the progressive death of the brain's neurons.

Fortunately, funeral directors don't have to worry about the disease very often. It is rare, occurring in only one out of one million deaths.[10] The United States, for example, will see only about 350 people die of CJD in any year. Many funeral homes never see a case. However, when a funeral director is asked to deal with a case the local coroner is certain to be called about handling the body during the period before cremation.

Funeral directors are quite worried about the possibility of one of their staff catching CJD as a result of handling an affected body. They can be reassured that this is unlikely. It is quite difficult to transmit CJD without getting prions into the bloodstream. The only possible way this might happen in a funeral home would involve embalming. The funeral industry knows this. To prevent transmission undertakers never embalm people with CJD. Most don't even want to bury their bodies — they just cremate them. Funeral directors should be reassured there is no risk when handling CJD cases if they wear protective gloves.

People afflicted with CJD start to notice problems with their memory. They act differently, lose their coordination, and start to have difficulties with their sight. Those with CJD are on a rapid path to increasingly severe dementia accompanied by anxiety, depression, paranoia, obsessive behaviour, hallucinations and even full psychosis.

Speaking becomes difficult. People who have CJD adopt a rigid posture when standing and lose their balance and develop a sloppy gait when walking. Involuntary jerky movements, blindness and weakness develop before coma sets in.

About 70% of people with CJD die within a year of diagnosis.[11] Most die six months after their first symptoms appear. Typically, fluid collects in the lungs because the cough reflex diminishes, and a fatal pneumonia develops. Nobody seems to have survived Creutzfeldt–Jakob disease for more than two and a half years.[12]

Multiple Sclerosis

At some point their careers, coroners who work in the world's northern temperate zone will probably investigate the death of a person, most likely a woman, known to have been diagnosed with multiple sclerosis (MS). Since MS is a disease that increases in prevalence the further away one gets from the equator, it is no surprise that Canadian coroners investigate some of these deaths.* However, MS rarely occurs in the Inuit population.

People who develop MS live for many years after its onset. Their nerve sheaths gradually deteriorate, triggering different sensations depending on which nerve is involved. Symptoms are mild and transient at first. Some people's MS flares intermittently. In others MS symptoms gradually worsen over the years. Patterns change too, so the next onset of unpleasant MS symptoms is never predictable.

Most people experience tingling or a feeling of pins and needles accompanying loss of sensation in some part of the body. When the nerves involved lead to the eyes, MS can cause blurred or double vision. Sometimes sight temporarily disappears from one eye. When the nerves involved supply the throat or vocal cords it becomes difficult to swallow or speak.

MS that affects the bowels causes periods of diarrhoea or constipation. Some with MS can't stop urinating while others need catheterization because they cannot pass urine at all. MS can cause muscle

---

* The prevalence rates per 100,000 people in 2015 were as follows: Canada 291, Denmark 227, Sweden 189, United Kingdom 164, and Norway 160. https://www.statista.com/statistics/372361/prevalence-rate-of-ms-in-select-countries/

pain anywhere in the body. Some people become weak and develop an awkward wobbly gait when walking.

The effects of MS on the brain are many. Moods can fluctuate between anxiety and depression. Poor concentration in advanced cases of MS often makes it tricky for people to recall things quickly. Finding the right word can become difficult. Doing things may take longer, and some people with MS start to find it hard to solve problems. Above all, multiple sclerosis usually fatigues people so easily that they feel tired all day long.

It is often said that people do not die of MS but simply with MS. The disease itself does not actually cause death in an afflicted person. However, one study found that, on average, people with MS in Manitoba die seven and a half years earlier than those in the province who do not have the disease. (Death occurring at 75.9 years vs. an expected 83.4 years lifespan.)[13] So multiple sclerosis seems to play a role in shortening life.

Some diseases are statistically more often fatal in people who have multiple sclerosis. This makes sense when you consider that MS eventually makes people so weak that they become bedridden by the disease. Those bedridden are prone to develop bed sores that can become infected. They also develop urinary tract infections. Swallowing difficulty leads to food aspiration, which leads to the development of pneumonia.

All three of these types of infections can cause septicaemia followed by shock and ultimately death. These infections, and respiratory diseases especially, were found to have caused more deaths in MS patients than in the Manitoba population at large. The terminally weakened state of people with severe cases of MS may explain the statistical difference in death rates between those with MS and everybody else.

A coroner who signs a death certificates for a person who died of MS may describe the primary cause death as a particular infection or perhaps damage caused by a fatal injury. In such instances, MS can be considered a contributing factor. An equally correct alternative is to describe the terminal disease as simply "a complication of multiple sclerosis." In either case, though, life's end was due to something other than multiple sclerosis itself.

There are many other degenerative nerve diseases that are considered fatal.* Some, like spinal muscular atrophy, are primarily found in children. However, in all of these instances, neuronal death will have worsened the body's ability to avoid death from infection, heart failure or respiratory failure. Depending on the neurological condition, death may come quickly or not happen for years. Coroners almost never investigate any of them.

NOTES

1 Thurman, D. J., Hesdorffer, D. C., & French, J. A. (2014). Sudden unexpected death in epilepsy: Assessing the public health burden. *Epilepsia, 55*(10), 1479–1485.

2 See note 1 above.

3 World Health Organization. (2020, September 21). *Dementia.* https://www.who.int/en/news-room/fact-sheets/detail/dementia

4 National Institute of Neurological Disorders and Stroke. (2020, June). Amyotrophic Lateral Sclerosis (ALS) Fact Sheet. https://www.ninds.nih.gov/Disorders/Patient-Caregiver-Education/Fact-Sheets/Amyotrophic-Lateral-Sclerosis-ALS-Fact-Sheet

5 Elbaz, A., Carcaillon, L., Kab, S., & Moisan, F. (2016). *Epidemiology of Parkinson's disease. Revue Neurologique, 172(1), 14–26.*

6 Marras, C., Beck, J. C., Bower, J. H., Roberts, E., Ritz, B., Ross, G. W.,...Tanner, C. M. (2018). Prevalence of Parkinson's disease across North America. *npf Parkinson's Disease, 4, 21. doi.org/10.1038/s41531-018-0058-0*

7 Cheng, H.-C., Ulane, C. M., & Burke, R. E. (2010, June). Clinical progression in Parkinson disease and the neurobiology of axons. *Annals of Neurology, 67,* 715–725.

8 Dayalu, P., & Albin, R. L. (2015). Huntington disease: Pathogenesis and treatment. *Neurologic Clinics, 33*(1), 101–114.

9 Heemskerk, A.-W., & Roos, R. A. C. (2010). E04 Causes of death in Huntington's disease. *Journal of Neurology, Neurosurgery and Psychiatry, 31,* A22.

10 U.S. National Library of Medicine. (n.d.). *Creutzfeldt-Jakob disease.* https://medlineplus.gov/ency/article/000788.htm

* Examples include Alpers disease, Batten disease, Cerebro-Oculo-Facio-Skeletal syndrome, corticobasal degeneration, Gerstmann–Straussler–Scheinker disease, kuru, Leigh's disease, monomelic amyotrophy (MMA), multiple system atrophy (MSA), opsoclonus-myoclonus syndrome, and progressive multifocal leukoencephalopathy (PML).

11 National Institute of Neurological Disorders and Stroke. (2018, May). *Creutzfeldt–Jakob disease fact sheet.* https://www.ninds.nih.gov/Disorders/Patient-Caregiver-Education/Fact-Sheets/Creutzfeldt-Jakob-Disease-Fact-Sheet

12 Mizutani, T., Okumura, A., Oda, M., & Shiraki, H. (1981). Panencephalic type of Creutzfeldt-Jakob disease: Primary involvement of the cerebral white matter. *Journal of Neurology, Neurosurgery, and Psychiatry, 44,* 103–115.

13 Marrie, R. A., Elliott, L., Marriott, J., Cossoy, M., Blanchard, J., Leung, S. & Yu, N. (2015). Effect of comorbidity on mortality in multiple sclerosis. *Neurology, 85*(3), 240–247.

9

Deaths in Children

Unfortunately, children do die, but in today's developed world they die infrequently. Coroners are especially thankful for that because they find the process of investigating child fatalities quite unpleasant. A child's death heavily impacts everyone involved. The only type of death more emotionally distressing is a mother's death during or after labour.

Coroners find it particularly hard to investigate the death of a child who is the same age and sex as one of their own. Throughout these uncomfortable investigations, coroners can forgive themselves for constantly thinking "Thank God that's not my child, but it could be." That thought is a subconscious trick their minds play to maintain composure while preparing to talk with the parents.

To appear professional, a coroner must put aside all the personal feelings that result from viewing the child's dead body. Those already at the death scene will have worked out how to manage their emotions. By the time the coroner comes, most police officers guarding the child's body have their feelings well under control.

When a child's death is accidental, some family members cry throughout their conversation with the coroner. When a child's death is anticipated, the family has often had a long time to become resigned to it. Coroners investigating an expected childhood death frequently arrive to find a mother tearlessly cradling or hugging a dead child while the rest of the family sits nearby, silently staring.

A coroner who has difficulty maintaining composure while viewing a child's dead body need not worry. Tears in a coroner's eyes may seem a bit unprofessional, but since most other people present at a child's death scene are terribly upset too, they don't mind. The coroner can simply wipe the tears away and gently start to ask questions.

Coroners do not investigate children's deaths very often. The province of Ontario in Canada has population of over 14 million. Figure

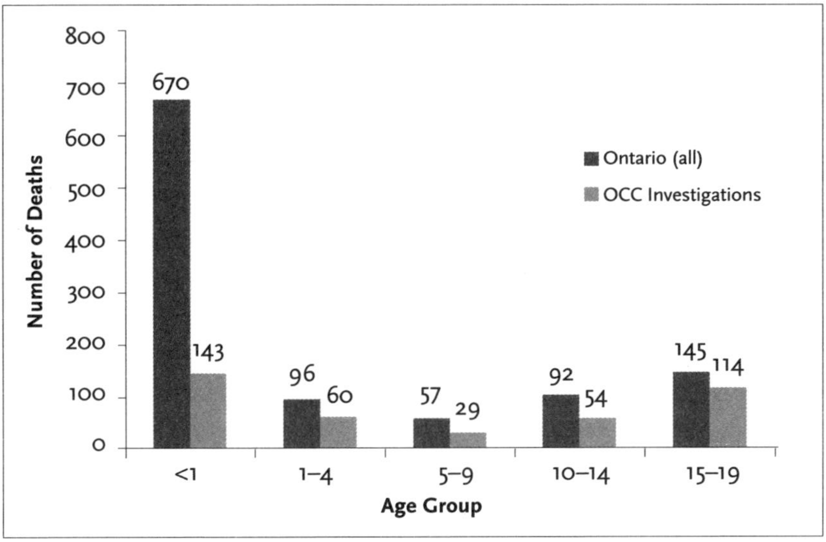

Figure 9.1: The number of children's deaths investigated by the Office of the Chief Coroner, Ontario, 2016.[1]

9.1 shows the proportion of children's deaths that Ontario coroners investigated in 2016.

Note how few children died in a province of over 14 million people — just over 1000. Coroners only investigated 400 of them. This means that many Ontario coroners did not investigate a child's death during that year, and probably none was involved with more than three or four child deaths at most. That will likely be true throughout the developed world.

Age of Child

Causes of childhood deaths vary with age. Children's capacities and activities expand as they grow older, but under the age of one year a child is completely dependent on parents for everything. Abnormalities present at birth often prove fatal in the first year of life. For that reason, both the World Health Organization (WHO) and coroners separate the first year of life from the rest of childhood.

The incidence of death varies greatly during that first year on different continents. Child death rates are much higher in developing than in more developed countries. The WHO estimated 4.2 million children around the world died before their first birthday in 2016.[1] That seems an enormous number, but it's a significant decrease from the 8.8 million deaths that took place in 1990. To give you an idea of geographic variation, Africa — at 52 deaths per 1000 live births — had a death rate more than six times higher than that in Europe (8 deaths per 1000 live births.)

In 2016, the United States recorded only 22,241 deaths of children under one year of age in the whole country.[2] The top 10 causes of American children's deaths that follow change little from year to year.

RANKING	CAUSE OF DEATH	TOTAL NUMBER
1	congenital anomalies	4,816
2	short gestation (prematurity)	3,927
3	Sudden Infant Death Syndrome (SIDS)	1,500
4	maternal pregnancy complications	1,402
5	unintentional injury	1,219
6	placenta, umbilical cord, membranes problems	841
7	bacterial sepsis	583
8	respiratory distress	488
9	circulatory system disease	460
10	neonatal haemorrhage	398

Table 9.1: Leading causes of death in children aged <1 year, United States, 2016[3]

Table 9.1 shows that most of these deaths arise from natural occurrences or diseases. Coroners consider deaths to also be natural when they arise from a known complication of a disease or its treatment. Coroners do not investigate natural deaths.

Fewer than a quarter of all these deaths would require a coroner's investigation. That number includes all deaths from Sudden Infant Death Syndrome (SIDS) because they are totally unexpected. Coroners also investigate an infant death caused by accidental injury. Only in very unusual circumstances is a coroner asked to investigate any of the other eight leading causes of death.

Institutions have different protocols for notifying a coroner about a child's death, even when death was natural, and no investigation is required. Some hospitals notify a coroner about every child or infant death. When that's the case, a coroner receives reports that a natural infant death has occurred. A coroner simply listens to the informant, usually a physician or nurse, recite their patient's medical history in a condensed form. Once it is clear that the cause of the infant's death was a natural one, the coroner should politely decline the case. Then ask the informant to arrange for a care provider to sign the child's death certificate. When talking to a resident physician, both as a courtesy and for education purposes, close the conversation with a short explanation of how the coroner would complete the death certificate if an investigation were required.

When a child has died the family usually don't want to see any unfamiliar faces, including the coroner's. When the family believes the child's medical care was inadequate, they will have to explain their concerns to the coroner as part of the review of the child's treatment. Most often, the coroner concludes that the care provided was quite unremarkable. Many of these coroners' investigations are actually a type of psychotherapy that society has agreed to pay for in order to partially assuage the grief of a dead infant's distraught family.

Coroners also investigate natural deaths in infants less than one year old whenever parents did not seek appropriate medical care for their deceased child. Parents don't do this a lot, but it happens more often than one would think. Religious beliefs or distrust of orthodox medical therapy may lead to less than timely medical care for their infant or, in many cases, none at all. The press becomes very interested in these deaths and gives them a high profile locally. National statistics for these types of deaths are hard to locate.

The WHO's second childhood death grouping comprises children from 1 to 5 years of age. Throughout the world this group has only about one third the number of deaths found under one year of age. The United States collects its statistics a bit differently. It counts deaths from 1 to 4 years old, one year less than the WHO. America's top 10 causes of child deaths during this three-year period are outlined in Table 9.2.

RANKING	CAUSE OF DEATH	TOTAL NUMBER
1	unintentional injury	1261
2	congenital anomalies	433
3	malignant neoplasms	377
4	homicide	339
5	heart disease	118
6	influenza and pneumonia	103
7	septicaemia	70
8	perinatal period problems	60
9	cerebrovascular conditions	55
10	chronic low respiratory disease	51

Table 9.2: Leading causes of death in children aged 1 to 4, United States, 2016[4]

Note that most of the types of death listed in Table 9.2 are natural. Coroners routinely only investigate deaths in this age group when the death is due to unintentional injury or homicide. Again, in this age group, a coroner investigates natural deaths when the death took place without medical care or when a deceased child's family believes inappropriate care contributed to the child's death.

Unintentional injuries trigger a coroner's investigation in the one to four years age group. Coroners investigate all accidental deaths – deaths that arise from an occurrence, incident, or event that happens without foresight or expectation. Unintentional injuries fit this definition.

Ontario coroners investigate two thirds of all deaths in 1- to 4-year-olds, but investigation numbers aren't high. Ontario, which accounts for 40% of all the children in Canada, recorded only 95 deaths in this age group in the eight-year period from 2005 to 2012. Coroners investigated 63 of them.[5]

The third WHO child death group spans the ages from 5 to 14. After 14 years of age, epidemiologists deem the causes of child death to approximate those of adults. Consequently, older teenager death causes need not be separated from those causing adult deaths. Fourteen years of age is adult in death statistics.

The WHO estimated that 900,000 children between the ages of 5 and 14 died in 2018. That's about 2,500 per day.[6] Though this figure may seem high, it is much lower than the incidence in 1990, when 1.7 million children aged 5 to 14 died. This age group's mortality dropped 42% during that quarter century.

Most of these deaths occurred in Africa. A lesser number died in Asia, South America, and Russia. In Europe, Australia, New Zealand, Canada and the United States, substantially fewer 5- to 14-year-olds died. As shown in Tables 9.3 and 9.4, the United States divides its deaths in this age group into two different periods. One age group is from 5 to 9, and the other is from 10 to 14 years of age.

RANKING	CAUSE OF DEATH	TOTAL NUMBER
1	unintentional injury	787
2	malignant neoplasms	449
3	congenital anomalies	203
4	homicide	139
5	heart disease	77
6	chronic low respiratory disease	68
7	influenza and pneumonia	48
8	septicaemia	40
9	cerebrovascular conditions	38
10	benign neoplasms	31

Table 9.3: Leading causes of death in children aged 5 to 9, United States, 2016[7]

RANKING	CAUSE OF DEATH	TOTAL NUMBER
1	unintentional injury	847
2	suicide	436
3	malignant neoplasms	431
4	homicide	147
5	congenital anomalies	146
6	heart disease	111
7	CLR disease	75
8	cerebrovascular conditions	50
9	influenza and pneumonia	39
10	septicaemia	31

Table 9.4: Leading causes of death in children aged 10 to 14, United States, 2016[8]

These rankings are similar for most developed countries, although there may be a somewhat lower homicide percentage in countries where guns are less widely used than in the United States. Coroners need to investigate suicide among 10- to 14-year-olds. Otherwise, the requirement for a coroner's investigation does not differ from the 1- to 5-year-old age group.

Ontario did not follow the WHO's statistical reporting; it followed the American practice in separating death investigations into separate groups for 5- to 9-year-old's and 10- to 14-year old's. From 2008 to 2015 the numbers of deaths were even lower than in the 1 to 4 years old group. In that seven years period only 62 5- to 9-year olds died and 85 10- to 14-year old's died. Just over half the deaths in the 5 to 9 group and two thirds of the deaths in the 10 to 14 group were investigated.[9]

When looking at deaths in the last childhood age group, from 15 to 19, the difference between males and females has to be taken into account. At this age, boys become sexually active and girls can become pregnant. The WHO gives the breakdown shown in Table 9.5.

FEMALES	MALES
maternal conditions	road injury
self-harm	interpersonal violence
road injuries	self-harm
diarrhoeal diseases	drowning
tuberculosis	HIV-AIDS

Table 9.5: Leading causes of death in adolescents aged 15 to 19, worldwide, 2016[10]

Unsurprisingly, the highest levels of death in both sexes in this age group takes place in Africa. The United States collects death causes from the ages of 15 to 24 rather than stopping their assessment at 19. The causes are similar to those found in the 10 to 14 age group, except that septicaemia disappears and complicated pregnancy replaces it. There is a slight shift in order, the most noticeable change being that homicide increases dramatically.

To get a better idea of the problems in the 15 to 19 age group one could use the Ontario experience as a guide for coroners in developed countries. Over the eight years from 2005 to 2012 there were 287 deaths, more than three times the number in the 10- to 14-year-old age group (85). Coroners investigated 233 (81%) of these deaths consisting of high numbers of suicides, homicides and accidental deaths.

Natural Deaths

When death arises from natural causes of any sort, children experience similar symptoms to those felt by a dying adult. When the death is protracted, most parents will have observed their child's daily decline the whole time. Coroners rarely investigate these deaths. Mother and father both well understand their child's suffering. They don't ask anything about their dying child's feelings or how death occurred. Both parents witnessed their child dying. The whole family suffered through it together and know very well what the child went through.

If involved, all a coroner will offer in these cases, apart from a thorough investigation, is condolences.

Some natural childhood deaths coroners always investigate. Some jurisdictions require that all children living in group homes or who are wards of the state must have their deaths investigated. Sudden and unexpected deaths are also always investigated to see if they are due to Sudden Infant Death Syndrome (SIDS) or something else. These two types of death make up the majority of coroners' natural childhood deaths investigation.

A third group of natural deaths that coroners sometimes investigate arise when one parent (sometimes both) complains that inadequate care was provided to their dying child. This may turn out to be the case, of course, but frequently the investigation simply is triggered by excessive parental grief. Mother and father believe that a coroner's investigation will in some way slake it, but of course it only helps a little.

Spiteful behaviour between separated parents sometimes occasions a coroner's investigation into a natural childhood death. One parent of a deceased child is usually attempting to gain some benefit by alleging that negligent care on the other parent's part led to the child's death. The coroner becomes involved to try to determine what actually happened.

Sudden Infant Death Syndrome

Coroners investigate many cases of SIDS, which is also called crib death or cot death (in the United Kingdom). About 20,000 such cases are recorded worldwide annually.[11] Numbers vary in most developed countries from under 1 per 1,000 to 1 per 10,000 live births. (The American figure was only 0.54 per 1,000 live births in 2005.) However, the United States notes racial disparities in these deaths. In 2009, the rate of SIDS deaths among American and Alaskan Indigenous people was 119.2 per 100,000 live births.[12] African Americans had a SIDS death frequency 2.5 times higher than did Caucasian Americans.[13]

Children who die of SIDS need to be less than one year old. Ninety-five percent of them are found dead in their first six months of life, with the numbers peaking at two to four months of age.[14] To reach a SIDS diagnosis two other requirements must be met. First, an exhaustive death scene investigation has to unearth no explanation for dying. Secondly, an autopsy must reveal no cause of death. Most coroners investigate several SIDS deaths during their careers.

Nobody knows why SIDS occurs. A baby is unexpectedly found dead with no sign of any struggle. Death typically occurs in a crib, while asleep, between midnight and 9:00 a.m. In the not-very-distant past SIDS was usually attributed to suffocation. Babies commonly slept in bed with mothers who were thought to have rolled over and smothered the sleeping children. That mistaken assumption caused unimaginable guilt and despair in thousands, if not millions, of mothers whose children died of SIDS in years gone by.

People also theorized a mother might have intentionally smothered her child. Such smotherings do occur. Investigating police officers and coroners periodically get fooled into misconstruing an intentional smothering as SIDS, but probably less than 10% of the time.[15] Mothers have long committed infanticide, particularly when suffering from post-partum depression. Nevertheless, infanticide is much less common than SIDS. Most coroners never investigate a child homicide, while almost all deal with more than one cases of SIDS over the course of their career.

Coroners dealing with middle-class parents in the developed world often find the parents of dead children questioning their child rearing abilities whenever a SIDS death happens. At least subconsciously, both parents somehow feel responsible for the infant's demise. Many of these parents know and have followed all medical recommendations to minimize the chance of SIDS occurring:

- The infant was sleeping on his back.
- The house was devoid of tobacco smoke.
- The temperature in the baby's room was just right.
- The infant was not overdressed, and the cot did not contain too many stuffed animals or bumper pads.

Still, their infant died.

It's important to reassure the parents they had nothing to do with their baby's death. Tell parents they can formulate theories about why this death happened if they wish. (They will.) Point out to them that if anyone had figured out the cause of SIDS there would, by now, be a widely known method to prevent it. Genetics probably has something to do with SIDS. One known fact is that the male: female ratio is more than 3:2; boys are more likely to die of SIDS than are girls.[16]

Investigators think about SIDS using the "triple risk model."[17] The first risk is an underlying vulnerability, possibly due to some brainstem abnormality. The second risk is something happening at a critical period of the child's development, usually the first six months of life. The third risk is stress — pre- and post-natal environmental stressors such as overheating, nicotine exposure or side or prone sleeping. Those are three areas for coroners to consider when assessing whether a death was due to SIDS.

It is slight comfort for SIDS-bereaved parents that the infant does not suffer. The child's heart simply stops beating while asleep, leading to a painless death five minutes later. Pointing that out is the only solace a coroner can offer distraught parents of a child who died of SIDS. When leaving the death scene, it is worth reiterating one last time that there is no reason for the parents to blame themselves. Say this nicely, and the message will eventually sink in. Both parents will ruminate for a long time on every word the coroner said that day.

Sudden Unexplained Deaths in Childhood

Children also die suddenly and unexpectedly after they reach their first birthday. This sudden unexplained death in childhood (SUDC) is an uncommon condition. SUDC has to pass three tests before it can be diagnosed.[18] Just like in SIDS, all potential causes of death have been ruled out — an exhaustive examination of the site where death occurred must discover no possible cause of death. A detailed personal and family history cannot reveal any disease that might trigger a sudden death. Finally, a pathologist must conclude, after autopsy, that a thorough investigation of the child's tissues revealed no cause of death. The U.S. Centers for Disease Control and Prevention reported that in the United States only 393 children died of SUDC in 2015.[19]

SUDC usually occurs between the ages of 1 and 4. In 2018, U.S. incidence of SUDC was 1.4 deaths per 100,000 toddlers.[20] The condition remains unexplained. As yet unrecognized causes may include cardiac arrhythmias due to genetic disorders, neurological disorders that may cause death in a similar manner to the unexplained death in epileptics, and infections that cannot be detected. Some children with SUDC have been noted to die after experiencing a seizure. Most coroners never see a case of SUDC. Should it happen, remember: there is no use speculating on its cause, so don't.

Accidental Deaths

The U.S. Centers for Disease Control and Prevention published a childhood injury report in 2008[21] looking at fatal childhood injuries in the United States that occurred in the period from 2000 to 2006. This is the summary of their findings:

- On average, just over 12,000 children (0 to 19 years of age) died each year from an unintentional injury.
- Overall, the death rate for males aged 0 to 19 years was almost twice the rate for females. The death rates for males were higher than for females in all childhood age groups.
- Combining all unintentional injury deaths among those between 0 and 19 years, motor vehicle traffic–related deaths were the leading cause. The highest death rates were among occupants of motor vehicles. There were also a substantial number of pedestrian and bicyclist deaths among children.
- The leading causes of injury death differed by age group. For children less than a year old, two thirds of injury deaths were due to suffocation. Drowning was the leading cause of injury death for those 1 to 4 years of age. For children 5 to 19 years of age, most injury deaths resulted from occupying a seat in a motor vehicle crash.

- Risk for injury death varied by race. Injury death rates were highest for American and Alaskan Indigenous people and lowest for Asian or Pacific Islanders. Overall death rates for whites and African Americans were approximately the same.
- Injury death rates varied by state depending upon the cause of death. Overall, states with the lowest injury death rates were in the northeast. Fire and burn death rates were highest in some of the southern states. Death rates from transportation-related injuries were highest in some southern states and some states of the upper plains, while lowest rates occurred in states in the northeast region.
- For causes of injuries occurring in low numbers, death rates greatly varied by age. For example, the poisoning death rate for those older than 15 years was at least five times the rate of the younger age groups, and the suffocation death rate for infants was over 16 times the rates for all older age groups.

These injuries cause death in children in the same way as they do in adults except that children tend to die more quickly. How people die from accidents or poison are dealt with in the chapters on trauma (Chapter 15) and poisonings (Chapter 18). Coroners investigate all accidental deaths in children the same way as they investigate adult deaths.

Homicide

In simple English, the word *homicide* means the killing of one person by another. Killing a child is the worst possible form of child abuse, and, unfortunately, child abuse happens everywhere. How children are killed varies with their ages. The different ways children die is largely dependent on a child's age-related ability to avoid injury. Until the age of five most children can't get out of harm's way very quickly. Angry people, usually family members, can kill very small children quite easily.

Most little children are battered, strangled or suffocated by relatives. The killers use their hands or feet as lethal weapons. An equal number of very young male and female children die in this fashion. More men than women tend to kill children under the age of six, though in most countries the percentage difference between the sexes is slight.

Only in the under six years old group is there a high percentage of child killers who are women. The reason for this may be in some way related to post-partum depression. In many countries the relationship of depression with post-partum homicide is recognized in the criminal law. Many countries' criminal codes have a special term for a woman killing an infant – infanticide.

Infanticide

Canada and the United Kingdom are two countries that differentiate the crime of women (only) killing infants from that of anyone killing older children. In both countries, women killing young children are prosecuted for the crime of infanticide. The United States does not have such a crime. The rationale for the concept of infanticide is that some mothers of newborns develop such severe psychological distress that they are unable to manage their new maternal role.

The Canadian Criminal Code defines infanticide in complicated legalese as follows:

"A female person commits infanticide when by a wilful act or omission she causes the death of her newly-born child, if at the time of the act or omission she is not fully recovered from the effects of giving birth to the child and by reason thereof or of the effect of lactation consequent on the birth of the child her mind is then disturbed."[22]

Coroners need only know that this sort of crime exists. Dealing with it is the province of police, courts and lawyers. However, the word *infanticide* is commonly used in conversation. Colloquial usage of the word simply describes the killing of an infant, usually by its mother.

Child Abuse

There are many ways that children can be abused, but some abuse can actually be fatal. Parental abandonment may lead to death. Abandoned children may be accidentally or intentionally killed, starved or die of exposure. Neglected children may unwittingly encounter a dangerous situation beyond their capacity to manage. They may be hit by a car or fall off a cliff. An abandoned child may be kidnapped and killed, often after the kidnapper has abused the child in some way.

These deaths unfold just as they do in adults, but death happens more rapidly. Children have less physiological reserve than do adults, and thus have less endurance. Fortunately, such deaths are relatively uncommon. They are of great interest in every society, and in the developed world receive wide publicity. A coroner will undoubtedly investigate every one of them, but most coroners will never be called upon to do so.

Childhood abuse deaths are not the same as traumatic adult deaths. Childhood abuse deaths usually arise from a parent or caregiver's forceful action. Many types of physical child abuse occur, and not infrequently. Their causes are multifactorial. Often the abuse has been going on for a long time, producing repeated injury before death finally occurs.

The coroner only becomes involved when childhood physical injury or neglect was so great that it became lethal. Child protection agencies or a Children's Aid Society (CAS) may have been involved previously. In jurisdictions such as Ontario, coroners are required to investigate any death in which the local CAS has been involved to determine whether child abuse played any role in the death.

Physical abuse of a child comes in many forms. A couple of types have names that have become part of common parlance. Coroners use them when speaking with the child's relatives because the names aptly describe the mechanism of lethal injury. One such term is the shaken baby syndrome.[23] Another is battered child syndrome.[24]

Shaken Baby Syndrome

This type of fatal child abuse happens only in very young children because they have large heads and weak necks. Severely shaking infants causes bleeding to occur within their skulls (see Figure 9.2).

Only when children are small enough for their tormentors to easily pick them up and vigorously shake them can such deaths happen. For that reason, death from shaken baby syndrome is usually found in children under the age of five.

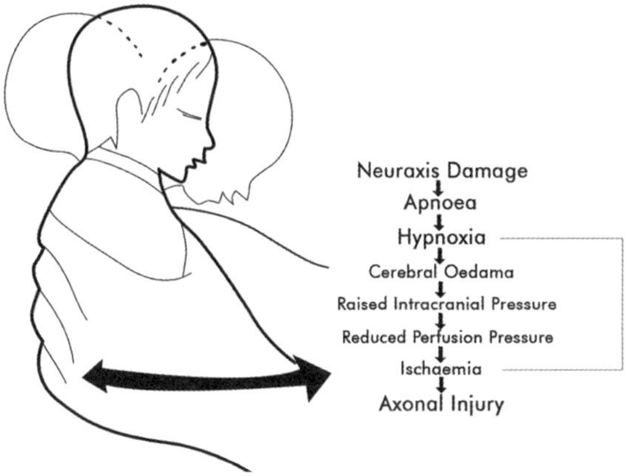

Figure 9.2: Shaking babies can be fatal when children are very young.

Quite often a coroner examining the site where a baby has died sees no obvious cause of death. Police information about previous involvement with a Children's Aid Society may raise suspicions about possible child abuse. Failing a perpetrator's admission or a witness' report, it will be the pathologist who first discovers death arose from shaking the child.

The pathologist may deduce shaking from discovering retinal haemorrhages and a subdural haematoma. The coroner should discuss the pathologist's conclusion with the police (who may be considering criminal charges) to ensure they are aware of it before passing that information on to the family. Those two findings should be enough for a provisional diagnosis of a fatal shaken baby syndrome. Other relevant evidence may appear later in the autopsy report. Providing no fall occurred, the fatal bleeding arose from shaking the infant's head backwards and forwards very forcefully. While it's possible for one single shake of the head to cause a fatal bleed, more often there will have been many.

The pathologist's findings will raise the question why a parent, or anyone else, would shake a baby so much. Police investigators find many reasons. The suspected abuser may suffer financial stresses, or he may simply be an unpleasant person with poor impulse control who drinks excessively or uses drugs. If you are questioned about motivations, don't speculate. Simply acknowledge that many are possible.

While the cause of death arises from bleeding produced by shaking the head, the pathologist may also discover a number of other injuries. For example, X-rays often show many fractures at different stages of healing. The injuries are then considered to be part of a battered child syndrome, even though the cause of death is still bleeding inside the head.

Battered Child Syndrome

The full extent of the battered child's injuries only becomes apparent after an autopsy. These children usually are infants too. But the age range for lethal child battering is quite a bit greater than that for fatal baby shaking. One American child battering study included battered children from one month to 13 years of age. Its authors believed that a "battered child" death could occur at any time until the teenage years.

Coroners are supposed to look carefully at the body of any deceased person. This duty is technically called *viewing*. Comprehensive study of a dead child's body is especially important. Parents usually tell a coroner that their child was just found dead. This happens, but external bruising or an obviously broken bone should make the coroner suspect child abuse. Then, rather than being natural, the child's death has a chance of turning out to be a homicide.

Similarly, a child, small for their age or wasted, can raise the suspicion that death is in some way unnatural. Battered child syndrome is usually a concern of family physicians and paediatricians. It is only when the battering becomes fatal that the coroner and the police both become involved. Defining the extent of the injuries and opining on whether they are likely related to child abuse is the job of pathologists. They have extensive literature to help formulate that opinion.[25]

When a child has been battered the fatal bleeding can arise somewhere other than the head. However, most often the fatal bleed will be an intracranial haemorrhage of some sort. It is not until the pathologist confirms evidence of bruising, evidence of new or old fractures, or the dead child's wasted state that the diagnosis of a battered child should be considered certain.

Even though a coroner may investigate children's deaths for years, dealing with these investigations will never become easy. Whether it is the vulnerability of being a child, the unfairness that death has come so prematurely, or the emotional effect a child's death has on everyone in their life, some factor in the investigation makes the coroner (and the investigating police officers) very upset that it has happened. Only after departing the scene should a coroner expect any mood improvement and a return of emotional equanimity.

NOTES

1 World Health Organization (WHO). (2017). Global Health Observatory GHO Data. http://www.who.int/gho/child_health/mortality/neonatal_infancy/en/

2 Ely, D.M., & Driscoll, A.K. (2019). Infant mortality in the United States, 2017: Data from the period linked birth/infant death file. *National Vital Statistics Reports, 68*(10). Retrieved February 15, 2021, from https://www.cdc.gov/nchs/data/nvsr/nvsr68/nvsr68_10-508.pdf

3 National Center for Injury Prevention and Control, Centers for Disease Control and Prevention. (n.d.). *10 leading causes of death by age group, United States — 2016*. Retrieved February 15, 2021, from https://webappa.cdc.gov/cgi-bin/broker.exe

4 See note 4 above.

5 Paediatric Death Review Committee and Deaths Under Five Committee, Office of the Chief Coroner of Ontario. (2016). *2015 annual report*, Chart 3.

6 World Health Organization (WHO). (2019, September 23). Mortality among children aged –14 years. Retrieved February 20, 2021, from https://www.who.int/news-room/fact-sheets/detail/mortality-among-children-aged-5-14-years

7 See note 4 above.

8 See note 4 above.

9 See note 6 above.

10 World Health Organization (WHO). (2016). Causes of death among adolescents. Retrieved February 20, 2021, from https://www.who.int/maternal_child_adolescent/data/causes-death-adolescents/en/

11 Abubakar, I. I., & Banerjee, A. (2015). Global, regional, and national age-sex specific all-cause and cause-specific mortality for 240 causes of death, 1990–2013: A systematic analysis for the Global Burden of Disease Study 2013. *Lancet, 385*(9963), 117–171.

12 Powers, D. A., & Song, S.-E. (2009). Absolute change in cause-specific infant mortality for blacks and whites in the US: 1983–2002. *Population Research and Policy Review, 28*(6), 817.

13 Pollack, H. A., & Frohna, J. G. (2001). A competing risk model of sudden infant death syndrome incidence in two US birth cohorts. *Journal of Pediatrics, 138*(5), 661–667.

14 Duncan, J. R., & Byard, R. W. (2018). Sudden infant death syndrome: An overview. In *SIDS Sudden infant and early childhood death: The past, the present and the future* (Chapter 2). Adelaide (AU): University of Adelaide Press.

15 Milroy, C. M., & Kepron, C. (2017). Ten percent of SIDS cases are murder — or are they? *Academic Forensic Pathology, 7*(2), 163–170.

16 Mage, D. T., & Donner, E. M. (2007). The fifty percent excess of infant respiratory mortality *Acta Paediatrica, 93*(9), 1210–1215.

17 Guntheroth, W. G., & Spiers, P. S. (2002). The triple risk hypotheses in sudden infant death syndrome. *Pediatrics, 110*(5): e64.

18 Krous, H. F., Chadwick, A. E., Crandall, L., & Nadeau-Manning, J. M. (2005) Sudden unexpected death in childhood: A report of 50 cases. *Pediatric and Developmental Pathology, 8*(3), 307–319.

19 National Organization for Rare Disorders (NORD). (2020). *Rare disease database: Sudden unexplained death in childhood. Retrieved February 26, 2021, from https://rarediseases.org/rare-diseases/sudden-unexplained-death-in-childhood/*

20 Rare Disease Database. (2020). Sudden unexplained death in childhood. *National Organization for Rare Disorders (NORD).* https://rarediseases.org/rare-diseases/sudden-unexplained-death-in-childhood/

21 Retrieved on February 18, 2021. https://www.cdc.gov/safechild/child_injury_data.html

22 *Criminal Code*, R.S.C. 1985, c.46, s.233.

23 Healthwise Staff. (2020, January 31). Shaken baby syndrome. *Alberta Health.* https://myhealth.alberta.ca/health/pages/conditions.aspx?Hwid=hw169815

24 Kempe, C. H., Silverman, F. N., Steele, B. F., Droegemueller, W., & Silver, H. K. (1962). The battered-child syndrome. *Journal of the American Medical Association, 181*(1), 17–24.

25 Maguire, S. (2010). Which injuries may indicate child abuse? *Archives of Disease in Childhood — Education and Practice, 95*(6), 170–177.

10

Maternal and Foetal Deaths

Both mother and child have found birth to be dangerous throughout recorded history. English parish records show that in the 1700s and the 1800s between 0.5% and 1% of all mothers died at childbirth. In the United States at the turn of the twentieth century, roughly 10% of children died during that era's rather long (by current standards) perinatal period of one year.

In today's developed countries, both statistics have improved dramatically. The maternal mortality rate in low-income countries in 2017 was 462 per 100,000 live births versus 11 per 100,000 live births in high-income countries.[1] The risk is highest for girls under the age of 15. Even taking the whole world into account, death within the first month of life occurred in only 17 per 1,000 live births in 2019 — mostly in Africa or Southeast Asia.[2]

In Europe, North America and Australasia, maternal deaths don't happen very often. The numbers have been increasing in the last 30 years though, perhaps because mothers are getting older when giving birth. For example, in Canada, the number of maternal deaths per 100,00 live births in 2018 was 8.3 — or 31 mothers in the whole country.[3] That low number means few Canadian coroners will ever have to investigate a maternal death.

The death of a mother or her child impact people differently. Sorrow accompanies both events, but all birth attendants, as well as many parents and their families, know that some foetuses simply will not survive either the trauma of birth or the neonatal period that follows. Infants dying at or just before birth do upset everyone associated with them, of course. The parents are the saddest of all, but like birth attendants and other relatives they eventually overcome their grief. It is almost always dispelled with the birth of another child.

Maternal deaths, on the other hand, hit people much harder. Everyone in the delivery room, the hospital, in fact everyone in society at large understands the consequences to a family when a mother dies while attempting to give birth. The coroner who arrives at a delivery room or obstetrical floor shortly after a maternal death will meet teary-eyed nurses, despondent physicians, a desolate family and a pervading atmosphere of gloom.

The hospital staff worked terribly hard to save the life of a healthy young woman whose life was about to be enriched by a newborn child. Her death was totally unexpected. Everybody involved recognizes the impact her death will have on the remaining family. Everybody looking after her knows they could not keep their patient alive. A lot of them feel very guilty. The constant reminder of their failure, usually covered over with a white sheet, lies nearby awaiting a coroner's visit.

The entire team knows this mother's death will shatter her family. Some blame themselves for this happening. Case room staff choose obstetrics because they enjoy delivering babies and participating in the joy of a new birth. A coroner needs to keep their feelings in mind before starting to talk to anybody present about the death.

In developed countries, maternal deaths almost always occur in hospitals. The occasional home maternal death without medical care undoubtedly happens, but rarely. Should a coroner be asked to investigate an unattended home death, there will be no medical staff to talk to. However, the coroner will undoubtedly find police officers trying to retain their composure, a couple of unhappy paramedics and perhaps a disconsolate father trying to comfort children in varying degrees of distress depending on their ages. The father will be the only person who can say for sure what happened.

In such an emotionally charged environment a coroner must choose every word very carefully. Say nothing judgemental. Ask only those questions needed to discover what happened. To comfort the family after the coroner (and perhaps the police) depart, someone will have to remain. When the death occurs in a hospital, social workers will be available to help. If a death occurs at home, neighbours or relatives need to be located. Police may be able to offer crisis counsellors.

Two different types of obstetrical procedures that have completely opposite objectives cause maternal deaths. One is the delivery of an infant. The other is the abortion of a foetus. Maternal deaths occur in several different ways.

Maternal deaths are usually defined as deaths at the time of delivery or within 42 days thereafter.* Foetal deaths occur either before delivery, in which case they are called stillbirths, at the time of delivery, or just afterwards. The dead foetus, once delivered, is called a stillborn. A baby's death at any time within the first 28 days following birth is classified as neonatal.

Causes of Maternal Death

Maternal death at birth or after delivering a baby occurs in one of the following six ways:

- bleeding
- infection
- eclampsia
- amniotic fluid emboli
- obstructed labour
- pulmonary emboli

These will be discussed in that order.

Bleeding

Normally, after birth, the mother's uterus (shown in Figure 10.1 containing a foetus), which is basically a muscle lined with blood vessels, shrinks rapidly and significantly. As a rule, the uterus contracts enough after expelling the baby to prevent its endometrial lining from continuing to bleed more than a manageable trickle. When the uterus remains enlarged and flabby it cannot compress uterine blood vessels very much. Continued uterine bleeding leads first to haemorrhagic

* In this chapter, The time periods used for maternal and neonatal deaths are those defined by the World Health Organization.

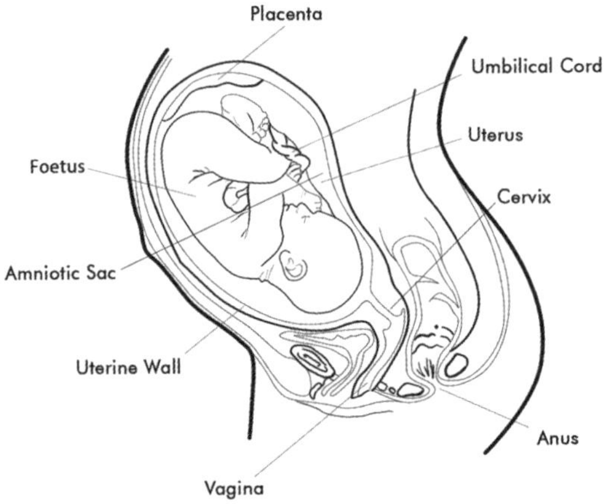

Figure 10.1: During pregnancy, the uterus stretches to accommodate the foetus. After the birth, the uterus shrinks back down.

shock and then death. Post-partum bleeding accounts for between 25% and 60% of maternal deaths around the world.[4]

Before bleeding can stop following the baby's delivery, a mother's uterus also must expel the whole placenta (colloquially called an afterbirth) into her vagina. The placenta's only purpose was to transfer nutrients from the mother to help the foetus grow. Once the baby is born, a placenta has no more use. It needs to be expelled from the mother's body. When the uterus does not eject the whole placenta, pieces remaining can cause ongoing bleeding or infection. The uterus may haemorrhage a lot right after delivery, but equally heavy bleeding can occur hours later. There are several reasons for both these occurrences.

Sometimes a placenta, positioned at the mouth of the uterus, blocks the baby's way out. In other instances, the afterbirth is actually embedded deep into the wall of the uterus. Some placentas even grow through the uterus and into the bladder. When delivery proceeds without these problems being recognized, a lot of bleeding can result at the time of a vaginal birth.

The uterus can also rupture while the baby emerges. This is known to happen when women who had an earlier baby delivered operatively through Caesarian section choose natural childbirth for a subsequent child. Bleeding from such a tear can be quite heavy. Usually only the baby dies when the uterus tears this way, but sometimes the mother does too.

When a mother's blood will not clot while she continues to bleed after a delivery mayhem erupts in the delivery room. The heavy bleeding may result from a woman's body lacking some factor needed to make blood clot, but it can also be a paradoxical complication of haemorrhagic shock.

In both cases the fatal uterine bleeding continues long after delivery. This haemorrhage may start while still in the room where birth took place. The risk of such heavy bleeding continues for the next 24 hours.

When nothing else comes into play, apart from fright, the sensations a mother feels while bleeding to death change as she loses increasing amounts of blood. The woman will feel nothing untoward until she has lost half a litre to a litre of blood. At that point the woman will begin to feel a bit cold. Then, as her heart beats faster, the woman may become aware of her heart beating in her chest. The mother's blood pressure starts to drop, so she finds standing or even propping herself up makes her faint. Finally, as the dying woman continues to bleed she loses consciousness and enters her terminal coma.

In a hospital, the moment post-partum haemorrhage is detected urgent measures are instituted to manage the bleeding. Medicines are administered to induce her uterus to contract. They may make the woman nauseated or cause her to vomit. If the medicine proves effective, forceful uterine contractions often cause severe abdominal cramping. This discomfort is felt only while she remains awake. Once unconscious, of course, all pain disappears. In most fatal bleeds, any such discomfort is short-lived because the bleeding continues.

Post-partum haemorrhages may be quick, may be massive and may require packing of the uterus in an effort to stop the bleeding (see Figure 10.2). Packing a womb is quite uncomfortable and is usually a prelude to a hysterectomy. This surgical procedure is painless when the patient is anaesthetized, but in most of the fatal haemorrhages coroners investigate it has not worked, and the mother has died on the operating table or shortly thereafter. Since the woman will have been unconscious for some time, death was painless. That is also true when nothing at all was attempted to stop the bleeding.

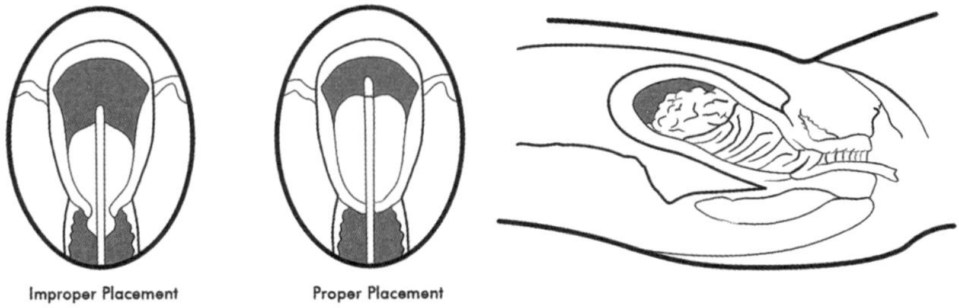

Figure 10.2: Proper technique is required for uterine packing to be successful.

Infection

Maternal death from infection after the birth of a baby has been recorded as far back in time as ancient Egypt. For a long time this post-partum infection was called puerperal sepsis, and it continued to be fatal until antibiotics were discovered in the twentieth century. Nowadays these deaths are, thankfully, rare. Worldwide, however, sepsis still probably accounts for 15% of maternal deaths. The percentage is a bit lower in the United States, at 12.5%.[5]

These infections usually start a day or two, and even possibly up to a couple of weeks, after delivery. Signs and symptoms start with a tender painful lower abdomen. Women with infected uteri often develop a foul-smelling vaginal discharge and perhaps light vaginal bleeding. Then they start to feel hot, develop chills and perspire.

Modern antibiotics can usually cure any infections that occur following giving birth. Post-partum uterine infection only becomes fatal after sepsis develops when bacteria spread into the woman's bloodstream. In coroners' cases sepsis has turned into lethal septic shock. Dying from post-partum septic shock is no different from dying from septic shock in any other circumstance.

Most coroners in the developed world never investigate a death from a post-partum infection. Coroners in Ottawa, where I work, occasionally do though. Ottawa hospitals are the referral centres for the territory of Nunavut, an enormous, sparsely populated Arctic area. Many Canadian Inuit live there in tiny, isolated hamlets hundreds of kilometres from any other populated area. To understand Nunavut's vastness (2 million square kilometres), think of it as having the same area as all of western Europe.

Nunavut has fewer than 40,000 residents and they are served by only one small hospital in Iqaluit, the capital. Women who have their babies at home in a hamlet are hours away from Iqaluit even if flying there. Pregnant women are in trouble if they develop sepsis. It often takes a long time to get to Iqaluit for treatment. The only way to get to Iqaluit quickly is to fly. Planes can't take off or land in snowstorms, which are common events in Nunavut. Even if the hamlet is lucky enough to have a physician on-site, any therapy on offer is very limited.

Even in Iqaluit, all that can be done is start some antibiotics. The woman will still have to spend several hours more until an air ambulance can deliver her to a tertiary care hospital in Ottawa where proper intensive care starts. This unavoidably lengthy delay has resulted in post-partum septic deaths in Ottawa. Coroners have investigated them very carefully, with the result that all births are now supposed to take place in the Iqaluit hospital. Still that does not always happen.

Unfortunately, the geographical and climactic barriers to speedier and better care won't disappear. This means post-partum septic deaths will continue until all births take place in hospital in Iqaluit. Though desirable, that's unlikely to happen soon. These deaths are investigated primarily in Nunavut, but Ottawa coroners and pathologists will likely continue to play their role in investigating this Arctic territory's post-partum septic deaths for years to come.

Eclampsia (Blood Pressure Problems)

High blood pressure is a risk in all pregnancies. Obstetricians regularly look for high blood pressure in pregnant women because appropriate treatment usually prevents death. In the United States and the United Kingdom, the percentage of recent maternal deaths due to eclampsia has ranged from just under 6% to almost 12%. Figures for developing countries vary but are higher. An average of 14% of all their maternal deaths are due to eclampsia. In different parts of the Third World eclampsia causes between 10% and 25% of all maternal deaths.[6]

A pregnant woman has no way of knowing her blood pressure is high until it becomes very elevated. Potentially fatal blood pressure starts with a syndrome called pre-eclampsia. If there are any abnormal sensations, they are minimal — perhaps just a headache and feeling anxious. More frequently nothing is felt at all. Most pre-eclampsia is diagnosed at a doctor's visit by discovering a rise in blood pressure and protein in the woman's urine.

The discovery of pre-eclampsia usually triggers aggressive therapy to return the woman's blood pressure to normal until delivery. Pre-eclampsia that turns into eclampsia at the time of birth sometimes ends in the mother's death. A couple of centuries ago this fatal progression was common. Better medical care makes eclampsia rare in the developed world nowadays, though it does still sometimes happen. Coroners in underdeveloped countries investigate eclamptic deaths more often.

The progression of pre-eclampsia to eclampsia is accompanied by severe headaches, nausea and vomiting. The woman's arms, legs — or, in fact, any part of her body — swell. Her vision blurs, and some eclamptic women become temporarily blind.

An eclamptic woman may feel a sense of foreboding similar to the aura epileptics experience just before they convulse. This sensation, though painless, will be puzzling. The woman won't know what it means unless she experienced a seizure before she became pregnant. The convulsion that follows is the same as with any other seizure. The woman is unconscious and has no idea she convulsed once she awakens.

An eclamptic woman's seizure can be quite dramatic. In eclampsia her body often adopts an arched position, as depicted in Figure 10.3, before the convulsion subsides. A seizure in eclampsia, like any other seizure, may cause sudden death. An eclamptic seizure involving opisthotonos and the woman's subsequent death should be painless even though alarming to onlookers. Most coroners in developed countries can be fairly confident they will never investigate an eclamptic death.

High blood pressure has another route to death at the time of delivery, or even before the pre-eclampsia diagnosis. Between 3% and 5% of all women have a bulge in one of their cerebral arteries, called a berry aneurysm.[7] These aneurysms have thin walls.

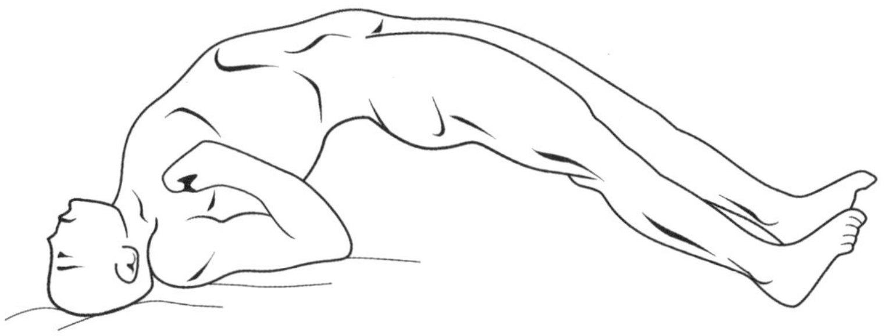

Figure 10.3: The arched position caused by muscle spasm during a seizure is called opisthotonos.

High blood pressure may cause an aneurysm to develop a leak. The pressure of the leaking blood causes the same sort of terribly severe headache that occurs in any other haemorrhagic stroke. The speed with which blood flows out of the aneurysm determines the severity and duration of the headache.

The speed of blood loss also determines how long a woman lives. Small leaks from a berry aneurysm are survivable. Big leaks are not. Since most women are unaware of their berry aneurysm until it ruptures, a headache is the first warning of something going wrong with it. The process of dying starts with this very severe headache, followed by a loss consciousness for minutes to hours before death.

A pregnant woman will die from a ruptured berry aneurysm not only at the time of her delivery, of course. Elevated blood pressure could cause the aneurysm to burst at any time during her pregnancy.

Amniotic Fluid Emboli

Amniotic fluid, foetal cells, hair or other foetal debris sometimes become part of a mother's circulating blood at the time of delivery. These materials enter through a cervical laceration, the placenta or a ruptured uterus. If this debris gets stuck somewhere, it becomes "amniotic fluid emboli." Fortunately, these do not form very often. This phenomenon is more common in women with multiple children or those who had a Caesarian section to deliver the baby, but nobody knows why.

About half of amniotic fluid embolism deaths occur within an hour of the first embolic material entering a woman's bloodstream.[8] These early deaths are a form of suffocation. The woman finds it harder and harder to breathe until she loses consciousness. Amniotic fluid embolism deaths that occur later on result from continued uterine bleeding caused by a flabby uterus and blood that will not clot. Some women die after a sudden cardiac arrest. Regardless of how the amniotic fluid emboli kill her, the woman becomes unconscious and she dies painlessly.

For the first few moments a woman dying from amniotic fluid emboli feels very anxious while she cannot catch her breath, but very often that sensation only lasts for seconds before she passes out. A woman who stays alert longer will know something is going wrong. Amniotic fluid emboli cause flushing; her breathing speeds up and it becomes hard for the woman to draw air into her lungs. The woman begins to cough, gets really short of breath, and becomes restless, agitated and confused before she falls into a terminal coma.

Amniotic fluid emboli can lead to some women having a seizure before dying. It is painless, of course, and the woman will never know she had one. An amniotic fluid embolus triggers a fatal shock that may result from an anaphylactic reaction. Notice the word *may* – death from amniotic fluid emboli is still poorly understood.

It is a good idea to tell inquiring relatives that it is common for a woman unlucky enough to experience a post-partum amniotic fluid embolus to die. Amniotic fluid embolism occurs in 1 in 20,000 live births, but it accounts for 10% of maternal deaths worldwide. In developed countries only 13% to 26% of women who experience it die nowadays.[9]

Obstructed Labour

The inability to expel a foetus from her body still kills women in the developing world. About 19,000 of these pregnant women died in 2013, most because an obstruction caused them to rupture their uterus.[10]

Nowadays this virtually never happens in developed countries. Still, globally it accounts for 8% of all maternal deaths.[11]

In centuries past, throughout the world an untold number of women died when unable to deliver their babies. The agony their failed labour produced must have been terrible. Their uteri would have contracted in an increasingly painful fashion for hours before finally rupturing. At that point the women would have quickly lost consciousness and bled to death.

Any woman who has experienced childbirth may be able to recollect the pain of the strong uterine contractions needed to deliver a baby. With an obstructed birth, the pain is the same, but more intense and longer lasting.

Modern obstetrical practices, involving the use of forceps, vacuum extraction or Caesarian section to deliver a foetus, whether dead or alive, makes this problem mostly an historical one in the developed world. Unless birth takes place at home without medical assistance, no coroner in the developed world is likely to investigate a death from obstructed labour.

Pulmonary Emboli

Depending on what statistics you look at, anywhere from 3% to 10% of maternal deaths arise from blood clots, called pulmonary emboli, that block blood flow into the lungs' arteries. Death from these clots can come at any time during the pregnancy or after the baby is born. Obese women, hypertensive women and those who had Caesarian sections tend to develop pulmonary emboli more often than do other mothers. Nevertheless, pulmonary emboli could kill any pregnant woman.

Blood clots in a woman's veins more often when pregnant than at other times in her life. The reason why is not really known,* so avoid any discussion about how pregnancy changes the blood's clotting factors. Should the deceased woman's family persistently inquire about how the clot developed, plead ignorance (that's usually honest) and

---

* One theory is that the elevated incidence results from a temporary increase in the blood's ability to clot – nature's attempt to protect against post-partum haemorrhage following childbirth. However, that's just a theory.

refer them to their own physician for more information. Alternatively, recommend a web search to understand the many factors involved in blood clot development.

If relatives go to the internet, factors they might discover that influence clotting include abnormalities in the blood vessel wall, blood flow changes, a pregnant woman's decreased mobility, and the consistency of a pregnant woman's blood. Different coagulation factors and proteins play a part in the coagulation cascade. This is far too complicated for a coroner to discuss with families. They need to talk to a haematologist for a fully informed conversation. Even most family physicians or obstetricians have trouble discussing the intricacies of coagulation.

What the woman felt before death will depend on the size and location of the fatal emboli in in the lung's arteries. When a massive "saddle" embolus blocks the main pulmonary arteries, death is sudden. The woman collapses, loses consciousness and dies without any sort of pain at all.

Where the clots are smaller or become wedged in more peripheral arteries, the woman will notice her breathing speeds up, and each inhalation or exhalation causes a sharp pain in her chest. Breathing becomes more difficult; coughing starts. The clots usually come from a calf or thigh that was swollen or painful before the embolus broke loose. A quarter of these women also notice their hearts beating rapidly. These symptoms may not last long, but more often they continue for hours before the loss of consciousness preceding death occurs.

Abortions

By one account, abortions account for 13% of maternal deaths globally.[12] This number increases to 50% in sub-Saharan Africa. Whether an intentional effort to terminate a pregnancy or simply a natural unavoidable event, all abortions can end a woman's life in the same way as can any successful pregnancy. Bleeding after an abortion can be so heavy that it is fatal. This commonly happens when a "backstreet" abortion ruptures a woman's uterus. If a hospital cannot be reached in time, irreversible shock prevents both blood transfusions and surgery from saving her life.

Instruments that are not sterile will introduce fatal infections into the uterus that move into the blood. Deaths can still occur this way when an untrained "community" abortionist ends a pregnancy, though it is much less common in Canada today than it was 40 years ago. In those days a fatal uterine infection often resulted from using a dirty wire coat hanger as the abortion tool. Africans still frequently use them to perform abortions, but twigs and chicken bones also have been pressed into service when no coat hanger is available.

Women in developed countries now usually terminate their pregnancies in sterile settings. Legal changes have made medical abortion much more accessible. New medicines can induce labour and prematurely expel a foetus. These developments have reduced the risk of fatal infection from miscarriages too.

Nowadays incomplete removal of some part of the placenta or foetus by the abortion is the major risk for infection following abortion. In countries with easy access to hospitalization, removal of the retained tissue and vigorous antibiotic therapy usually cure post-partum infections. Where hospital care is unavailable or delayed, these women can still quickly develop a fatal septic shock that will lead to a coroner's investigation.

Problems with obstructed labour almost never occur in a miscarriage. A woman's uterus has no difficulty expelling a small foetus. Obstruction might occur in a late-term abortion induced medically rather than by vacuum extraction or dilation and curettage, the common surgical procedure. Though death is theoretically possible from obstruction after a medically induced late-term abortion it is highly unlikely.

Recurrent miscarriages cause more clotting in leg veins. Once these clots become large enough and break loose, they turn into fatal pulmonary emboli.

Stillbirths

While not a maternal death, pregnancy has another fatal consequence. A foetus delivered dead it is said to be stillborn, and the death is a stillbirth. Stillbirths are a relatively common outcome of pregnancy. As a rule, coroners don't investigate them. Their occurrence is considered a natural event. It's even a moot question whether a coroner actually has the jurisdiction to investigate one.

Peoples' views differ on when life begins. For coroners, law has resolved this question. The exact resolution varies with different statutes in different jurisdictions, but the gist of each law is similar: a foetus has to leave the mother's body and take a breath before it can be said to have been born alive.

If stillborns are considered to have never lived they can never die, and coroners only investigate deaths. The one time a coroner may investigate a stillbirth is when a family believes that inadequate medical care in the case room prevented delivery of a live baby.

Almost all stillbirths are natural. Perhaps 30% of the time they are due to problems with the pregnancy. Those include pre-term labour, twins, triplets, or the placenta tearing away from the uterine wall. When the cause of stillbirth is to be found in the foetus, many of these causes can be explained:

- About 10% of the time a congenital anomaly, which may result from fatal chromosomal abnormalities that impair proper development, causes death.
- In another 10% of stillbirths, an umbilical cord wrapped around the neck is considered to have cut off blood supply to the foetus.
- A third 10% arise from infection of the foetus or the placenta.
- In another 25% of cases, the placenta is also the culprit when very premature deaths arise from insufficient placental blood flow to stay alive.

Around 25% of stillborn deaths still cannot be explained, even with autopsy. In all stillbirths the cause of death is the realm of the pathologist. Rarely does a stillbirth result from problems during the delivery. Sometimes maternal illnesses like diabetes mellitus, hypertension, or smoking play some role in stillbirths, but that happens in fewer than 10% of cases.[*13] A coroner does not need to know anything about other possible causes of stillbirth. The only stillbirth that I investigated (at the instruction of my regional supervising coroner) resulted from excessive prematurity.

---

* All these percentages come from the Stillbirth Collaborative Research Network.

In my medical school days, a foetus needed to live for seven months to be expected to survive birth. That age has now fallen to about five months thanks to advances in paediatric intensive care. Even so, still-births continue. According to current Ontario law, a test with two parts applies when considering the question of whether a pregnancy has resulted in producing a foetus. To meet the requirement of the first part of the test, at least five months of development in the mother's uterus needs to have elapsed. A second way a foetus can be said to exist is when a weight 500 grams has been attained. If either of these two requirements are met, a stillbirth is considered to occur. Failure to meet either one means the tissue expelled from the mother's uterus is simply considered "products of conception." These tissues are simply disposed of in the same way a hospital disposes of tissue removed at surgery. Other jurisdictions' definitions of a foetus will either be identical to Ontario's or resemble it with only slight variation.

NOTES

1 World Health Organization. (2019, September 19). *Maternal mortality.* https://www.who.int/news-room/fact-sheets/detail/maternal-mortality

2 UNICEF. (September 2020). *Neonatal mortality.* https://data.unicef.org/topic/child-survival/neonatal-mortality/

3 Statistics Canada. (2019, November 26). *Deaths 2018.* https://www150.statcan.gc.ca/n1/daily-quotidien/191126/dq191126c-cansim-eng.htm

4 World Health Organization. (2005). *World health report 2005: Make every mother and child count.* https://www.who.int/whr/2005/en/

5 Centers for Disease Control and Prevention. (2020, November 25). Pregnancy mortality surveillance system. https://www.cdc.gov/reproductivehealth/maternal-mortality/pregnancy-mortality-surveillance-system.htm

6 Douglas, K. A., & Redman, C.W. (1994). Eclampsia in the United Kingdom. *British Medical Journal, 309*(6966), 1395–1400; Sibai, B. M. (2005). Diagnosis, prevention, and management of eclampsia. *Obstetrics & Gynecology, 105*(2), 402–410; Sibai, B. M., Sarinoglu, C., & Mercer, B. M. (1992). Eclampsia VII: Pregnancy outcome after eclampsia and long-term prognosis. *American Journal of Obstetrics & Gynecology, 166*(6), 1757–1763.

7 National Institute of Neurological Disorders and Stroke. (2020, March 13). *Cerebral aneurysms fact sheet.* https://www.ninds.nih.gov/Disorders/Patient-Caregiver-Education/Fact-Sheets/Cerebral-Aneurysms-Fact-Sheet

8 Conde-Agudelo A., & Romero, R. (2009). Amniotic fluid embolism: An evidence-based review. *Americal Journal of Obstetrics and Gynecology, 201*(5), 445.e1–445.e13.

9 Kiranpreet, K., Bhardwaj, M., Kumar, P., Singhal, S., Singh, T., & Hooda, S. (2016). Amniotic fluid embolism. *Journal of Anaesthesiology Clinical Pharmacology, 32*(2), 153–159.

10 GBD 2013 Mortality and Causes of Death Collaborators. (2014). Global, regional, and national age–sex specific all-cause and cause-specific mortality for 240 causes of death, 1990–2013: A systemic analysis for the Global Burden of Disease Study 2013. *Lancet, 385*(9963): 117–171.

11 Khan, K. S., Wojdyla, D., Say, L., Gulmezoglu, A. M., & Van Look, P. F. (2006). WHO analysis of causes of maternal death: A systemic review. *Lancet, 367*(9516), 1066–1074.

12 Say, L., Chou, D., Gemmill, A., Tuncalp, O., Moller, A.-B., Daniels, J., … Alkema, L. (2014). Global causes of maternal death: A WHO systemic analysis. *Lancet Global Health, 2*(6) e323–e333

13 National Institute of Child Health and Human Development. (2016). What are the possible causes of stillbirth? https://www.nichd.nih.gov/health/topics/stillbirth/topicinfo/causes

11

Deaths from Exposure

Most people who live in the world's temperate and polar zones know cold weather can be harmful and sometimes even lethal. In many countries, for up to half the year, the first commandment is to stay warm at all times. The cold certainly influences Tibetan spiritual beliefs. Their image of suffering the eternal punishment their God will mete out to the newly dead, who led a life of repeated malfeasance, is a freezing hell.

For centuries inhabitants of the global north have struggled to survive in cold weather. They wore the warmest possible clothing, limited their outdoor exposure to wintery weather and kept their dwellings as warm as possible. These precautions remain necessary today, but not everybody takes them. Every year many Canadian coroners investigate deaths of people who have died from exposure to the winter's cold.

Doctors refer to the state of cold in the body as hypothermia. When mild, hypothermia is not fatal, but when severe it becomes lethal. Hypothermia is not just a wintertime problem either. In any month of the year, with the right physical environment, hypothermia can lead to death anywhere in the world. However, statistically, most hypothermic deaths happen in northern climes during the colder months of the year.

Throughout the world, very young children, who don't know any better, wander away from their parents. They get lost in the woods. In a northern winter these children cannot survive cold weather exposure very long. Their survival in below zero temperatures is measured in hours. Quite often, after a couple of days' searching, the children's bodies are found frozen in the snow. When their bodies are discovered in the spring after the snow has disappeared, they are decomposed and sometimes partially eaten by animals.

Nowadays, most adults only die from hypothermia when some impairment prevents them from being able to get out of a lethally cold environment. Three common impairments that too often result in death are alcohol intoxication, being "high" on drugs, or suffering some sort of mental illness that makes it difficult to appreciate the danger cold weather presents.

In Ottawa every winter, coroners view frozen bodies under bridges, in snowbanks or lying in snow-covered parks on the ground or on benches. Sometimes coroners are called to look at ice-encrusted bodies on the bank of one of its rivers after police diving teams have recovered them from under the ice.

When compared with other causes of death, relatively few people die from exposure to the cold. In the United States, about 25,000 people die of hypothermia each year. In Canada the number is 8,000, and in the United Kingdom it's about 20,000 annually.[1] These statistics probably exclude elderly people whose death occurred from a longstanding medical condition that was worsened by the cold.

Freezing weather is not a requirement for a body to cool enough for the cold to be a killer. No single temperature is always lethal for everyone. People's body sizes and shapes vary so much that a lengthy exposure to any temperature below 10 degrees Celsius (10°C, or 50 degrees Fahrenheit, 50°F) can trigger a fatal hypothermia.[2]

A person's skin temperature is often quite a bit lower than the body's core temperature (the temperature of the internal organs). When talking about a hypothermic death, skin temperature is relatively unimportant. The body's core temperature has to drop in order for death to occur. Everyone's capacity to survive when their core temperature drops is different because the rate at which it declines depends upon a person's body size and composition. No single temperature is the dividing line between life and death. Rarely can anyone survive core temperatures lower than 26°C, though.[3]

Extreme cold causes death when it lowers the core temperature of the inner organs of the human body. That temperature results from the balance between heat production and heat loss. Even at rest, the body's metabolism generates heat as a by-product of its functions that keep all the body's tissues viable. Every function — for example, eating and digesting food — produces heat. Even the blink of an eyelid produces a little bit. Voluntary muscle activity and involuntary shivering both rapidly increase heat within the body.

Skin loses heat through perspiration. Breathing blows water vapour out of the lungs, and with it heat also escapes from the body. The more rapidly breaths are taken the faster heat is lost. When a body's temperature control mechanism breaks down, different parts of the skin lose varying amounts of heat. While these are interesting facts, when talking about dying from exposure, try to avoid discussing the mechanism of dying from heat loss.

Older adults and children constitute the bulk of people killed by hypothermia. A child's body loses heat faster than an adults' because a child's surface-to-mass ratio is larger than that of an adult. Young children, still unaware of the danger of the cold, always risk being unable to get to a place of warmth once hypothermia starts.

Hypothermia quickly becomes fatal in the very elderly. The reason is straightforward. Mentally competent old folks who stop exercising soon discover that their muscles atrophy and weaken. Weakness decreases their overall activity. Eventually, the very weak, frail elderly become immobile. Less muscle activity generates less heat. Older adults' bodies also tend to lose heat rapidly,

Thin elderly people have little fat beneath their skin to act as an insulator to prevent heat loss. Thin people become cold much more quickly than those who are overweight. Thyroid glands frequently function poorly in the elderly, especially women. Less thyroid hormone generates less body heat. People with hypothyroidism freeze to death more quickly than others.

Many serious illnesses diminish the body's ability to properly manage heat loss or its thermoregulatory control. The skin and its adjoining tissues act as protective barriers to prevent the inner human body from losing heat at its core. When disease damages the skin's integrity some of its layers flake off. The result is that heat loss is more rapid.

Injuries do the same thing. A similar loss of heat accompanies head and spinal injuries. Ingesting drugs such as barbiturates and phenothiazines (a group of drugs commonly used to treat mental illness) causes the body to lose heat more quickly too.

However, in cases coroners investigate, alcohol is the most common cause of fatal loss of thermoregulation.[4] An intoxicated person who falls asleep out of doors in cold northern climes faces lethal hypothermia. Alcohol dilates superficial blood vessels. Heat then dissipates faster than when veins retain their usual size. Death occurs when the speed of body cooling is faster than the speed with which sobriety returns.

The Process of Dying

People in temperate zones experience the effects of milder hypothermia in different ways. Cold water coursing through the trenches where regiments of First World War soldiers bivouacked led to trench foot. It wasn't fatal, though. Usually death arose from "lead poisoning" after "going over the top."

Shins develop chilblains when inadequately protected from windy wintery blasts. Dry, cold winter wind also produces frostbite on skiers' cheeks. Discomfort from these types of minor cold injuries resolves once a person goes indoors and warms up. Coroners can assume these conditions may have existed transiently in many hypothermic deaths.

At first, a person dying of hypothermia feels the cold. Shivering begins, and the skin becomes increasingly pale while it cools. The heart rate speeds up as the body's thermoregulation tries to protect its tissues by constricting blood vessels, making the heart beat faster and the blood pressure rise. A person freezing to death starts to become consciously aware that their heart is beating.

That cold person also feels an urge to urinate. Blood vessels are constricting against a fixed volume of fluid contained within them. To allow the blood vessels to constrict, the volume within them must decrease. Excreting fluid out through the kidneys is the only way this can happen.

At this stage the frigid person is still conscious, more or less alert, but has difficulty speaking. Cold air passing over the vocal cords dries them. With each breath the voice becomes huskier until, eventually, the ability to talk completely disappears.

Along with vocal difficulties alertness steadily declines. Reasoning becomes difficult. Speech gradually slurs until it becomes senseless. For some reason, the hypothalamus no longer fulfills its role in regulating temperature; nobody knows exactly why.

A freezing person's skin becomes blue and puffy when the smallest blood vessels in the body (the capillaries) become inflamed. As their inflammation progresses, serum oozes out of the blood vessels, causing surrounding tissues to swell. Though these changes proceed steadily, a freezing person is unaware of them.

Hypothermia is sometimes responsible for a couple of odd behaviours in the elderly. When evidence of these behaviours occurs, police officers investigating the death — along with coroners who are unaware of them — suspect something sinister has happened. These unusual deaths frequently take place in a cold house rather than out of doors. Police become suspicious when a partially dressed body is discovered with discarded clothing lying nearby that had seemingly been taken off shortly before death. Most police officers consider it particularly strange that anyone would shed clothes in a very cold house. The coroner should reassure puzzled police investigators that this is just part of dying of hypothermia.

This behaviour is called "paradoxical undressing": the act of inappropriately removing pieces of clothing, or even completely undressing, when it is very cold. Investigators arriving at the death scene will be confronted by a naked or only partially clad body in surroundings that seem uncomfortably cool. It usually takes a bit of time to work out that the deceased person was probably fully clad until a short time before death.

Attempting to hide while dying is the second odd behaviour triggered by cold temperatures. Sometimes a police officer or coroner opens a cupboard in a very cold house and discovers a dead body curled up within. On other occasions, the body of a person who has died from hypothermia is discovered under a pile of household furniture. People dying from hypothermia may hide under a pile of clothing, books, rags or anything at hand. Sometimes these dying people crawl under the bed. There is no way of calculating exactly how long any material was piled up before the person actually died. All one can say is that the piling took place shortly before death. Most people dying this way are elderly, and it is hard to work out exactly why this happens. This odd activity has two names: "terminal burrowing" and "hide-and-die syndrome."

When the body's core temperature drops further, all activity slows. Weakness sets in. Any walking hypothermic stumbles at first, then repeatedly falls, and finally collapses in a stupor. Both head and limbs may involuntarily jerk a bit while the person is lying on the ground.

As stupor deepens breathing slows. Then the heart stops working properly. Nobody knows what cardiovascular changes actually take place, but they do trigger ventricular fibrillation that results in death roughly five minutes after it starts. At the time of a hypothermic death, the body is not frozen. Only when bodies remain undiscovered for a long time in frigid weather do the cells completely freeze.

Nobody can determine how long a hypothermic person remained conscious before dying from the cold. The range of possibilities makes it foolish to even speculate. However long it took, mental confusion in the final stages before losing consciousness makes dying from hypothermia not particularly painful. The general perception of a final dreamy period before freezing to death is probably correct.

Pain accompanies dying from exposure when the temperature is low enough that chilblains or frostbite develops early on. Frostbite makes the skin feel cold and makes the affected body part tingle with a pins and needles sensation before turning into throbbing. Frostbite usually affects the fingers, toes or face.

As the frostbite worsens and tissues freeze the pain disappears. Consequently, in hypothermic deaths, any pain occurs some time before death and does not last very long.

Delayed Death

Not every person dies of hypothermia right away. A number of extremely hypothermic people are discovered unconscious and half dead. They are then taken home or to hospital for rewarming and resuscitation.

Unfortunately, that process does not always work successfully. Rewarming is a long and difficult process, particularly when a person's core body temperature has dropped very low. Many different rewarming techniques are available to try to warm a person up to return their body's core temperatures to normal. Rewarming is usually performed on severely hypothermic patients, alive but unconscious, in a hospital intensive care unit (ICU).

Optimum hospital treatment can't always prevent fatal complications of hypothermia. Low blood pressure is often an intractable lethal consequence of the cold exposure. Aspirating vomit into the trachea or lungs becomes lethal when it totally prevents all airflow. More frequently, aspiration only partly blocks airflow but introduces bacteria that develop into a terminal pneumonia.

Hypothermia can also trigger heart failure and a fatal build-up of fluid in the lungs. Sometimes lethal pancreatitis develops. In hypothermia virtually any fatal infection is possible. Several other terminal events may end the prolonged ICU treatment of a person hospitalized with hypothermia. Bleeding from the gut, kidney failure, clots in blood vessels, muscle breakdown, gangrene and even brain damage are all possible life-ending events.

Until fully recovered from cold exposure the heart remains prone to rhythm abnormalities. Any complication along the path to recovery can easily trigger a fatal cardiac arrhythmia. Since these complications usually only occur while people are unconscious, death is painless. A Norwegian radiologist who was skiing went through the ice covering a creek. She was submerged for 80 minutes before discovery and subsequent resuscitation. She had the lowest known core temperature among adults who have survived hypothermia. At the time of her discovery, her core temperature had dropped to 13.7°C (56.7°F).[5]

NOTES

1 Reingardiene, D. (2003). Hypothermia. *Medicina* (Kaunas, Lithuania), 39(1), 90–97 (Article in Lithuanian). Summary available at https://medicina.lsmuni.lt/med/0301/0301-12e.htm

2 United States Power Squadrons. (2007, January 23). Hypothermia Safety. *Compass, 1*(1), 1.

3 British Medical Association. (1964, November 14). Accidental hypothermia in the elderly. *British Medical Journal.* https://europepmc.org/backend/ptpmcrender.fcgi?accid=PMC1817203&blobtype=pdf

4 Albiin, N., & Eriksson, A. (1984). Fatal accidental hypothermia and alcohol. *Alcohol and Alcoholism, 19*(1), 13–22.

5 MacDonald, F. (2016, October 14). This is how a Norwegian woman survived the lowest body temperature ever recorded. *Science Alert. https://www.sciencealert.com/this-woman-survived-the-lowest-body-temperature-ever-recorded*

12

Deaths in the Water

It is not surprising that many people die in water, since water covers almost three quarters of Earth's surface. Water may constitute most of the world's environment, but it is not the only liquid that kills humans. However, water's ubiquity makes it by far the most common of those liquids. *Drowning* is the word colloquially used to describe a death, or the mechanism by which a death occurred, when immersed in or caused by any type of liquid. Physicians prefer to talk about death by immersion, so the terms *drowning* and *immersion* are used interchangeably throughout this chapter.

Overview

Coroners focus on deaths in water since that is by far the most common liquid in which people drown. The number of people who drown varies around the globe. Mozambique tops the world with nearly 20 out of 100,000 people drowning each year. All the highest rates of drowning are in Africa. Of the 20 countries where immersion deaths are the highest, only Bolivia, Bangladesh and North Korea are not part of the African continent.

In 2014 the World Health Organization (WHO) estimated that 372,000 people a year drowned. Since more than 90% of those drownings occurred in low- or middle-income countries, the WHO considers drowning one of their more serious public health problems. But it is not the worst — malnutrition, much of which occurs in famine, kills twice as many as immersion in water. Poor statistics from many countries with a high risk of drowning make it likely their annual drowning numbers are grossly understated.

To understand the problem consider a few statistics. Worldwide, 42 drowning deaths occur per hour. Males drown twice as often as females, and half of those drowned are under 25 years of age. Drowning is one of the 10 leading causes of death for persons aged 1 to 24 years in every region of the world. Alcohol use is associated with both adolescent and adult drownings.[1]

In developed countries like Canada, the number drowned is not high. The Lifesaving Society of Canada recorded only 408 Canadian drownings in 2018, a substantial decrease from the 685 recorded in 1993. In Ontario, where the author lives, that year 100 drowned. Throughout Canada almost 80% of those drowned were male. Those over 65 years of age had the highest rate of drowning.

In Canada, 34% of drownings occurred in lakes, 28% in rivers or streams and 12% in bathtubs. In 2018, 9% of drownings took place in private pools. Over half of Canadian drownings occurred on the weekend, and almost two thirds took place in the warm summer months. Nearly 60% of drownings involved recreational activities, and 23% a motor vehicle accident.

The United States is a much more populous country than Canada. About one American drowns each day just from boating incidents. Almost 10 more drown daily for other reasons.[2] About 40% of Americans drown on weekends, more drown in the summer months (from May to August) than during the rest of the year, and more people drown in rural areas and in the southern and western states than the rest of the country. In California, Arizona and Florida, drowning is the leading injury causing death.[3]

Bangladeshis routinely bathe in ditches and streams and often drown in them. In countries with a similar level of development, most adolescents and young adults drown in natural water bodies. Britons drown at home approximately 10% of the time — most commonly young children and older adults. Most developed nations have similar statistics.[4]

Australia has many studies on drowning. Their statistics show that quite a few Australians drown in water tanks, but more drown in the ocean. Australian research has created a picture of the typical person who drowns while surfing. He is a young adult male who has consumed alcohol before going out to sea to surf and has usually swum too far off shore to return safely.[5]

Pathologists always refer to deaths in water as "immersion" deaths. They choose that term because people die in water in several different ways. Regardless of the exact mechanism, all deaths in water are colloquially referred to as drowning, and coroners can always use the word *drowning* when talking to relatives. If details of how the drowning occurred are sought, simply explain the type of drowning to them.

Types of Death

Drowning includes several categories of death in the water. Sometimes things are not what they seem. People may start on their death's trajectory by standing at the edge of a body of water. Then, they suddenly lose consciousness from a sudden fatal but natural event, like ventricular fibrillation or a massive pulmonary embolus. They fall into the adjacent water, where they stay until their dead bodies are subsequently found.

A reasonable first impression, on seeing a dead body floating on the water, is that the person drowned. In the cases described, of course that assumption would be quite wrong. These people lost consciousness and stopped breathing before they fell into the water. Water did not cause these deaths. It was simply the environment in which their dead bodies were found. These people never breathed while afloat or submerged. After a few minutes in or on the water while dying, death finally took place after all electrical activity ceased in their hearts and brains. The same is true when a blow delivered on land with lethal force knocks the dying body into the water where it is eventually discovered. In neither case did death arise from the water itself, so the official cause of death is not drowning.

People severely injured in the water often die before being able to return to land. Their injuries rather than water kill them even though they may have been said to have drowned. Cold water itself can be fatal. The human body cannot withstand low temperatures in cold water very long.

Divers sometimes succumb to air emboli while rising to the surface. Diving equipment can break down, stopping oxygen delivery from the scuba tank. Careless divers, who sometimes run out of oxygen while underwater, asphyxiate. Diving is an inherently dangerous sport. Even the best prepared or most skilled divers sometimes die in the water.

Even though none of these watery deaths mentioned so far are actually drowning, some people do truly drown.

Death before Entering the Water

Any sudden death starts with a loss of consciousness. A person standing on the water's edge can topple into it. Any cause of sudden death could be the trigger for this fall. Unless chest pain from a developing myocardial infarction preceded the collapse, such a death will probably be both sudden and painless. Relatives derive some slight relief to hear that.

Sometimes the previously mentioned lethal force knocks people into the water. A fatal blow to the head may tumble an unconscious body into a nearby body of water. Death follows in due course. The corpse usually continues to float until its eventual discovery.

An autopsy is required to determine whether death in or on the water resulted from an injury, natural disease or drowning. The pathologist's work is not always easy, since many people found dead in water have signs of a chronic, natural disease — such as severe coronary artery disease — that could have caused death by itself. The pathologist must then decide whether the person died before falling into the water or whether they drowned.

It's no different when the force of a fatal injury on land knocks a possibly lifeless body into water. A coroner can suppose the injuries were incompatible with life, but only a pathologist should decide, after autopsy, whether death occurred prior to entry into, or while in, the water. Without an autopsy, most people assume drowning to be the cause. To gently steer a reluctant family to agree to an autopsy, it is helpful to mention the role of the pathologist in such a case.

A live person floating on a body of water faces injury from many things other than water. Rocks, propellers, wood, and metal spikes, all assisted by the action of tides or waves, can be lethal. A coroner should only conclude a fatal injury occurred in the water after going over the incident thoroughly and determining a mechanism of death compatible with bodily injuries after an autopsy has excluded drowning.

Drowning

For drowning to occur water must trigger the death. It is possible to drown in any liquid of course, but non-water drownings are so unusual that coroners virtually never need to talk about them. In the unlikely event such a discussion becomes necessary, assume drowning happens in a similar manner to a death in water. You will find many people are well informed on how death occurs when drowning.

Unlike the way it may be depicted in films, drowning in real life is usually a quiet affair.[6] The instinctive drowning response is well known and routinely taught in lifesaving classes. Drowning people rarely call out or splash around. Their mouths alternately sink below and reappear above the surface of the water. The time above the water is not enough for them to inhale, exhale or call out for help.

Drowning people do not wave. Some may try to swim without making progress. More commonly they extend their arms laterally to try to press on the surface of the water to lift their mouths into the air. This arm movement is thought to be instinctive rather than voluntary and controlled. Drowning people hold their bodies upright in the water. They cannot kick with their legs.

The typical drowning person's head floats so low in the water that the mouth is at water level. Usually the head is tilted slightly backward with an open mouth, and hair hanging over the forehead or eyes. A drowning person's eyes are closed or glassy, empty and unfocused. Breathing while still above the water is either rapid or in gasps.

This stage usually only lasts for 20 to 60 seconds before the head submerges along with the rest of the body. Everyone has an automatic breathing reflex that causes a gasp whenever the level of carbon dioxide in the blood becomes too high. When the blood's carbon dioxide level causes a gasp with the head under water, some water will be drawn into the mouth and perhaps the lungs as well.

Drowning has four stages. In the first stage a drowning person voluntarily holds his breath until the urge to breathe becomes overwhelming. In the second stage a gasp aspirates water; sometimes a bit is swallowed too. During the third stage the brain becomes so deprived of oxygen that both breathing and aspirating water stops. In the fourth and final stage, the brain is so damaged by lack of oxygen that it stops functioning and the person dies.[7]

When asked by relatives about how a death by drowning occurred, a coroner should think about variations in these stages before answering. Once the drowning person sinks underwater, the second stage of drowning can develop in two different ways.

In the first type of case, water entering the windpipe (trachea) makes the vocal cords (larynx) close to prevent further water from entering the lungs. As a result, the drowning person can no longer make any sounds. Continuing spasm of the vocal cords also prevents the drowning person from breathing. As a result, the blood's carbon dioxide level rises and triggers a reflex gasp. At that point more water usually enters the lungs. Just before or after this gasp, the person loses consciousness.

In the second type of case, the drowning person does not take this final gasp. Between 7% and 10% (possibly even 15%) of drowning people never reopen their vocal cords before death.[8] In such cases the lungs do not fill up with water. This sort of death used to be referred to as "dry drowning", though the term is no longer considered correct by pathologists. Many people have heard this very descriptive term, so coroners find it a useful phrase if asked to explain these deaths.

Coroners should be aware that people drown differently in fresh water than in the sea, but this difference interests only academics. Lungs fill regardless of the type of water aspirated. The blood oxygen level drops low enough that brain damage begins. Stages three and four follow the same course in both ocean and freshwater drownings.

Aspirating a lot of water must be very unpleasant while a drowning person remains conscious. Inhaled water will cause both chest pain and some degree of panic from an inability to breathe. This state usually lasts less than a minute before the person becomes unconscious. A coroner should assure relatives that a drowned person probably did not suffer very long. How long it took to drown is a hard question to answer.

Dog studies show that dogs took longer to die in salt water than in fresh water. In fresh water dogs drowned in 4 to 5 minutes, while in sea water it took 8 to 12 minutes. Dog drownings do not accurately mimic human drowning though. There has been at least one case of a boy being submerged under water for 42 minutes and surviving.[9]

A coroner may be questioned about "secondary" drowning. This is a term once used to explain deaths, often from pulmonary oedema, that occurred in the period after a person was removed from the water following a period of immersion. Nowadays, these deaths are simply considered complications of drowning, and coroners should use that phrase. People understand the idea of complications very well.

Cold Water

The temperature at which humans consider water to be thermally neutral is 33 to 34 degrees Celsius (33°C–34°C), which is 91 to 93 degrees Fahrenheit (91°F–93°F).[10] At that point a nude person's body heat production balances the heat loss into the water. Most temperate zone bodies of water never achieve that high a temperature. All human bodies entering a lake, river or stream outside the tropics are bound to lose heat shortly after entering the water.

Exercise speeds up heat loss from the body in the following manner. The skin becomes cold first, but very cold water cools the tissues below the body's surface quite rapidly. A muscle's ability to produce force decreases after the muscle's temperature drops below 27°C (80°F).[11]

Studies of deaths in cold water have been carried out for more than a century. The successful sinking of so many Allied ships in the Battle of the Atlantic caused the United Kingdom to put a great deal of research effort into understanding cold water immersion to try to save sailors' lives. From that work came an understanding of the four methods of dying when immersed in cold water.[12,13]

Cold Shock

One type of cold water (25°C, 77°F) death is called "cold shock" or death at initial immersion. It has been known to happen when a seafarer, perhaps quite drunk, falls off the side of a ship into the cold ocean below. He may be pulled out of the water dead, even though only a couple of minutes have elapsed since his body entered the water.

In such a case, the initial immersion caused a sudden gasp, then rapid respiration or hyperventilation. The heart sped up and the blood pressure rose. Cold water probably stimulates nerve endings in the skin, nose, mouth or vocal cords and triggers some sort of fatal cardiac reflex ending in ventricular fibrillation.

Cold shock can occur at water temperatures below 25°C and is inevitable in water temperatures of 10°C to 15°C (50° to 59°F). It is likely a relatively painless death.

Swimming Failure

Short-term immersion, or swimming failure, is a second method of dying in cold water. Death in this stage happens between 3 and 30 minutes after a person has started to swim. Even good swimmers may be unable to swim for more than a few minutes in very cold water. The *British Medical Journal* reported the case of a 20-year-old male whose dinghy overturned in a reservoir filled with water at approximately 10°C (51°F) water. Although he was a good swimmer who was trying to swim just 50 yards (46 metres) to safety, the man sank in the cold water after trying for five minutes to swim that distance.[14] This cause of death may be a variant of cold water shock, or it may be what is called "a diving response."*

Hypothermia

The third type of death in cold water requires long-term immersion for 30 minutes or more. This cools the body, and the condition of hypothermia develops. A number of factors can affect the rate at which hypothermia develops. Factors speeding the onset of hypothermia include

- colder water
- higher waves or stronger currents
- lack of clothing (or any other insulating material) gathered around the body
- shivering and swimming, both a form of muscle exercise
- lack of body fat
- lack of physical fitness
- inadequate food intake prior to immersion
- poor body posture in water

* The diving response is characterized by breath-holding, slowing of the heart rate, reduction of blood flow to the limbs and a gradual rise in mean arterial blood pressure. The response is produced by water touching the face, and then the person either voluntarily or involuntarily (via reflex) stopping breathing. Water temperature, oxygen in the blood and anxiety all play a role in its development.

Hypothermia deaths result from either drowning or cardiac arrest. A core body temperature that drops below 24°C (75°F) makes cardiac arrest quite likely (though not certain).[15]

Post-Rescue Collapse

Unfortunately, just being hauled out of cold water alive does not guarantee survival. This has been known since at least 1875, when a Hamburg police surgeon recorded cases of sailors rescued from the harbour or canals who died within 24 hours of their rescue.[16] After the Second World War, the United States reported that 17% of shipwrecked survivors rescued from water at 10°C (50°F) or less died within 24 hours after rescue. Nobody rescued from water with a temperature above 20°C (68°F) died.[17]

Another common type of water fatality that coroners investigate is associated with diving.

Diving Deaths

People have probably been diving under the water without breathing assistance (free diving) since the first person learned to dive. Compressed air has been available to divers for well over a century now. Until the self-contained breathing apparatus (scuba) was invented, deep sea diving required wearing a heavy hood and a protective oxygen-containing suit connected by hoses to an oxygen source on a ship above.

Before the Second World War, diving deaths were infrequent industrial accidents involving unlucky professional divers wearing armour-like atmospheric suits working on the seabed. Since that time, scuba diving was developed, and each year since it has become an increasingly popular sport worldwide. Nowadays, scuba deaths occur in many countries each year. Since these deaths happen underwater, the diver, in common parlance, is said to have drowned. However, there are different reasons why scuba deaths occur.

The Royal College of Pathologists of Australia (RCPA) reviewed diving deaths in preparing a guideline for pathologists to follow when autopsying dead divers.[18] The RCPA concluded that between 52% and 86% of fatalities were actually due to drowning. Though drowning was the terminal event, the RCPA looked more deeply into the potential causes. They found these nine:

1. inability to swim
2. fatigue
3. panic
   - inadequate training
4. decreased level of consciousness
   - intoxication
   - nitrogen narcosis
   - seizures, such as an oxygen toxicity seizure
   - cerebral arterial gas embolism
   - hypercapnia (too much carbon dioxide in the blood)
5. natural disease, such as acute myocardial infarction, asthma, diabetes, epilepsy
6. trauma
7. entrapment in caves or wrecks
8. physical disability
9. equipment malfunction

Families are interested in all these possibilities, so a coroner should explain how the person drowned.

Most of these causes do not need explanation, but nitrogen narcosis does. This condition arises when nitrogen enters a diver's bloodstream. Symptoms of nitrogen narcosis usually only begin when a diver is deeper than 30 metres (98 feet). The symptoms follow a pattern, colloquially called "raptures of the deep", as they progress toward fatality.

The diver first becomes calm. This is likened to the sensation experienced when using cannabis, being drunk or taking a tranquillizer. The diver then begins to move more slowly. It becomes more difficult to multitask. The giddiness, overconfidence, anxiety or vertigo (a spinning form of dizziness) that may ensue will significantly impair the diver. At this point the unwitting diver may perform some foolish fatal act. Nitrogen narcosis is so rarely witnessed that it is usually only hypothesized, not proven.

Similarly, it is impossible to prove that a seizure took place underwater due to the effect of high oxygen pressure on the brain. Nor can anybody prove carbon dioxide toxicity was the reason for loss of consciousness before drowning. Death involving either of these two terminal events will always remain the subject of speculation.

Coroners need also to know that even snorkellers can experience fatal shallow water blackouts after hyperventilating, holding their breath and then diving. The snorkeller starts to develop inadequate oxygen in the blood while heading toward the surface, loses consciousness and drowns.

Another fatal problem can arise when using tanks of compressed air. In an uncontrolled ascent without inhaling, air is forced into the blood from the lungs, resulting in air bubbles in the arteries. These bubbles, called air emboli, move through the body's arteries until they end up in the brain.

The diver usually comes to the surface alert but then cries out and within minutes loses consciousness. Death shortly follows. Most of the time the diver ascended from a significant depth, yet this does not always have to be the case. Air emboli have been reported to occur in a depth as shallow as two metres of water.

Natural disease accounts for some deaths in older divers. Ischaemic heart disease and asthma account for 9% of diving deaths, but multiple factors usually cause the diver's death. The RCPA found that errors in judgement played a major role — 56% of cases involved low or no air in the tanks, while 52 % of deaths involved weight belt problems (either too much or too little).

Panic was found to have been involved 39% of the time. Salt water aspiration occurred in 37% of diving deaths. A surge of tidal currents was identified as a contributing factor in 36% of the cases. Diver fatigue played a role in 28% of the deaths. There were other findings, but these were the highest contributing cofactors in these Australian diving deaths.

All these factors are important to families who are trying to determine how their loved one's death occurred. Investigating police may be able to pinpoint some factors that contributed to death in the water. However, a coroner can safely talk about drowning as the cause regardless of what other factors led to death in a specific case. Most families understand diving is a dangerous activity in which death is a foreseeable risk.

NOTES

1 World Health Organization (WHO). (2014, November 17). *Global report of drowning: Preventing a leading killer.* https://www.who.int/publications/i/item/global-report-on-drowning-preventing-a-leading-killer

2 Centers for Disease Control and Prevention (CDC). (2020, October 7). *Unintentional drowning: Get the facts.* https://www.cdc.gov/homeandrecreationalsafety/water-safety/waterinjuries-factsheet.html

3 Safe Kids Worldwide. (n.d.). *Water safety at home.* https://www.safekids.org/safetytips/field_risks/water-and-drowning/field_type/fact-sheet

4 Cantwell, G. P. (2019, June 19). *Drowning.* Medscape. https://emedicine.medscape.com/article/772753-overview

5 Morgan, D., Ozanne-Smith, J., & Triggs, T. Direct observation measurement of drowning risk exposure for surf beach bathers. *Journal of Science and Medicine in Sport, 12*(4), 457–462.

6 Vittone, M. (2013, June 4). Drowning doesn't look like drowning. *Slate.* https://slate.com/technology/2013/06/rescuing-drowning-children-how-to-know-when-someone-is-in-trouble-in-the-water.html

7 Harle, L. (2019, August 26). Autopsy & forensics: Drowning. Wexner Medical Center, Ohio State University. https://www.pathologyoutlines.com/topic/forensicsdrowning.html

8 See note 4 above.

9 Palermo, E. (2015, June 2). *Surviving 42 minutes underwater ... How boy beat the odds.* https://www.livescience.com/51046-how-boy-survived-near-drowning.html

10 Alexiou, S. (2014). The biology of exercise. *Journal of the Biology of Exercise, 10*(2), 9–23. https://www.researchgate.net/publication/287415785

11 Veleskin, P. N. (n.d.) Hypothermia. In A. Prokhorov(Ed.), *Great Soviet Encyclopedia (1969–1978)* (3rd ed.).

12 Brooks, C. J. (2001, August 24). *Survival in cold water: A report prepared for Transport Canada.*

13 Golden, F., & Hervey, G. R. (1981). The "After-Drop" and death after rescue from immersion in cold water. In J. M. Adam (Ed.), *Hypothermia ashore and afloat.* Pergamon Press.

14 Keatinge, W. R., Prys-Roberts, C., Cooper, K. E., Honour, A. J., & Haight, J. (1969, February 22). Sudden failure of swimming in cold water. *British Medical Journal,* 1:480. https://doi.org/10.1136/bmj.1.5642.480

15 Gilbert, M., Busund, R., Skagseth, A., Nilsen, P. A., & Solbo, J. P. (2000). Resuscitation from accidental hypothermia of 13.7°C with circulatory arrest. *The Lancet, 355*(9201), 375–376.

16 Golden, F. (1974). Shipwreck and survival. *Journal of the Royal Naval Medical Service, 60*(1–2), 8–14.

17 Matthes, M. (1946). German air sea rescue services, World War II. USAF Surgeon General's Office, 1148.

18 Lawrence, C., & Cooke, C. (2006). *Fact file: Autopsy and investigation of scuba diving fatalities. https://www.researchgate.net/publication/290098466_Autopsy_and_the_investigation_of_scuba_diving_fatalities*

13

Deaths by Starvation

Refusing food is common at the end of many severely demented people's lives. Usually that's the only time physicians or coroners in most developed countries become involved with any death arising from starvation. Caregivers also find demented elderly folks will terminally refuse water as well as food. Technically, *starvation* can refer to a lack of either food or water. In its common usage, starving to death means only dying from a lack of food though. Death from lack of water is usually referred to as resulting from dehydration.

In years gone by, deaths from starvation were common around the globe. Periodic starvation has been humanity's lot, probably since the first humans roamed the planet. Famines continue to happen around the world periodically. Vivid images in the media constantly remind us of their effects. Famine still causes thousands, if not millions of people to starve and many to die. Widespread famine is now found in only the world's most underdeveloped countries, but this was not always the case.

Starvation does not always result from natural disasters. In the twentieth century some government policies created famines just as devastating as nature's worst. Two widely publicized examples occurred in the Soviet Union during Stalin's time and in North Korea periodically throughout its existence.

It is hard to get an accurate number of people who die from starvation annually. Statistics exist, but not all are reliable. The WHO 2014 hunger statistics reported that about 3.1 million children under five years of age died of malnutrition.[1] This is an educated guess, but the actual number may be quite a bit higher or lower. The reason: some governments do not tell the truth.

Countries that do not want the rest of the world to know their citizens are starving to death frequently report artificially low figures to cover up the problem. Various organizations raise money to feed refugees. Some forecast high numbers of likely starvation deaths hoping to raise money from sympathetic donors. These are the two common sources for starvation statistics.

In the developed world, the numbers of deaths from starvation are usually compiled by counting the diagnoses written on death certificates. Certifying how a person dies requires making a choice between different ways to describe the cause of death. Cognitively impaired people often stop eating or drinking for a period before they die, making starvation their final stage of dying. End of life starvation is also found among people with cancer, dementia or diseases that impair absorption of food or fluid. Starvation is one way to say these people died.

Nowadays most people who complete death certificates won't use starvation as the cause of death. They consider starvation and dehydration simply to be terminal events rather than the reason for death. The disease, injury or condition that led to the terminal failure to eat or drink is the real reason for dying. That is what is written on the death certificate as the explanation why a person died.

However, there are still those who do not see it that way. In 2013 *The Guardian* looked at death certificates in British hospitals and became quite exercised about the fact that 223 people were described as dying of dehydration and malnutrition each year.[2] This state of affairs was attributed by both the journalist and political commentators to neglect.

Neglect may indeed have been the case in some of these deaths. Still, a more in-depth examination of the dying process in each of these cases would probably have shown that for most, the term *starvation* simply described the terminal result of cognitive decline. In any case that number is not excessively high for a country with almost 80 million residents. Statistics Canada in 2018 attributed 220 deaths to "nutritional deficiencies",[3] which is another way of saying the same thing, and Canada has less than half the population of the United Kingdom.

Looking at the most recent malnutrition death rates per 100,000 population,[4] the UK's is 0.08, Canada's is 0.29, Australia's is 0.19, New Zealand's is 0.11, while the USA's is 0.90. Those countries are all at a similar stage of social development. Some of the difference in these statistics likely result from differing death coding techniques.

It is rare for people to actually die of starvation in any of these five countries.

That is not true of the tropics, where many more die from malnutrition than in developed countries. The 38 countries with the highest rates of deaths from malnutrition are all in Africa. The Democratic Republic of the Congo has the highest starvation death rate at 43.92 per 100,000 residents. The figures for countries in the developed world change little year after year, while statistics in less developed can vary significantly over time.

Causes

Starvation can become fatal in a short period of time. Famine is an unpredictable but (usually) unavoidable periodic natural scourge that results in many starving to death. For that reason, coroners don't investigate famine deaths. Another situation where starvation is considered natural is the cessation of eating or drinking at the end of a chronic disease. Coroners don't investigate these deaths either.

When a person eventually dies without eating or drinking for a period of time while slowly dying of cancer, dementia or any other degenerative disease, their deaths are certified by treating physicians or other practitioners. Experience tells them to avoid attributing their patients' deaths to starvation.

When surviving family members see "starvation" as a cause of death on a death certificate they often feel a sense of guilt and blame themselves for failing to prevent a loved relative from dying that way. That wording on the death certificate describes the cause incorrectly. The final period of starvation was the unavoidable terminal period of some lethal condition. The family's unhappiness is easily prevented by simply attributing such a death to "complications" of the problem that initiated it.

True deaths from starvation do occur when people are trapped in caves, pits or mines. People still occasionally starve to death when lost in the bush, especially in the far north. Fortunately, these deaths are infrequent, but when they do happen they need thorough investigation in an effort to see whether similar deaths could be avoided in the future.

Any death due to a parent's or guardian's neglect in providing or, more horribly, deliberately refusing to provide food to a child or an incapacitated adult must also be meticulously investigated. That does occasionally happen in developed countries. The willful refusal to take food or drink as a form of suicide is another starvation situation that will periodically occur. Whenever it does, a coroner will be required to investigate it.

Dehydration

Starvation can result from refusing food and also from refusing to drink. Without water, death occurs much faster than without food. It's not considered ethical to do studies to determine how long a human being takes to die when deprived of water. However, there is quite a bit of anecdotal evidence available about how long people can survive while dehydrated, and that information can be given to questioners.

Hospice literature suggests death from water deprivation can take up to five days, but the testimonials of relatives suggest that dying may take a week or more. It seems to be commonly believed that three days without water will kill most people. However, Andreas Mihavecz spent 18 days in 1979 forgotten in a prison cell and was still alive when discovered.[5] Usually "a few days" is an appropriate response to give in answer to a query about how long a person can survive without water.

Dehydration starts to bother people as the mucous membranes of their mouths begin to dry and they become thirsty. Thirst is a protective sensation nature accords to humans. Its message is find some water to drink quickly, or something bad is going to happen. The sense of thirst does not continue until death, though.

Thirst's disappearance may represent an evolutionary adaptation to the unfortunate truth that in millennia past death by dehydration was sometimes inevitable. After being deprived of water for a while, the human body gets the message that no more thirst-quenching fluid is coming. At that point thirst is useless, so the sensation disappears. Dehydrated older folks probably lose their feelings of thirst more speedily than do the young.

Loss of thirst probably arises because a person's body goes into a water conservation mode. The cells actually lose fluid, as does the blood within the blood vessels. As fluid in the blood decreases, the concentration of sodium in the blood increases. The combination of these changes somehow diminishes the brain's ability to appreciate pain, the discomfort of thirst and, for that matter, most other unpleasant external stimuli.

Most medical literature relating to what happens next is derived from people observing patients at the end of their lives. These dying patients receive sedation when uncomfortable. This allows them to die peacefully in a relatively serene state until the very end.

Even when sedation is not provided, palliative care nurses consider that their patients dying from dehydration experience a "good death." If you are asked to opine on the sensations felt when dying of dehydration, there is no need to make up an answer. An honest reply is that all good evidence we have points to death from water starvation or dehydration being a comfortable, painless one.

Food Starvation

When starvation arises from merely withholding food, death takes quite a bit longer than when water is denied as well. People who die of acute starvation are cases that a coroner might investigate. The only time a coroner will investigate a chronic starvation death is when some individual or institution is responsible for causing the chronic starvation. That is unlikely to occur in most countries that use coroners.

Acute Starvation

Nobody does studies to determine how long people can survive without food. There are varying estimates derived from fasting. Usual figures for survival range between two and three months.[6] The deaths of the IRA hunger strikers in 1981 proved that estimate to be correct. Much of the newspaper-reading world followed with a morbid fascination the declining health of 10 IRA hunger strikers in the Maze prison in Northern Ireland. These inmates drank water but refused food. The IRA commander of the group, Bobby Sands, eventually died after a fast lasted 66 days. His other nine colleagues survived for differing periods of time that ranged between 46 and 73 days.

Survival when starving requires the body to use its component material to replace nutrients normally derived from food. Consequently, fatter people survive starvation much better than do the thin because they have more bodily material to draw on. The pathway to starvation is quite well known. A quick summary follows, but coroners should feel quite confident they will never be asked about it.

Sugar (glucose) in the blood is derived from ingested food. This blood-borne glucose provides adequate energy as long as food continues to be eaten. Once the body stops receiving food to provide replacement glucose, glycogen stored in the body starts to be consumed instead. Once all the body's glycogen is exhausted, fatty acids are next. Metabolizing fatty acids goes on for quite a while because fatty acids exist in many tissues. People store up a lot of fat.

It is only at this point that the body begins to waste. Fat disappears first. After all fat is used up the body starts to destroy protein as it tries to produce enough glucose to keep going. A true state of starvation can be considered to exist at this point.

All fat reserves in the body have now been used up. Muscle mass decreases as it is broken down into proteins for metabolic use. Since proteins are also found in organs, continued starvation starts to deplete proteins in the body's essential organs too. Loss of protein finally damages an essential organ enough that its malfunction becomes fatal. Starvation's terminal event is usually a cardiac arrhythmia resulting from an electrolyte abnormality in the blood. Sometimes death comes from metabolic acidosis. [7]

Sensations experienced change as starvation worsens. Irritability, impulsivity or hyperactivity are felt initially. As fat and muscle become converted into compounds needed for survival, fatigue sets in, and the starving person becomes increasingly weak and apathetic. Weakness both decreases and slows any sort of movement. Starving people become totally self-focused. Women stop menstruating. The state of starvation usually starts after a person loses 30% of body weight and ends in death after 40% has gone.[8]

Chronic Starvation

A chronic starvation death ends in the same way as acute starvation. However, when chronically starved, a human body has not usually been deprived of enough nutrients to shut down quickly. Instead it adapts to its deficient state by changing the body's shape and function to survive. This state of chronic starvation is associated with diseases now usually only seen in Third World countries.

In developed countries chronic starvation still occurs in unusual circumstances. These involve negligent parents or guardians or deranged people imprisoning and providing so little food to their charges that they eventually starve to death. Fortunately, this rarely happens.

The effect of chronic starvation varies with age. A child deprived of food from birth will not grow as large as a child properly fed nutritious meals. This is termed "stunted growth." Very young children can develop diseases from chronic starvation. One such disease, called marasmus, notably features a wasted body and almost no energy. Another, kwashiorkor, is easily recognized because the starving child has a protuberant abdomen and red hair.

A lot of chronic starvation has a psychiatric basis. Eating disorders such as anorexia nervosa sometimes end in a (usually) woman starving herself to death. About 9% of people worldwide suffer from an eating disorder at some time in their lives,[9] and 10% of those with an eating disorder die.[10]

However not all these deaths result solely from starvation. One review of many papers written about death in people with anorexia nervosa found that almost 6% of people with the disease simply died prematurely.[11] A little over half of them died of complications from the disease as well as from starvation itself. Over a quarter of these deaths were suicides. The rest died in other or unrecorded ways.

Occasionally, people who have a digestive disorder that impairs absorption of food, who constantly vomit, or who have terminal cancer die of starvation. When neurological disorders — especially dementia — end life with a refusal to eat, this is usually not wilful. Instead, the person has lost the ability to remember how to eat. Starving is the terminal result of the underlying disease, so a coroner is unlikely to investigate these deaths.

There are also occasional, but fortunately rare, cases of parents, usually with some form of mental illness or unconventional religious or philosophical belief, who starve their children to death following some misguided principle. Examples of fatal childhood starvation include parents of a seven-month-old boy who owned a health food store in Belgium. Without apparent malice, they starved their son to death by feeding him a gluten-free diet that included quinoa milk. The court heard that his organs had shrunk to half their normal size. Both parents received a six months' suspended sentence.[12]

In an American case, vegan parents of an 18-month-old son starved their boy by feeding him nothing but raw fruits and vegetables.[13] In a different part of the United States, two parents were arrested after their two-year punishment of their six year old ended in the child's death from starvation.[14] In a third American case a couple in Michigan received life imprisonment for starving their five-year-old daughter to death.[15]

The problem of parents starving children to death, though rare, is worldwide. In Korea a jobless couple starved their three-month-old child while spending their days raising a virtual child on an Internet game.[16] A Polish couple in the United Kingdom starved their four-year-old son partly as misconceived discipline, but mostly because they were selfish, mean and totally incompetent parents.[17]

Equally unusual cases of death by starvation arise from imprisonment by mentally ill, very peculiar or just cruel people. Perhaps the most egregious institutional examples of this in the last century took place in Nazi concentration camps during the Second World War. More isolated incidents still occur around the world. These are so infrequent that the average coroner is unlikely to ever do more than read about such a case. All are widely publicized and result in criminal charges being laid.

NOTES

1 World Health Organization (WHO). (2018, February 19). *Millennium development goals (MDGS).* https://www.who.int/news-room/fact-sheets/detail/millennium-development-goals-(mdgs)

2 Rawlinson, K. (2013, December 2). Dehydration and malnutrition led to 2,162 deaths in care since 2003. *The Guardian.*

3 Statistics Canada. (n.d.). Table 1-1: Deaths and mortality rate, by selected grouped causes, sex and geography — Canada. https://www150.statcan.gc.ca/n1/pub/84f0209x/2009000/t001-eng.htm

4 World Life Expectancy. (n.d.). *Malnutrition death rate per 100,000.* https://www.worldlifeexpectancy.com/cause-of-death/malnutrition/by-country/

5 Kane, S. (2016, June 10). Here's the longest people have survived without air, food, water, sunshine, or sleep. https://www.sciencealert.com/here-s-the-longest-people-have-survived-without-air-food-water-sunshine-or-sleep

6 Bernhard, V. (2011). *A tale of two colonies: What really happened in Virginia and Bermuda?* Columbia, MO: University of Missouri Press, p. 112.

7 Toth, H. L., & Greenbaum, L. A. (2003). Severe acidosis caused by starvation and stress. *American Journal of Kidney Diseases 42(5), e22.1–e22.4.*

8 Elia, M. (n.d.) Effect of starvation and very low calorie diets on protein-energy interrelationships in lean and obese subjects. https://archive.unu.edu/unupress/food2/UID07E/UID07E11.HTM

9 Galmiche, M., Dechelotte, P., Lambert, G., & Tavolacci, M. P. (2019). Prevalence of eating disorders over the 2000–2018 period: A systematic literature review. *American Journal of Clinical Nutrition, 109*(5), 1402–1413.

10 Arcelus, J., Mitchell, A. J., Wales, J., & Nielsen, S. (2011). Mortality rates in patients with anorexia nervosa and other eating disorders: A meta-analysis of 36 studies. *Archives of General Psychiatry, 68*(7), 724–731.

11 Sullivan, P. F. (1995). Mortality in anorexia nervosa. *American Journal of Psychiatry 152(7), 1073–1074.*

12 Davies, G. (2017, May 16). Malnourished seven-month-old baby dies weighing just 9 lbs in Belgium after his father fed him a gluten-free diet which included quinoa milk. *The Daily Mail.*

13 Farberov, S. (2019, December 19). US vegan parents who eat only raw fruit and vegetables are charged with murder for the starvation death of their 18-month-old son who was found weighing only 17 lbs. *The Daily Mail.*

14 Eltagouri, M. (2017, November 7). Parents charged with murder for starving 6-year-old as punishment, police say. *The Washington Post.*

15 Boroff, D. (2016, March 10). Michigan parents sentenced to life in prison without parole for brutal starvation death of 5-year-old daughter. *New York Daily News.*

16 Campbell, C. (2014, April 15). Gamer dad arrested after toddler dies of neglect. .

17 Dolan, A. (2013, June 3). Boy, four, whose parents starved him to death suffered incomprehensible cruelty and looked like concentration camp victim. *The Daily Mail.*

14

Burn Deaths

Images of burning to death are vividly fixed in the popular imagination. Childhood comic books frequently depict terrified people trapped in blazing buildings and burning cars. In other cartoons characters are burned to death by terrorists or offered as sacrifices to gods in jungle rituals.

Fiery deaths in cops and robbers or gangster movies make great cinema. Vindictive criminals incinerate snitches. A flaming, explosive end to a car chase that once startled viewers has become unremarkable to twenty-first century movie-goers. Nowadays a screen full of flames is ubiquitous — in theatres, on TV sets and even on mobile phones.

Students learn about burning to death while studying the Spanish Inquisition, Joan of Arc, the Great Fire of London, or Nero's fiddling while Rome burned around him. Flames have immortalized some people in civic histories. It has long been believed that Mrs. O'Leary's cow started a fire in Chicago by kicking over a kerosene lantern while being milked in 1871. The actions of this ill-behaved animal set the whole city ablaze and indelibly linked Mrs. O'Leary's name with the history of Chicago.*

Preachers have long told their congregations to repent or face the horror of a fiery death in the afterlife. For centuries devout Christians believed the ultimate consequence of an evil life on Earth would be an eternal flaming torture in hell. The Bible was quite clear about it. Leviticus 10:2 reads "And there went out fire from the Lord, and devoured them, and they died before the Lord." Revelation 21:8 provides an equally horrible death for those who have failed to walk the path of righteousness. It reads:

* Mrs. O'Leary was probably a scapegoat. The official report of a commission of inquiry concluded that Mrs. O'Leary was not even in her barn at the start of the fire. The commission did not conclude the fire's precise cause but mentioned that a chimney spark from a nearby house on that windy night might have set her barn on fire.

But the fearful, and unbelieving, and the abominable, and murderers, and whoremongers, and sorcerers, and idolaters, and all liars, shall have their part in the lake which burneth with fire and brimstone: which is the second death.[1]

While society's increasing secularization makes these messages less believable, they endure as folk memory of how horrible burning to death can be.

In the Western world, men are burned to death twice as often as women — but death by burning does not occur very often. In 2014 throughout the whole United States of America only 3275 people died of burns. As expected, nearly two thirds were male.[2] The World Health Organization estimates that 180,000 people die of burns around the world each year. Most of them reside in low- or middle-income countries.

Two thirds of these burn deaths occur in Africa or Asia, where women die more often than men. A culture of open fire cooking, unsafe cook stoves and long loose flammable clothing is the reason.[3] In India brides are still occasionally burned to death when their families have not provided an adequate dowry. Indian widows still occasionally practise *suttee*, where a widow throws herself on her husband's funeral pyre to burn herself to death.

Some people do burn to death in fires. Dying from the heat of the flames is termed a thermal death, and it is one way that burning kills. Many thermal deaths take place in burning buildings. The heat generated by flames is only one way that fires kill, and heat is often not the lethal factor. Many, if not most, people killed by fires die of smoke inhalation. More about this later on in the chapter.

Flames are not required for a thermal death, though. Any type of dry heat can be substituted. Don't confuse thermal deaths with being burned to death. As we shall see, there are four other types of fatal burns; however, their incidence statistics are much lower than those for thermal deaths.

Scalding by a hot liquid produces a second type of fatal burn that more commonly kills small children and the elderly than fit, healthy adults. Water causes most fatal scalding, but any fluid warmed high enough is equally lethally.

Electrocution produces a third type of fatal burn. Charred spots on the skin mark the electrical current's entrance and exit sites on the body. All tissue between these points is burned instantly. When an electrical path of tissue destruction stops one or more vital organs from working, the body dies. Death comes quickly when electricity passes through the heart. Dying takes much longer when other vital organs (often the kidneys) fail.

A fourth source of fatal burns is ionizing radiation. With high enough exposure, death quickly follows irradiation. More frequently, it comes years after the exposure when a complication of the irradiation, such as cancer, appears.

Chemicals produce a fifth genre of lethal burns. Chemical burns are common but rarely fatal. Most coroners never investigate a death resulting from a chemical burn.

Thermal Deaths

Though burned buildings are the most common sites where coroners investigate thermal death, they are not the only ones. For example, some thermal deaths occur in forest fires. Coroners also look at deaths discovered in burned cars or trucks, ships and submarines, and even the occasional aeroplane. However, most human beings spend most of their day inside an edifice of one sort or another. That's the reason why the interior of a building is the most common location of thermal death.

A wall of fire is very hot. Flames in a burning building often reach 600° C (over 1100° F).[4] Heat of that intensity is more than enough to rapidly burn clothing. Cotton only requires a temperature of 210° C (410° F) before it bursts into flames. Nylons and polyesters resist heat longer. They only begin to burn at temperatures between 222° C and 277°C (432° F–532° F).[5] When clothing is vaporized this way, subsequent burns caused by the very hot flames hurt only momentarily. All the skin's nerve endings are destroyed by the heat almost instantly. Pain is over in a moment.

Doctors use several different systems to categorize burns, no one of which is "correct." Coroners need only consider three degrees of burns.

First degree is simply red and painful skin similar to a bad sunburn. Second degree burns mean blistered skin. Burns of these two degrees have little to do with death.

Fatalities result from third degree burns, termed "full thickness" because all the skin's layers are destroyed. Skin is often not the only tissue a third degree burn damages. Tendons, muscles, bones and all tissues supporting them are destroyed when a burn is deep enough. Burned bodies often exhibit all three degrees of burns in different parts.

When more than 90% of the body suffers full thickness burns, survival is uncommon. The Baux score, now revised to include more than its two original factors, was created as a method to predict a burn's mortality. The basis of the Baux score is that death is likely when the sum of the burned person's age and the percentage of the burned body exceeds 140.[6] That rule reflects the fact that young people tolerate severe burns much better than the elderly.* Improved care in urban hospital burn units has improved survival year after year, making the Baux system's 140 figure a somewhat inaccurate prognosticator. Still, the Baux score is a useful tool for coroners to use in discussions with relatives about the likelihood of survival when the percentage of the body that was burned is known.

Everyone knows from their own experience that burns hurt. The pain felt when burning to death would be similar in type, though much more severe even if not long-lasting. The terminal pain felt may be momentary. Third degree burns only hurt as long as the skin's nerve endings remain alive. Since nerve endings die almost immediately when exposed to great heat, many thermal deaths are likely less uncomfortable than one would imagine.

Fires damage more than just skin. Heat, hot smoke particles, and occasionally flames themselves can also burn nerve endings in both the throat and the lungs. The process of burning them is more likely to be painful. If a pathologist reports that a person's mouth and lungs were burned prior to death, a coroner should try to avoid discussing this with relatives. When that conversation cannot be avoided, agree pain was probable but minimize its duration.

---

* The percentage of burned body can be calculated using the rule of nines. The head and arms each comprise 9% of a body's area. The front of the chest and abdomen, the back, the left leg and the right leg each constitute another 18%. The scrotum and penis in a man or the vulvar area in a woman make up the remaining 1%.

Burned bodies found at the scene of a fire represent the minority of thermal deaths. Most occur long after the blaze was extinguished, in hospital after life has slowly ebbed away. In developed countries, this often happens in specialized hospital burn units. Since coroners only investigate fatal burns, these are the starting places for many coronial thermal death investigations.

Most people who have been burned survive, but even with top-notch care in American burn centres 4% of them die.[7] The inability to keep breathing with burned mouths or lungs is sometimes the cause. At other times the body loses so much fluid that its kidneys can't keep working. Infection causes many deaths too. This is particularly common when pneumonia in damaged airways causes terminal respiratory failure. Burned skin and fat often become fatally infected, and urinary tract infections developed in hospital can end in renal failure. Bacteria entering the bloodstream end life once sepsis develops.

By the time a person with severe thermal burns finally expires, family members have had frequent conversations with hospital staff. Relatives tend to be well informed and require no explanations about dying. Only uninformed relatives ask questions about thermal deaths occurring in hospital. A coroner questioned about the dying process should defer any discussion about it to hospital staff.

When conversation is unavoidable, a coroner is wise to generalize. People are often satisfied to know that in severe burn deaths, a lot of fluid typically moved from the circulatory system into the burned area, and that infection may have occurred resulting in fatal renal failure.*

Relatives often wonder whether survival might have been possible had a rescuer arrived sooner. Some, who feel they might have helped their burned relative, blame themselves. Learning from a neutral third party that death was inevitable often helps family members better accept their loved one's death.

However, heat or flames don't usually cause deaths in burning buildings. Smoke inhalation, not the fire itself, kills most people. Lots of burned materials produce carbon monoxide (CO). It's a by-product of incomplete combustion. Smoke is filled with carbon monoxide.

---

* Whenever the body swells a lot, when many muscle fibres burn, or if heat destroys too much blood, death follows in days. Products of the decomposing burned tissue clog up the kidneys' filtration system. If the burn becomes infected, death may be rapid. Otherwise the kidneys gradually shut down for days or months before the renal failure causes death.

When inhaled CO attaches itself to the blood protein called haemoglobin, a problem arises. Haemoglobin usually transports oxygen around the body by attaching an oxygen molecule to itself. Unfortunately, haemoglobin prefers attaching to a carbon monoxide molecule rather than an oxygen molecule. The resulting compound, called carboxyhaemoglobin, does not release oxygen to tissues.

Carbon monoxide, a gas lighter than air, develops when burning materials smoulder. When a basement furnace catches fire, lots of carbon monoxide rises to the top of the house. People usually sleep upstairs. Sleeping people, particularly children, are often discovered lying dead in their beds due to inhaling carbon monoxide from a fire in the basement. The fire is often extinguished before flames reach the upstairs rooms, but by then it is already too late for children to survive.

While it is little comfort to survivors, their relative's death from inhaling carbon monoxide was painless. A sleeping person poisoned by CO simply never wakens. In cases where a person wakes, breathing in CO is not distressing, but hot soot particles in smoke might burn the throat. When people are awake and exposed to carbon monoxide, their symptoms depend on how much CO has attached to their haemoglobin to create carboxyhaemoglobin.

Carboxyhaemoglobin levels correlate with the type of symptom experienced (see Table 14.1). People are unaffected by small amounts of carbon monoxide.

CO BLOOD LEVEL	SYMPTOMS
< 10%	none (level in smokers' blood)
20%	mild headache, difficulty catching one's breath
30%–40%	throbbing headaches; difficulty in focusing, reading a book, or solving any form of puzzle
40%–50%	all initiative lost; movements slow; confusion and severe disorientation
> 50%	death can occur; brain receives so little oxygen that it stops functioning properly; seizures may follow
70%	loss of consciousness; death ensues

Table 14.1: Symptoms associated with levels of CO in the blood.

These are the relationships that are traditionally used, but some authors believe the correlations between CO levels and symptoms are pretty weak.[8] Carbon monoxide is only one product of combustion. Any smoke has hundreds of chemicals in it. Cigarette tobacco, perhaps the world's most studied combustible material, is known to produce over 7,000 different chemicals when set aflame.[9] Some 50 of these compounds can cause cancer. That means cigarettes kill in two different time frames. A burning cigarette tip causes instant death when it ignites a fatal house fire. A slower, later death occurs when years of cigarette smoking trigger a fatal heart attack or malignant cancer.

Two factors must be considered to answer a question about how much discomfort a person feels when burned in a fire. One is pain. The other is time. Exposure to the 600° C heat created by a wall of flame causes momentary searing pain when the skin's nerve endings notify the brain of their destruction. That pain is instantaneous and immediately forgotten.

Heat destroys nerve endings so speedily that pain cannot last. Fire consumes all the air's oxygen somewhat less quickly, but inhaled air steadily contains increasing amounts of carbon monoxide and smaller amounts of oxygen. It only takes a minute before high carboxyhaemoglobin levels in the blood make people comatose. Death follows a few minutes later. Though the body may end up being horribly charred, any pain felt while dying was likely to have been of very short duration. That information offers some consolation to grieving families.

When a person is enveloped by smoke in a burning building but is some distance from the flames, the situation differs. The air initially contains enough oxygen to allow a person to stay alert, but they are probably coughing a lot while trying to find a way out. In coroner's cases, no escape route was ever found. A coroner cannot ever know how long consciousness lasted before the person collapsed. When talking to the family, don't lie, but suggest the time might have been quite short.

Scalding

The percentage of the body that must be scalded to cause death is identical to that required for burns arising from flames or dry heat of any sort. Note that the term *scalding* is used for deaths caused by wet heat, whereas thermal deaths are dry. Coroners usually investigate scalding deaths of children, or elderly people who cannot get out of the bathtub when the water becomes too hot. If a person's skin is exposed to a liquid with a boiling point higher than water, such as cooking oil, greater heat than that produced by water can be applied to the skin. Burns can be potentially more severe, and death may happen faster.

Full thickness burns are the key to all burn deaths, scalding included. Table 14.2 summarizes what happens in bathtubs. The speed with which the burn develops depends on the temperature of the water surrounding the body.[10]

WATER TEMPERATURE	TIME TO FULL THICKNESS BURN
65° C (149° F)	2 seconds
60° C (140° F)	5 seconds
55° C (131° F)	25 seconds

Table 14.2: Time taken for full thickness scalding to develop

Water temperature rarely stays constant. Should a first responder be able to measure it on arrival and find temperatures in the range of 55° C to 65° C, these times could be used to estimate how long the person might have experienced pain before a full thickness burn developed, ending all discomfort. Water temperature is rarely known, though. Often the bathtub is drained before the coroner or any other first responder arrives.

When a scald arises from something other than immersion in a tub of liquid, the whole body is not usually affected. In these cases, just the side of the body exposed to the boiling liquid is scalded. These victims are usually taken to hospital for treatment. If the scalding material (say liquid creosote) has attached itself to the skin, this will have to be removed as part of the burn management.

Coroners only investigate failed treatments. The families of hospitalized scalded patients tend to understand the degree of suffering their relative experienced in hospital. They don't usually ask coroners any questions about dying because their questions were answered previously by treating physicians.

Most people have felt the initial pain of a relatively minor scald. When the area scalded is large enough to be fatal, multiply the pain of a scalded finger a hundredfold. The only saving grace in severe scalding cases is that the duration of pain might be quite short. That is one comforting thought relatives might like to hang on to.

Electrocution

Long before electricity was harnessed by humans, bolts of lightning struck people outside in the open during thunderstorms. Many died, and people still do today, though less frequently than in the past. Only about ten people a year die of lightning strikes in Canada, a country of 37 million.[11] In Zimbabwe, with a similar population, 150 are likely to die before the rainy season ends each year.[12]

The reason for Zimbabwe's higher number is its weather. Subtropical weather allows Zimbabweans to live outdoors comfortably much more of the year than can Canadians. The fatality rate from a lightning strike varies between 10% to 30%.[13] A lightning bolt knocks a person instantly unconscious and delivers a painless death.

Nowadays, electronic materials or devices — everything from high-tension wires to cellphone chargers — are more lethal than lightning. Everyone is exposed to alternating current throughout the house. Amperage measures current flowing through an electrical wire. A flow of 10 milliamperes of electricity into a person's body is much less than the normal household current. Still, it's enough to cause muscle spasm of such force that a person weighing 70 kg (154 lb) cannot relax the tensed muscle. Electricians call it the "let go threshold." That amperage forms the basis for many preventive measures in the electrical industry.[14] Heavier people can tolerate a bit more current before irreducible muscle spasms occur than can those who weigh less.

Household electricity in North America is provided at 60 Hz (50 Hz in Europe). Voltage measures the force that drives electricity. The amount of voltage necessary to electrocute someone varies with skin resistance, meaning opposition to the flow of electricity. Skin resistance varies from person to person and by time of day. The skin's biggest variable when transmitting electricity is whether the skin is moist. Wet skin is 100 times less resistant to electricity than dry skin.

An analysis of an electrical current fatality considers four factors. Amperage is one — the higher the current, the more lethal the shock delivered. How long the current continues to flow is important too — the longer the duration, the greater the risk of death. The third factor is the electrical force. The higher the voltage, the more skin breaks down. Skin damage lowers its resistance, so the increased current flow is more likely to be fatal. Skin breakdown starts to happen with more than 500 volts.[15]

Finally, the pathway of the current matters. Electrical current that flows through the heart muscle is likely to be lethal, which is what usually happens in electrocutions. An electrical current that passes between the arms or between an arm and a foot tends to follow a pathway through the heart. The electrical shock converts the normal sinus rhythm of the heart muscle into ventricular fibrillation. Death follows within five minutes.

Electrocution is a hazard in many workplaces, and these are the electrocution deaths that a coroner is most likely to investigate. People who work with electricity are well aware of the ever-present risk of death, but nevertheless accidental electrocution deaths occur every year, killing 166 workers in the United States in 2019.[16] Defective household devices or their improper use can be lethal too. The method with which they cause a fatality is the same as any other electrocution. These deaths are uncommon but do happen when an electrical device used in a bathtub falls into the water. People are still electrocuted using the electric chair in the United States. How that device kills is discussed in Chapter 22.

Thermal burns may also occur when a worker is exposed to an arc flash while working with electricity. Dying this way is similar to dying from a thermal burn or a scald. Arc flash burns have been quoted as killing one or two people per day in the United States, but this number is disputed by industrial associations. The correct figure should become clear in the next few years.

Radiation

Radiation may be ionizing or non-ionizing. X-rays and the gamma rays from nuclear explosions are examples of fatal ionizing radiation. Non-ionizing radiation found in microwaves, radar and cellphones causes virtually no deaths. Most of the ionizing radiation deaths that occurred to this day probably resulted from the two atomic bombs dropped on Hiroshima and Nagasaki in the Second World War.

Since then nuclear reactor incidents, like the one at Chernobyl, state-sponsored assassinations (as occurred with Alexander Litvinenko), and deaths following exposure to radioactive waste are more modern examples of ionizing radiation deaths. Only if nuclear war breaks out, or a nearby nuclear reactor melts down, will future ionizing radiation deaths be likely. Most coroners will probably never investigate one.

An unstable atomic nucleus emits three types of rays — alpha, beta and gamma. Gamma rays are the best at penetrating the body and are often fatal. Exposure to gamma rays only kills when the dose is high enough though. The SI units now used to measure radiation dosage are called Grays (Gy), and the likelihood of death can be measured using those units.

Death can occur once a person's entire body (whole body) has been exposed to as little as even 1 Gy or 2 Gy. When the exposure increases to more than 30 Gy, death will likely occur within 48 hours. Unfortunately, most radiation deaths don't happen as quickly as that. More often death from a radioactive substance resembles that experienced by Mr. Litvinenko. The television images of him slowly dying make a good mental guide for a coroner who becomes involved in any conversation about radiation deaths.

When the whole body is exposed to 1 Gy, the number of white blood cells decreases and the likelihood of a fatal infection increases. Initial symptoms are just fatigue and weakness. Up to half of the people with this level of exposure become nauseated. Most also develop a slight headache. For a while these people can carry on normally, most of them for a long time. However, up to 5% die within six to eight weeks.

At a higher exposure of 6 Gy to 8 Gy, nausea is accompanied by diarrhoea, a worse headache, fever, mental fuzziness, dizziness and finally disorientation. Those exposed lose all their body hair, bruise easily and can bleed from any part of their bodies. Frequently their deaths arise from a fatal infection, often in the lungs or kidneys. These people can also bleed to death from the gut, lungs or even their kidneys. Regardless of how they die, and even with the best medical care, 50% to 100% of people exposed to 6 Gy to 8 Gy die within two to four weeks.

With an even higher exposure of somewhere between 8 Gy to 30 Gy, the same symptoms occur but incapacity and then loss of consciousness are more rapid. Dying lasts anywhere from two days to two weeks following exposure. Exposures over 30 Gy trigger seizures and tremors followed by death in two days or less.[17]

When exposure to ionizing radiation is not immediately lethal, the resulting cellular damage it causes may eventually lead to death. Leukaemia was the cancer first associated with exposure to radiation. Now, many other malignant tumours are also known to develop ten years or more post–radiation exposure. People die from these ionizing radiation–caused cancers in the same way as from identical cancers with different origins. The cause of any cancer is irrelevant to how it causes death.

Non-ionizing radiation is found in ordinary kitchen microwave ovens. Its wavelength spectrum overlaps with the spectrum that is detected by military radar. Most oven users know microwaves heat from the inside out. Cellular injury or death occurs whenever body tissue temperature exposed to this radiation is maintained more than five degrees above normal.[18] The higher the temperature the quicker the death. It is unfortunately not an urban legend that infants have been killed in microwave ovens, but thankfully these deaths happen rarely.[19]

Radar waves are generally considered harmless. However, there has been a case where a man near a tower emitting radar waves had his intestines heated to such a point that he needed hospital admission. The intestines became gangrenous, so surgery was undertaken to cut out all the gangrenous bowel. It was unsuccessful, and the man died post-operatively. This sort of death is very rare, but when it occurs a coroner needs to investigate it.

Chemical Burns

While heat is the most common cause of the fatal burns that coroners deal with, other substances do the same thing. Chemicals are one such substance. Simple acids, alkali materials such as lime (alkalis are the opposite of acids), mustard gas in warfare, phosphorus, and other chemicals such as phenols and creosols all produce fatal burns. All these compounds' lethal effects result from their acidic or alkaline qualities. Murderers have used both acids and alkalis to completely dissolve the bodies of their victims.

Chemical burns cause death differently depending on the route by which acid or alkali enters the body. In most coroner's cases acids or alkalis are swallowed, but in accidents where a truck or train overturns chemicals may spill onto people's skins. Fortunately, in developed countries, cases of both such swallowing or spillage are quite unusual. The average North American or European coroner is unlikely to ever investigate either sort of death.

Dying from a chemical burn is initially very uncomfortable. Pain continues until the lethal compound burns through enough tissue to destroy all the nerve endings of whatever body parts it touches. Time until death varies. In an unlucky case, severe pain might continue for hours, days or even weeks.

Ingested alkali or acid is extremely uncomfortable. Both cause a pain that resembles the sensation produced by ingesting very hot food, but ingested chemicals hurt much more than food of any sort. Only when all nerve endings along the digestive tract touched by the chemical die does the pain cease. Death may take hours, so dying is very painful in these cases. Any similar chemical introduced in the body through the anus would cause an equally uncomfortable death.

Death from inhaling these chemicals is more rapid. Lungs fill with fluid, making breathing very difficult. After a minute or so the person loses consciousness. A person covered with a chemical that cannot be quickly removed may only experience pain a short time before all the skin's nerve endings are destroyed. That is the only good thing a coroner can say about the injury. The period of dying that follows may involve a lengthy hospitalization, repeated infections and an eventual protracted organ shutdown that causes death.

Cremation

There is one other form of body burn that comes after death that only peripherally involves the coroner, but people frequently ask coroners about it. However, cremation is a subject more properly in the realm of an undertaker. Most coroners know very little about cremation and try to avoid talking about it. Still, they sometimes have to say something before more detailed questions can be properly answered at a future meeting with a funeral director. All a coroner should do is try to prevent any misunderstanding about what actually happens when a body is cremated.

Most relatives do not know that almost all the body's tissues, other than bone, vaporize when cremated. Crematoria's retorts (sources of heat in the furnace) raise the temperature to around 900° C (1652° F).[20] At this high temperature almost all tissue, other than bone, turns into gas. Occasionally faint traces of powder remain after the retort is cooled down. That powder cannot be called *ashes.* The so-called ashes of a cremated body that funeral directors place in an urn for relatives are actually burned bone fragments.

Most jurisdictions have rules about where these ashes may be scattered. Many cemeteries or crematoria contain legally designated sites for a scattering ritual to take place. But many relatives do not want to use these sites for scattering their ashes. A cottage, lake or place with a significant view or other meaning to the deceased is often their preferred location. Funeral directors are well aware relatives often scatter ashes at unauthorized sites, though such actions are not sanctioned by any law.

Funeral directors won't report a potentially improper scattering of ashes to the police. As a rule, police don't charge any relative for this act either. Both police and funeral directors consider the improper scattering of ashes at most no worse than jaywalking. It's technically illegal, everybody does it, and most of the time no harm comes of it. Only if a problem arose would an illegal ash scattering even be noted.

A newer, less fiery variation in cremation requires no heat at all to dispose of a body. This "green cremation" involves a chemical process called alkaline hydrolysis. The solution into which the body is immersed totally dissolves everything — including bones. Some people consider a green cremation more environmentally friendly than incineration.

Right now, green cremations are not available everywhere. At some future time, hydrolysis may become more popular than incineration as a method of disposing of cadavers. However, there is some municipal opposition to green cremations when their effluent flows out of a cremation tank into municipal sewers. Until that opposition is overcome, incineration will likely continue to be the cremation method of choice. Defer questions about any form of cremation to funeral directors whenever possible.

NOTES

1 *The Holy Bible,* Authorized King James Version.

2 American Burn Association. (2016). *Burn incidence fact sheet. https://ameriburn.org/who-we-are/media/burn-incidence-fact-sheet/*

3 World Health Organization (WHO). (20018, March 6). *Burn fact sheet.* https://www.who.int/news-room/fact-sheets/detail/burns

4 City and County of San Francisco Fire Department. (n.d.) *Home fire facts. https://sf-fire.org/home-fire-facts*

5 Graf, S. H. (1949). *Ignition temperatures of various papers, woods, and fabrics* (Bulletin No. 26). Oregon State University. https://ir.library.oregonstate.edu/catalog?utf8=%E2%9C%93&search_field=all_fields&q=Ignition+temperatures+of+various+papers

6 Osler, T., Glance, L. G., & Hosmer, D. W. (2010). Simplified estimates of the probability of death after burn injuries: Extending and updating the Baux score. *Journal of Trauma and Acute Care Surgery 68*(3), 690–697.

7 See note 2 above.

8 Smollin, C., & Olson, K. (2010, October 12). Carbon monoxide poisoning (acute). *British Medical Journal of Clinical Evidence.* Article 2010: 2103. https://www.ncbi.nlm.nih.gov/pmc/articles/PMC3217756/

9 Rodgman, A., & Perfetti, T. A. (2009). *The chemical components of tobacco and tobacco smoke.* Boca Raton, FL: CRC Press.

10 Armstrong, P. L. (1978, September 15). *Technical bulletin 34: Burn rate. Available at https://www.statewaterheaters.com/lit/bulletin/bulletin34.pdf*

11 Government of Canada. (2021, January 14). *Lightning fatality and injury statistics in Canada.* https://www.canada.ca/en/environment-climate-change/services/lightning/safety/fatalities-injury-statistics.html

12 Holle, R. L. (2008, April). *Annual rates of lightning fatalities by country.* Paper presented at the 20th International Lightning Detection Conference, Tuscon, AZ. https://www.researchgate.net/publication/267855823_Annual_rates_of_lightning_fatalities_by_country

13 Elsom, D. M. & Webb, J. D. C. (2017). Lightning deaths in the UK: A 30-year analysis of the factors contributing to people being struck and killed. *International Journal of Meteorology, 42(401), 8–26.*

14 Cadick, J., Capelli-Schellpfeffer, M., & Neitzel, D. (2005) *Electrical handbook* (3rd ed.).McGraw-Hill.

15 Fish, R. M., Geddes, L. A. (2009). Conduction of electrical current to and through the human body: A review. *Eplasty 9,* e44

16 Electrical Safety Foundation International. (n.d.). Workplace injury & fatality statistics. https://www.esfi.org/workplace-injury-and-fatality-statistics

17 Bushberg, J. T. (October 2020). Radiation exposure and contamination. Merck Manual Professional Version. https://www.merckmanuals.com/en-ca/professional/injuries-poisoning/radiation-exposure-and-contamination/radiation-exposure-and-contamination

18 McLaughlin, J. T. (1957). Tissue destruction and death from microwave radiation (Radar). California Medicine 86(5), 336–339.

19 Sumter, A. N. (2019, May 15). China Arnold: The mother who killed her 3-week-old baby, Paris Talley, by cooking her in a microwave. *The Criminal Journal.* https://www.thecriminaljournal.com/murder-of-paris-talley-by-china-arnold-mother-killed-her-3-week-old-baby-girl-by-cooking-her-in-microwave/

20 "How is a body cremated?" (2019). *Cremation Resource: A Guide.* https://www.cremationresource.org/cremation/how-is-a-body-cremated.html

15

Traumatic Deaths

Severe, traumatic injuries are frequently lethal, even with the most advanced medical therapy. Many prove fatal long before help of any sort can possibly arrive. How one dies depends on which parts of the body are injured. A single organ injury can be fatal, but often simultaneous injury to multiple parts of the body causes death. Lethal injuries to several organs make it difficult to describe dying precisely — two or more body functions stop working at the same time. A large enough force striking anywhere in the body has the potential to cause death. The head is particularly vulnerable.

One type of traumatic death coroners frequently investigate is a fall from a height. Details of how one dies when falling are provided in the jumping section of Chapter 20. Falls and motor vehicle accidents represent the majority of trauma investigations an average coroner will ever undertake; these are discussed later in this chapter.

Head Injuries

While it is often the case that the skull fractures in cases of fatal head injuries, it is a brain injury beneath the bone that is lethal. In a couple of circumstances, the mechanism of death does involve parts of a broken skull. One is a depressed skull fracture, which occurs when something blunt delivers a forceful blow to a small area of the skull and presses bits of broken bone into the brain. (See Figure 15.1.)

The other circumstance in which death does involve parts of a broken skull is a fall from a height when the person lands feet first. Once the soles of the feet strike the ground, the force of their impact on the ground is transmitted up the spine to the base of the skull. The skull fractures in a circular ring around the foramen magnum. (See Figure 15.2.) Death results from that circular ring of skull bone and the cervical spines below ramming upwards into the brain.

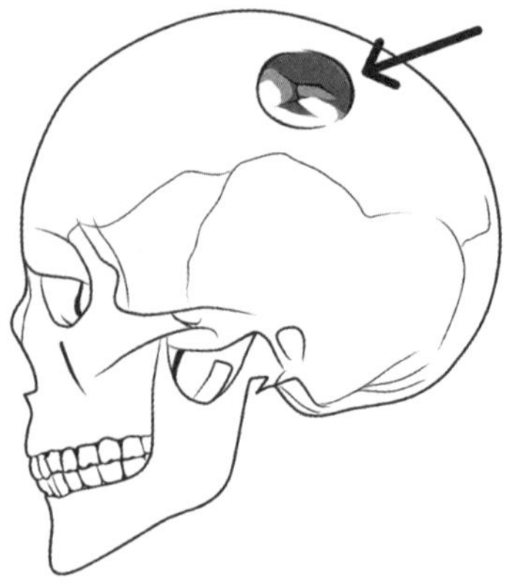

Figure 15.1: A forceful blow from a blunt object can cause bits of bone to penetrate the brain.

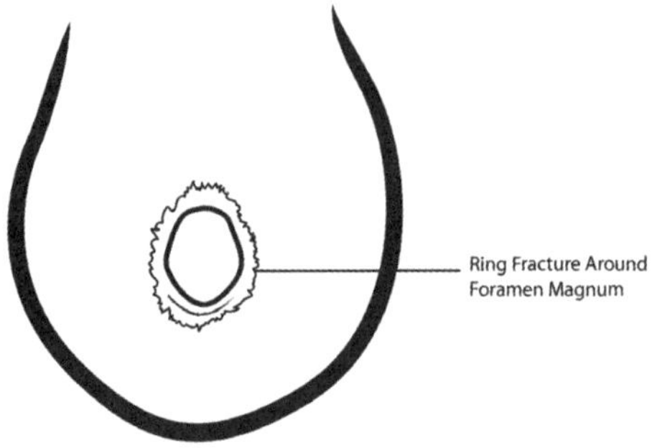

Figure 15.2: A ring fracture occurs in the spine at the base of the skull.

When talking to relatives about any type of fatal brain injury, remember that the brain is covered by three linings or maters called *meninges*, as shown in Figure 15.3. The dura, or outer lining, is attached to the undersurface of the skull. The inner lining, or pia, is attached to the brain. The arachnoid mater, or middle lining, is separated from the other two meninges by fluid. Between the arachnoid and pia mater is the subarachnoid space, which is full of clear cerebrospinal fluid. The subdural space between the arachnoid and dura mater is filled with veins.

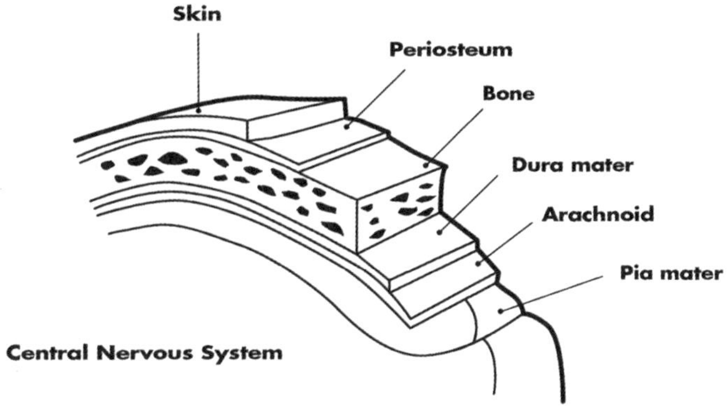

Figure 15.3: The meninges lining around the brain is made up of the pia mater, the arachnoid, and the dura mater.

A head injury with no wound penetrating the dura mater (on the underside of the skull) is called a closed head injury. Once a wound penetrates through the dura for any distance at all the injury becomes open. Brain tissue that bulges out through a hole in the scalp and skull is called an extrusion. A coroner can tell relatives that once the brain extrudes death is almost certain. Skull fractures are discussed in more detail in Chapter 1.

The type of bleeding within the skull is another way to describe fatal head injuries. To make it simple, discuss only the four major types that are shown in Figure 15.4:

1. Bleeding between the dura mater and the skull is an epidural haemorrhage. Fatalities from this type of haemorrhage are uncommon, unlike the other three.
2. Bleeding in the subdural space between the dura and arachnoid mater is called a subdural haemorrhage.
3. Bleeding in the subarachnoid space between the arachnoid mater and the pia mater covering the brain itself is called a subarachnoid haemorrhage.
4. Bleeding within the brain itself is described as an intracerebral haemorrhage.

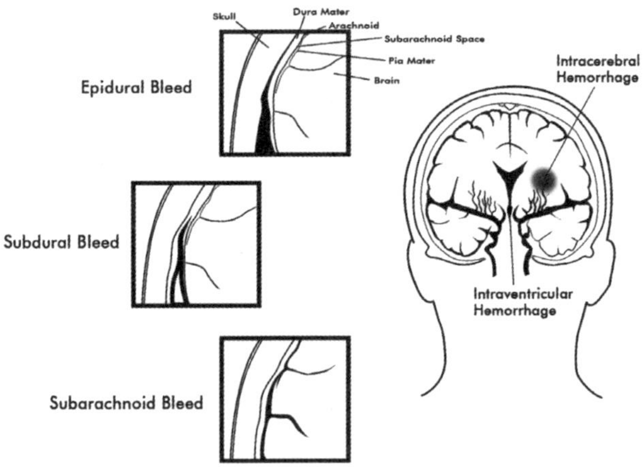

Figure 15.4: The four major types of fatal head injury.

Any blow to the head can cause a concussion, but fatal blows injure tissue. Most lethal blows to the head rupture either veins or arteries in the skull. Others lacerate the brain and drive bone fragments, dirt and germs into the brain. Prior to loss of consciousness, the symptoms of fatal head injury vary. Everyone should experience, at least momentarily, a headache, nausea, confusion, loss of balance and trouble tolerating bright lights.

The duration and severity of these sensations varies while conscious, but they disappear once comatose, never to return. Death follows anywhere from minutes to months later. Without observing the period before loss of consciousness, it is impossible to form a useful opinion on what the person felt or how long any head injury sensation might have lasted. The correct reply when asked about what was felt before death is the honest admission that you don't know, and no other coroner nor anybody else ever will. Add that death might have come rapidly. That observation is likely to be more right than wrong and might provide the questioner some comfort.

Ruptured blood vessels within the skull bleed steadily. As the volume of blood inside the skull increases, a headache worsens. Pain only disappears once the person is unconscious. This is the usual pattern in fatal subdural haemorrhages. In epidural bleeds a period of feeling better may follow the initial headache before it starts to worsen again. Subarachnoid bleeds can prove fatal within minutes or lead to a protracted course of dying.

Relatives present at the time of the haemorrhage witnessed the pain of dying. They don't ask questions. Questions come only from relatives who weren't there. The coroner can reasonably suggest a headache and nausea prior to loss of consciousness were likely. Also mention that the duration may have been brief. Dying from these bleeds is fully discussed in Chapter 1.

Traumatic Asphyxia

Injury to the chest is a second common type of fatal trauma. Whenever something blocks the ability of a chest to expand enough to breathe in air the result is traumatic asphyxia. This manner of dying arises in many different scenarios. A common one occurs when a heavy object, such as a piece of masonry, a large tree, or a steel girder, falls across or simply presses so heavily on someone's chest that they can't breathe.

Workers in trenches suddenly covered with falling earth when a wall caves in, people caught in landslides and farmers buried by grain in their silos die the same way. The mechanism of death is identical when a vehicle or heavy object pins a person against the wall, or a tractor topples on top of a farmer. In not all fatal tractor accidents does the farmer die from traumatic asphyxia, however.

Note that a tractor may pin a farmer's body to the ground without causing asphyxia. The farmer will be able to breathe but unable to move or stanch bleeding from any unreachable lacerations. That means a slow death from exsanguination. In one famous Canadian case in 1948, while pinned to the ground the dying farmer lived long enough to scratch with his pocket knife on his tractor's bumper "In case I die in this mess I leave all to the wife. Cecil Geo. Harris." This bumper was successfully probated in court as his last will and testament and is now on permanent display at the University of Saskatchewan law school.

Traumatic asphyxia is not always brought on by objects. Throngs of people cause it too. The same sort of chest compression has occurred when rowdy crowds at British, European or African football games trampled over or fell on top of people on the ground.[1] Aggressive crowds at rock concerts have crushed concert goers, knocked people over, trampled on them and suffocated them too.[2] Traumatic asphyxia has killed hundreds of Islamic pilgrims when crushed on their Hajj in

Mecca.[3] Any human stampede can cause fatal traumatic asphyxia by trampling on the fallen or simply squashing people together so tightly that they can no longer breathe.

All individuals who die from traumatic asphyxia do so in a similar way. Some males, usually drunk and obese, have been known to suffocate female partners by lying on them for a protracted period during and after sexual intercourse. The women were able to breathe initially, but the continued pressure of the men's heavy bodies against the women's chests tired them out. Once they no longer had the energy to draw breaths the women suffocated.

Two or more people are not needed to cause deaths by traumatic asphyxia. People do it to themselves. In recent years individuals have suffocated themselves by diving into used clothing donation boxes.[4] Their necks or chests become trapped by the clothing chute, preventing inhalation. These people become unconscious before they can withdraw themselves from the boxes.

Pathologists now call this latter type of traumatic asphyxia postural or positional asphyxia. They also use those terms to categorize the deaths of elderly people who fall out of their beds and wedge themselves between the side of the bed and the wall. Positional asphyxia is also the cause of death of thieves who die wedged in windows in an unsuccessful attempt to enter or exit a house. Sheet metal workers who trap themselves in ventilation ducts they are trying to install or repair sometimes suffer the same fate.

Motor Vehicles

Since the start of the twentieth century, the ever-increasing number of cars and motorcycles have caused vehicular deaths to rise year after year. Automobile drivers, front seat passengers and rear seat passengers die in different ways. Motorcyclists die from still differently applied forces. Both automobile drivers and motorcyclists also strike and kill pedestrians.

Most motor vehicle collisions are accidents, but not all. Occasional deaths result from suicides or even homicides, and these are often tricky for police and coroners to determine. A driver with his wife in the front passenger seat has been known to crash the passenger side of car, kill his unwanted spouse and collect insurance proceeds on her death. It is equally horrific when some drivers deliberately and maliciously strike pedestrians with their cars, killing them.

The introduction of first seat belts and then air bags in the last half of the twentieth century decreased the numbers who die inside the car in automobile collisions. Motorcycle deaths continue at the same pace as ever. In some places, they may actually be increasing.

American motorcycle deaths since 1975 have varied in number from just over 2,000 to just over 5,000 per year.[5] However, in the decade from 2010 to 2020, the numbers have generally been at the higher end of that range. These deaths also now involve more people over the age of 30. Accidental automobile deaths are primarily caused by distracted driving nowadays. Drivers usually have their seat belts on. As an example, in 2018 Newfoundland police reported that in the previous five years only about 35% of deaths in that province involved unbelted drivers.[6]

The mechanisms of motor vehicle accidents have been well researched. Police and pathologists both know what usually happens to a driver in a frontal collision, which is the most common cause of fatal automobile accidents. Death results from the rapid deceleration that occurs when the vehicle suddenly stops. The body of an unbuckled driver slides forward on the seat. That movement drives the legs against the lower part of the dashboard. At virtually the same time, the driver's abdomen and lower chest slam against the steering wheel. The driver's upper body then bends over the steering wheel and rises up off the seat. The driver's head bends forward and hits the windscreen. Injuries also arise when bits of the automobile break off and strike different parts of the body.[7]

Fatal traffic accidents can break bones in the driver's legs virtually anywhere. The liver usually ruptures, and the spleen, kidneys and intestines are often severely damaged too. Skull fractures cause fatal bleeding within. Fractured cervical spines may fatally damage the spinal cord. Commonly the aorta is lacerated, producing such massive haemorrhage that death follows in short order.

Cases like this make it hard for a pathologist or a coroner to ascribe death to any one fatal injury. When the only significant damage is to the head, it is possible to ascribe death to that injury alone. The same can be done with a torn aorta. Quite often neither situation is the case though. Several injuries will be discovered at autopsy, each potentially fatal, making it impossible to solely attribute dying to any one of them. In those cases death is then said to arise from "multiple injuries."

Frontal collisions may be the most common, but they are not the only type of fatal automobile accident. Collisions with both the side and the rear of the car also produce fatalities. So do rollovers. Death is especially likely once a person flies out of the vehicle. When, shortly after the accident, the driver is discovered dead in the front seat or outside on the ground after being ejected from the vehicle, it is safe to assume an immediate loss of consciousness and death shortly thereafter.

Seat belts help avoid, but cannot always prevent, motor vehicle accident deaths. In 2011 in the United Kingdom, 95% of people seated in the front of the car and 89% of those in the back used seat belts or child restraints. There were still 816 car occupant fatalities — 552 were drivers and 264 were passengers. The chance of survival of people sitting in the front seats but not wearing seat belts would have improved 45% had they buckled up.[8]

In automobile accidents drivers, front seat passengers and those sitting in the rear experience similar fatal injuries. The probabilities of death vary though. In the developed world many more drivers than front seat passengers die in car accidents, largely because one third of their fatal vehicle collisions have only the driver in the car. Usually, rear seat deaths occur when those passengers are unbelted, and are the result of multiple injuries. In developing countries many more passengers die than drivers because their vehicles are frequently overcrowded.[9]

Ejection from an automobile makes death more probable. Drivers are eight times more likely to die when ejected from the car during a rollover than if they remain seated when the vehicle comes to a stop. The front passenger is seven times more likely to die in the same scenario.

Air bags create a barrier between the driver's or front seat passenger's body and the steering wheel or dashboard. These bags work quite well and usually prevent serious harm. Injuries from bags deploying are rare, but both adults and children have been killed when bags inflate. Children usually die from head or neck injuries. In one scenario, their skulls fracture and fatal bleeding within the skull develops. In the other scenario, cervical spines break and lacerate their spinal cords, often at the base of the skull. Loss of consciousness is instant, and death occurs not long afterwards. Adults can die the same way. Yet the first adult to die from a Takata air bag deploying bled to death when flying pieces of metal lacerated a carotid artery in her neck.[10] The U.S. National Transportation Safety Agency calculates that 284 deaths occurred from air bags deploying from 1990 to 2007. Most were in earlier model cars.[11]

Motorcycles

In the United States motorcyclists are 29 times more likely to be killed in a motor vehicle accident than automobile passengers.[12] In 2012 in the United States about 15% of motor vehicle accidents involved motorcyclists.[13] Unless the rider is impaled (a rare event), a motorcyclist's head eventually strikes the ground, another vehicle, or something else in the process of the motorcycle falling flat. Unsurprisingly, most motorcyclist deaths are due to head injuries.

In most countries (if not every country) in the world, all motorcyclists are required to wear helmets to forestall this event. While helmets are usually worn at the time of fatal motorcycle accidents, only 37% of the time will headgear prevent death when a head strikes a solid object forcefully at high speed.[14] Sometimes chinstraps unbuckle and helmets fly off the head at the time of the collision, meaning the head loses any protection the helmet could have provided at the critical moment.

Many other injuries occur when the motorcyclist collides with the surface of the road. Both arms and legs are often fractured. Those injuries alone may not be fatal. One accident that causes immediate death happens when a motorcyclist who is following a truck too closely rides under its tailgate. The collision results in lethal head or neck injuries. Sometimes the motorcyclist is decapitated.

Bicycles

People riding bicycles collide with automobiles quite often too. Many times, the collision is fatal for the cyclist. Contact with a car is not always necessary for a cyclist to die accidentally though. In 16% of bicycle fatalities the rider simply loses control of his bike.

The United Kingdom experience probably provides a typical picture for any developed country. The Royal Society for the Prevention of Accidents reported a total of 102 cyclist deaths in 2016/2017. Further,

- 15% were children under the age of 15 years
- 80% were male
- roughly 65% were killed near intersections, most commonly near a T-junction
- roundabouts (traffic circles) were also sites of many bicycle fatalities
- more deaths happened where the speed limit was high
- 80% took place in daylight
- 75% died of head injuries.[15]

Pedestrians

Around the world, many pedestrians die when walking on the road. Low- and middle-income countries have a much higher ratio of pedestrian/motor vehicle occupant deaths than does the developed world. Worldwide, pedestrians and cyclists account for 26%[16] of all traffic deaths. Injuries to people on foot vary depending on the type and size of car or truck that hits them.

When an automobile with a low bumper strikes a man head on, the bumper knocks his legs out from under him. One of two things follow. A vehicle with a hood that is low and sloped lifts (scoops) the pedestrian up onto the hood. The man's head strikes the front windscreen, and his body them moves in one of two directions. The man may fall off to the side of the vehicle, or his body may flip over the roof, slide down the back window, slide over the trunk (boot), and often the person lands on his head. Alternatively, the person struck is flung sideways. Death comes from the body's impact on the road's hard surface or when it is run over by another vehicle.

With a higher bumper strike, a pedestrian's body will either be thrown forward and up into the air or knocked down to the ground. A pedestrian's body that lands on the road directly in front of a vehicle while it is still moving may be caught on its undercarriage or run over by its wheels.[17] In the case of large trucks, pedestrians hooked onto the undercarriage can be dragged for miles before the driver stops to investigate a knocking sound and finds a body underneath his vehicle.

Repeatedly banging the body against the ground fractures bones over and over again. It squashes organs and all body tissues to the point that the body compresses into a large ball. That makes identification difficult. In one case in which the author was involved, a truck drove 20 miles along a Toronto closed access highway before the driver realized he had struck a pedestrian. It apparently was very difficult to extricate the body from the semitrailer's undercarriage. Two police officers delivered the body in a green plastic garbage bag to me while I was working as a casualty officer in the nearest hospital emergency department. The body was pounded into a nearly perfect sphere.

In cases of such severe injuries, death occurs very rapidly. Unless the injury is confined to the head, or possibly a solitary lacerated aorta, there are too many injuries to attribute death to any one of them. In such a case, relatives clearly understand that the combined multiple injuries caused death.

Trains

Trains kill in two different ways. In the more common scenario, a train strikes an individual on a railway track or an automobile at a level crossing. These may be accidental deaths, but quite often they are suicides. In 2017, 888 people were killed walking or lying down on rails in the United States.[18] In 2018, the United Kingdom reported that 300 people die annually on British railway lines. 17 of them would be trespassers and all the rest suicides.[19]

Those killed by trains usually suffer multiple injuries when they are struck while standing. Their bodies may be torn apart by the train's impact, even when the engineer has slowed the train while attempting to stop. Body parts can be strewn along the tracks for many metres. Such a death is virtually instantaneous and likely painless. Sudden rending of the body into many parts makes appreciating pain impossible.

The body of a person lying down across train tracks is severed into parts. The wheels decapitate the head from the body when the person lies down beside the tracks with only the head between the rails. This type of death is just as instant and painless as a guillotine decapitation. When a train simply amputates body parts, such as limbs, death is painful while the person is still conscious. Severed nerves hurt and large vessels bleed copiously, causing a fairly rapid loss of consciousness and death minutes later.

A train that strikes a car stalled at a level crossing invariably kills its occupants. Fatal injuries received resemble those caused by automobile collisions. Deaths will likely be attributed to head injuries, lacerated aortas or multiple injuries. The coroner's major job in these cases is to try to determine whether these are accidental deaths or suicides. Families do not often inquire about the mechanism of death when a train collides with a car, but they do want to know whether the death is a suicide. Most coroners investigate at least one "suicide by train" if they work long enough.

The second type of railway death occurs when two trains collide, or when one derails and tips over. In both these cases, engineer and passengers may experience similar deaths to those found in motor vehicle crashes. The lack of seat belts in a train results in the engineer and passengers being tossed around within or ejected from the train. Their mobile bodies are likely to strike some part of a passenger car, engine or the ground with great force.

Many trains derail and collide every year around the world. Most of the time people are simply injured but not killed. Few coroners will ever investigate the death of a passenger resulting from a train derailment or collision. However, if called for one such death a coroner will probably need to investigate others. Severe train accidents commonly kill multiple passengers.

Aircraft

In 2018 there were 197 plane crashes around the world. Thirteen were commercial and caused 534 fatalities.[20] The rest were small planes, most of which killed only the pilot, who was the sole occupant of the plane. The largest number of deaths in a single crash in 2018 was 189. The last plane crash death I investigated involved a floatplane. The wind flipped the plane upside down at the time it hit the water, and the pilot drowned.

Three factors play a role in aircraft deaths. First is the magnitude of the forces experienced by passengers at the time of impact. Death is inevitable when the force of impact with the ground exceeds the tolerance of a human body. A plane diving and crashing from 36,000 feet makes survival impossible. Fortunately, most aircraft crashes involve much lesser forces than that, meaning that not every passenger necessarily dies.

The second factor that affects survival rates is the degree to which the plane's structure remains intact. When most of an aircraft is destroyed in a crash, its occupants may be killed by flying parts as the plane bursts apart; passengers may be ejected from the plane; they may collide with part of the plane while being ejected; or they may strike something outside its structure, thereby injuring themselves. Passengers and crew may burn to death when fire in the plane prevents their exit.

The third feature that plays a role in aeroplane deaths is the location of the crash. When occupants survive the plane crash but are injured, deaths are likely if the occupants are unable to reach hospital within the necessary period of time. Crash survivors may die from excessive bleeding, infected wounds, starvation, dehydration, drowning or simply exposure. A person injured in a plane crash near Toronto is much less likely to die than when the crash happens in the barren lands of the Northwest Territories, the Sahara Desert or the Pacific Ocean a thousand miles from Tuvalu.

In the same accident people die in different ways. One Colorado investigation[21] of 28 deaths when a commercial airliner crashed concluded that nine passengers died from asphyxia. One died from a penetrating cranial injury. The rest died from blunt trauma similar to the type of injuries seen in motor vehicle accidents. Most died from a fatal head injury, 36% of whom had associated spinal fractures. Others died primarily from chest injuries, though 27% of them also had spinal fractures.

One important feature of investigating the death of a pilot rests solely in the realm of the pathologist. Investigators must determine whether a pilot died of natural causes before the plane crashed, or whether the crash killed the pilot. This is determined by a pathologist who dissects the pilot's wrists looking for carpal bone fractures.

A pilot who is alive and trying to bring the plane out of a terminal dive usually holds firmly onto the joystick until impact with the ground. The force of the aircraft's collision with the ground or water is transmitted through the tightly clutched joystick to the pilot's wrists, causing one or more carpal bones to fracture. A pilot who loses consciousness before the crash lets go of the joystick, so at the time of the crash no carpal bones break. Discovery of carpal bone fractures in the wrist is considered definite evidence that a pilot was alive at the time the plane struck the ground or water.

Explosions

Explosions come in three types — mechanical, chemical and nuclear. Deaths from explosions occur quite often in wars, but coroners are almost never involved in investigating those fatalities. Most countries leave review of armed forces' explosion deaths to a military panel. Terrorists kill some civilians with explosive devices though, and coroners do investigate those deaths. More common sources of explosion deaths that coroners investigate are due to dynamiting accidents in mines or quarries, stored chemicals detonating in a factory, and boilers that break due to excess pressure build-up.

Death sometimes results simply from the impact of the blast's force on the body. Explosives are categorized as low order or high order. Coroners investigate low order explosives deaths when gunpowder, petroleum bombs or dynamite blow up. Nobody but the military uses high order explosives.

For civilians to die from a mechanical explosion, they need to be quite nearby for its force to be lethal. A terrorist whose bomb inadvertently explodes while deploying it will often die from the blast. Someone on the other side of the road might suffer only minor injuries.

Full force of the blast will cause bleeding along the gastrointestinal tract and in the lungs because both organs are full of air. Often the explosion victim's damaged lungs rapidly fill up with blood, causing suffocation. Air emboli resulting from the blast are another route to sudden death. Sometimes the force of the explosion ruptures some intestines. The injured person may survive the initial blast but die later from gastrointestinal bleeding or infection. In whatever manner they may happen, these deaths are primary effects of the explosion.

Many more explosion deaths result from the blast's secondary effects. When an explosive device shatters it produces projectiles, flying many times faster than a bullet, that can pierce vital organs. The explosion also turns loose objects or debris into missiles. These can kill immediately when striking the lungs or heart. Wounds created by piercing other parts of the body may lead to a later death from bleeding or sepsis. People in buildings are often fatally struck or crushed by falling bricks or beams when the force of the explosion causes part of a building to collapse. Most explosion deaths arise from these secondary blast injuries. The longer it takes to extricate an injured person from rubble caused by the explosion, the less likely is survival.

Chemical explosions are much less common than mechanical ones. All explosions create a blast of superheated air that can ignite inflammable material to cause fatal burns. Burning chemicals resulting from an explosion may produce hundreds or even thousands of poisonous gases or toxins. To read about the most common types of poisonous gas deaths, see Chapter 18 (on deaths due to poison) and Chapter 20 (suicides). Whatever the gas or toxin, death is quicker for people with respiratory impairment such as chronic obstructive lung disease. Coroners should investigate all these deaths, but few are ever required to.

Nuclear explosions are fortunately rare. If radioactive material is involved in any explosion, death may be instant, or a later death may result from delayed complications of exposure to a high level of radiation at the time of the blast. More information about this type of death can be found in Chapter 14 (on burns). A coroner is unlikely to ever be called upon to investigate such a death.

NOTES

1 Fisher, D. (1989, April 16). 93 killed in soccer game: Victims trampled at English Stadium: 200 reported hurt. *Los Angeles Times*. https://www.latimes.com/archives/la-xpm-1989-04-16-mn-2494-story.html

2 Bailey-Milado, R. (2019, December 4). The Who announce first Cincinnati concert since fatal stampede in 1979. *New York Post*. https://nypost.com/2019/12/04/the-who-announce-first-cincinnati-concert-since-fatal-fan-stampede-in-1979/

3 Robinson, J. & Tomlinson, S. (2015, September 24). Horror at the Hajj: At least 700 people are crushed to death and hundreds injured in stampede during Muslim pilgrimage in Mecca just two weeks after crane collapse killed 109. *The Daily Mail.* https://www.dailymail.co.uk/news/article-3247269/At-310-people-crushed-death-450-injured-stampede-Muslim-Hajj-pilgrimage-Saudi-Arabia.html

4 Beale, A., Chavez, N., & Rossmann, R. (2018, November 28). Body of Petaluma homeless woman found dead at donation box. *The Press Democrat.* https://www.pressdemocrat.com/article/news/body-of-petaluma-homeless-woman-found-dead-at-donation-box/

5 Insurance Institute for Highway Safety (IIHS). (March 2021). *Fatality facts 2019: Motorcycles and ATVS.* https://www.iihs.org/topics/fatality-statistics/detail/motorcycles-and-atvs

6 The Telegram. (2018, July 26). N. L. RCMP warns lack of seatbelt use causes death. *The Telegram.* https://www.thetelegram.com/news/local/nl-rcmp-warns-lack-of-seatbelt-use-causes-deaths-229059/

7 Saukko, P., & Knight, B. (2016). *Knight's forensic pathology* (4th ed.). Boca Raton, FL: CRC Press, 277–280.

8 Road Safety Observatory. (2018, January 12). *Seat belts.* https://www.roadsafetyobservatory.com/HowEffective/vehicles/seat-belts

9 Nantulya, V. M., & Reich, M. R. (2002). The neglected epidemic: Road traffic accidents in developing countries. *British Medical Journal 324*, 1139.

10 Brook, B. (2018, February 28). The face behind the airbag deaths that caused the world's biggest car recall. https://www.news.com.au/technology/motoring/motoring-news/the-face-behind-the-airbag-deaths-that-caused-the-worlds-biggest-car-recall/news-story/f7f556655e49b50d26de72b1ff22b1b4

11 National Center for Statistics & Analysis of the National Highway Traffic Safety Administration. (2007, July 1). Counts of frontal air bag related fatalities and seriously injured persons. https://crashstats.nhtsa.dot.gov/Api/Public/ViewPublication/AB0707

12 Dimovski, A. (2021, January 28). *35 alarming statistics on motorcycle accidents — 2020 overview.* https://carsurance.net/blog/motorcycle-accidents/

13 U.S. Department of Transportation, Federal Highway Administration. (2019, December 2). *Motorcycle.* https://highways.dot.gov/research/research-programs/safety/motorcycle

14 U.S. Department of Transportation, National Highway Traffic Safety Administration. (May 2018). *Traffic safety facts: Lives and costs saved by*

Motorcycle Helmets, 2016. https://crashstats.nhtsa.dot.gov/Api/Public/ViewPublication/812518

15 Royal Society for the Prevention of Accidents. (November 2020). *Road safety factsheet: cycling accidents. https://www.rospa.com/media/documents/road-safety/cycling-accidents-factsheet.pdf*

16 World Health Organization (WHO). (2018). Global status report on road safety 2018. https://issuu.com/globalncap/docs/who-status-report-eng

17 Saukko, P., & Knight, B. (2016). *Knight's forensic pathology* (4th ed.). Boca Raton, FL: CRC Press, 288–290.

18 McCausland, P. (2018, March 11). *Railroad trespassing fatalities in the U.S. reach a 10-year high.* NBC News. https://www.nbcnews.com/news/us-news/railroad-trespassing-fatalities-u-s-reach-10-year-high-n852881

19 Government of the U.K., Department of Transport. (n.d.). Transport statistics Great Britain: 2020. Available from https://www.gov.uk/government/statistics/transport-statistics-great-britain-2020

20 Young, A. (n.d.) *To70's civil aviation safety review 2018.* https://to70.com/to70s-civil-aviation-safety-review-2018/

21 Lillehei, K. O., & Robinson, M.N. (1994). A critical analysis of the fatal injuries resulting from the Continental flight 1713 airline disaster: Evidence in favor of improved passenger restraint systems. *Journal of Trauma 37*(5), 826–830.

16

Hospital Deaths

Since they first evolved, human beings usually became sick and died out of doors or inside their homes. The ancient Greeks developed healing temples, and Romans had some military hospitals, but civilian hospitals in the Western world began with Byzantium. Their number increased as monasteries began providing health care, something they did for centuries.[1] The Western world's hospital of today only started during the Enlightenment. Asian and Middle Eastern hospitals followed a different path in their creation.

Though hospitals had become commonplace, most people throughout the world died in their own dwellings until at least the end of the nineteenth century. Decade by decade, fewer people died at home until this most recent millennium arrived. Nowadays most people die in hospitals. Their numbers vary depending on the source of the statistic, but Stanford University's palliative care website estimates that 60% of Americans die in hospital.[2] The relatively recent trend to palliative care encouraging dying at home or in a hospice may eventually lead to fewer in-hospital deaths. This has not happened at the time of writing; most people still die in hospitals.

Most people only die in hospital when very ill or seriously injured. Their deaths are not unexpected. Only the timing is unpredictable. Coroners don't investigate most in-hospital deaths unless they occurred as a result of fatal accidents, suicides or homicides. Natural or expected deaths are only occasionally the subject of a coroner's investigation — when attending staff or the dead person's family question some aspect of the care provided. Otherwise any review of in-hospital care is provided by the hospital staff members themselves.

Statistics Canada tracks the percentage of deaths that occur in Canadian hospitals. Between 2007 and 2017 that number never varied more than a 1% or 2% from the 60% mark.[3] The hospital death percentage in the United States is perhaps 1% or 2% higher than that in

Canada. The United Kingdom was also near the North American level a couple of decades ago, but in recent years fewer than 50% of Britons die in hospital. That's the same situation as in Australia.

During the first decade of the twenty-first century, most people who died in hospital were elderly. In the United States about three quarters of hospital inpatients who died were aged over 65. One quarter were actually older than 85. This will continue to be the case. People live much longer nowadays than in years gone by. At the start of the twentieth century British men only lived to the age of 48 and women to the age of 54. In 2018 the United Nations predicted that British men should live, on average, 79.5 years and British women to the age of 83.[4]

Reasons for dying in hospital vary with a country's state of development. In India during the 20 years from 1995 to 2014, hospital admission rates doubled.[5] Care in Indian hospitals differs depending on whether the hospital is private or government-run. Some Indian private hospitals operate at developed country standards; many government-funded public hospitals do not. For example, some Indian public hospitals have only one physician. As a result, Indians fear that diagnoses and treatment in public hospitals will be incorrect. In addition, the staff may be insensitive, and the hospitals are frequently dirty. Nobody was surprised when the *Deccan Herald* reported The Lancet had found out that 4,300 people a day die in Indian hospitals.[6] Like everywhere else, most were natural deaths or fatal complications of accidents.

Exactly why people die in hospital varies by country. Those who die in developed countries' hospitals have different reasons from patients dying in the third world institutions. More people in lesser-developed countries' infirmaries die of infectious disease than do patients in hospitals in the first world.

In Canada in 2017, 160,000 people died in hospital.[7] Most died from stroke, heart attack, heart failure, cancer, pneumonia, chronic obstructive lung disease and sepsis. In India deaths in a tertiary care hospital offer a similar picture. However, in smaller Indian hospitals a higher percentage of deaths arises from diarrhoea, tuberculosis, preterm birth and neonatal conditions such as septicaemia, birth asphyxia and birth trauma.[8] In most developing countries more people die in hospital from infections and childbirth than in the rest of the world.

Most people enter hospital grudgingly, very ill or in need of therapy that only a hospital can provide. All treatments involve some degree of risk that varies by type of patient and type of therapy. As a prelude to treating patients, physicians explain risks before obtaining their consent to proceed. The circumstances under which treatment takes place makes the risk of death vary dramatically.

Consider hip surgery. Elective surgery to replace an arthritic hip proves fatal in only three to four cases per thousand operations.[9] Repairing a fractured hip is much more dangerous. Most people who fall and break hips are elderly and in poor health. By one estimate, after surgical repair of a fractured hip 5% of people die within the next 30 days, and 25% of them will be dead within a year.[10] Their subsequent death rate from any cause (usually heart disease or dementia) remains three times as high as people the same age who did not have a hip fracture.[11]

Even so, most people who break their hips opt for surgery. The alternative is a short, painful life of almost complete disability. The broken hip will leave a person bedridden, requiring help for practically every life activity. The prospect of an independent mobile existence makes surgery the only reasonable choice for most. Coroners investigate hip fractures as accidents. They only occasionally make useful recommendations to prevent future falls. Unfortunately falling is a predictable consequence of advanced age and frailty.

Infection

Until Covid-19 struck, many people were only dimly aware that hospitals abounded with germs that only partly arose from their very sick occupants. Rigorous cleaning decreases their numbers but cannot eliminate all harmful micro-organisms. Patient infections are so frequent that hospital-acquired infections have their own name — nosocomial. Other patients, any surfaces in rooms, linen, used bandages and operations can all be a source of a nosocomial infection. Nurses, physicians or anyone else treating a patient may originate a nosocomial infection too. Consequently, the risk of a fatal infection is constant throughout any hospital admission. Lethal nosocomial infections, which sometimes follow surgery, are a foreseeable complication of a hospital stay. Before an operation, patients are warned of the relatively uncommon but quite foreseeable post-operative complications of bleeding and infection. Most of these problems are successfully managed, but severe post-operative infections may be fatal.

The number of hospital-acquired infections is more than one would think. The United States may have 98,000 annual deaths from these nosocomial infections.[12] A Norwegian study reported the death within 30 days of almost 5% of people who acquired infections in hospital.[13] But only when some form of malpractice is suspected in a nosocomial infection death does a coroner investigate one.

Urinary Catheters

There are many reasons why hospitalized patients need urethral catheterization. (See Figure 16.1). Some catheters stay in place for only a few hours. Others remain for a day or two. Less fortunate patients require an "indwelling" urinary catheter indefinitely. The longer a catheter is in place, the more likely it is to become infected. Each day a catheter remains in place increases the chance of an infection by around 5%.[14] Initially only the urine is infected. However, once those germs move into the bloodstream a potentially fatal bacteraemia develops.

In a study in the United Kingdom,[15] 35% of people who developed bacteraemia from a urinary infection developed septic shock and died within 30 days — 20% died within the first week. Men and women

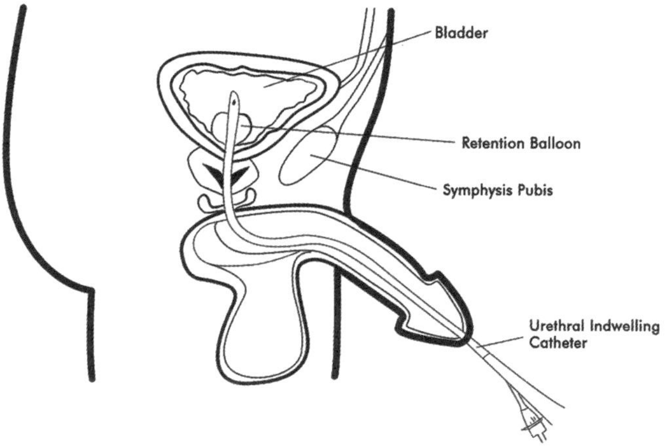

Figure 16.1: Urinary catheters can be a source of infection.

develop bacteraemia equally often. Over half of the cases of bacteraemia progressing to septic shock, or urosepsis, are in people aged over 70. As a result, deaths from catheter infections occur mostly in the elderly.

Central Venous Line Catheters

In emergency departments or intensive care units, hospital staff often need to insert a plastic catheter into one of a patient's large veins for rapid fluid administration. This catheter establishes a central venous line. (See Figure 16.2.) Skin around the insertion site is always carefully cleansed before the needle pierces it. Still, pushing the catheter through the skin and underlying tissue can drag any bacteria that cleaning did not eradicate into the bloodstream. Central line infections are 64 times more likely to occur than when the normal needle and tube are inserted into an arm or leg vein to run in intravenous fluid.[16]

It is hard to get accurate figures for how many Americans actually die from central line septicaemia. However, the CDC reports that between 12% and 25% of all central venous line bloodstream infections are fatal.[17] In 1998 one American surgical intensive care unit cultured 232 central venous catheters. Of these, only 49% were found only to be germ free, 17% were colonized with too few bacteria to be considered infected, and 34% were infected.[18]

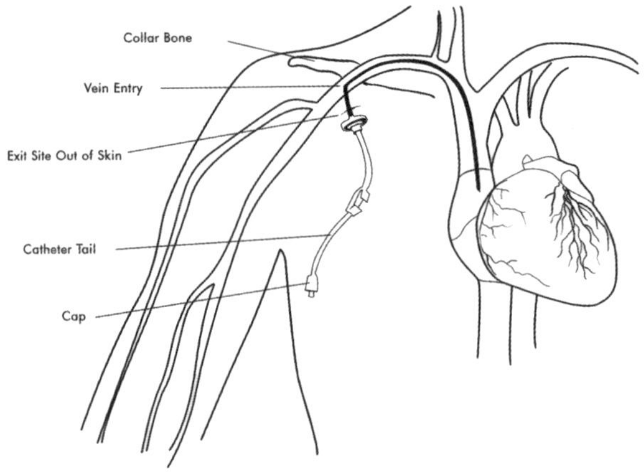

Figure 16.2: A central venous catheter inserted into a major vein in the chest.

In that study, 15 of the 78 infected patients died from infection-related causes. They all died within two weeks of the catheter insertion, with two of them dying within three days. So, nearly 20% of those infections led to death. What does that mean? All those catheterized in the study were very ill post-operative patients. These deaths are foreseeable complications of their illnesses or injury. Coroners rarely investigate these deaths since they cannot really be said to be unexpected.

Statistics change over the years as processes improve. A coroner asked to look into a central line death should consult an intensive care physician to obtain up-to-date data on the likelihood of death from central line infection in that community's hospitals. This will add an important mathematical perspective to the interpretation and explanation of the results of the death's investigation.

Surgery

We have already noted that infection is commonplace after any type of surgery. Post-operative infection can be expected 5% of the time. Fortunately, most people who develop an infected surgical site do not die. Still, wound infection makes post-operative death twice as likely. In 2002, 8,205 Americans died of surgical site infections.[19] Coroners consider these deaths unfortunate, but natural, complications of an operation. Few are investigated.

These fatal infections have many possible origins. The patient's own body, an operating room table, surgical instruments, the surrounding air, and the attending operating room staff are all potential sources. Predisposing factors make an infectious death of some patients more likely. Age is one of these factors. Fatal surgical infections disproportionately kill the very old and the very young. Others who are disproportionately affected include diabetics, smokers, steroid users and those taking immune-suppressant drugs. In fact, a poor immune system in anybody increases the risk of death from a post-operative infection.

The longer the hospitalization, the more likely an infection. That means lengthy preoperative hospital stays become risky. Infection is also more frequent when a person undergoing surgery has a bacterial infection somewhere other than at the operative site. For example, pneumonia or an abscess will increase the risk of an operative infection. Weight matters too. The obese and the malnourished develop more wound site infections than do patients of average weight. Unsurprisingly, surgical post-operative deaths also increase when the area of the body to be cut through is already infected at the start of the operation.

Both surgeons and anaesthetists classify the infection risk of any proposed surgery. A high risk does not mean an operation cannot proceed, though. Patients frequently give their surgeons the go-ahead even with a very high risk of infection. All surgeons and operating rooms follow a system to minimize infections. With slight variations between different operating rooms, all systems resemble one another. Basic components include preoperative antibiotics, lengthy surgical scrubbing of hands, antiseptic cleansing of the surgical site, good operating theatre ventilation, sterile instruments, and techniques to keep operative times as short as possible.

Elective patients may be told to avoid smoking the month before surgery, to shower before coming to hospital and possibly to cleanse with chlorhexidine. If diabetic, good blood sugar control right up to the date of surgery will be requested.

When the hospital, family or staff involved believe that a fatal infection arose from hospital error, a coroner may be asked to review the system as part of a death investigation. This review should include looking at the need for hospitalization, treatment, central line insertion, catheterization, surgery and the hospital processes associated with care during the terminal admission.

It is impossible to know how long people scrubbed their hands, of course. The coroner's investigation is primarily a paper review. Most investigations are likely to find the required precautions, preoperatively, intraoperatively and post-operatively were taken even though the patient died of an infection. The coroner's conclusion will usually be that the patient died a natural death of infection, a common complication of the surgery. Quite often the family remains upset to hear these findings. All the coroner can do in such a case is to reiterate that the post-operative infectious death was a natural one, and not the result of any discernable malpractice.

Falls

In spite of nurses being located throughout hospitals patients fall more than one would think. Though their numbers may be decreasing a bit, falls still occur in about 2% of hospital stays. In the United States, the incidence of falls ranges from 3.3 to 11.5 per 1,000 patient days in hospital. Most falls are quite innocuous. In only a quarter of falls is the patient even injured. A mere 2% of falls result in a broken bone, and only 0.0005% of in-hospital falls are fatal. So people do die from falls in hospital, but rarely.[20]

Errors

Patients are cared for by staff who, at the time of writing, are all human beings except perhaps in Japan. Human beings all make mistakes. Sometimes, mistakes involving a patient's health can be fatal. How many people die each year because of hospital errors in the United States is a subject for debate. In 2016, Johns Hopkins estimated there were 250,000 such deaths each year.[21] Others have guessed the number to be as high as 440,000.

Possible errors are many. Here are a few.

1. Adverse drug reactions. Almost everyone who enters hospital takes at least one type of medication. Most patients take more. Whenever multiple medications are prescribed, the combined interactions may make the drugs act differently than when administered individually. Probably 7,000 Americans die from adverse drug reactions each year, though not all in hospital. Hospitals have systems in place to prevent these sorts of events from happening. Still, occasionally staff are unaware of a medication a patient is taking that might cause a fatal reaction when combined with a hospital-administered drug. At other times a hospital is unaware a patient previously reacted to a medication the hospital plans to administer. Sometimes the fatal drug reaction happens for the first time during a hospital stay.

2. Probably the most potentially fatal error is misdiagnosis.
3. Unnecessary treatment can actually cause death. The more that is undertaken, the more likely it is that treatment will be fatal.
4. Virtually all hospital patients have laboratory tests performed. Most will be normal. Some abnormal test results indicate speedy action may be needed to help the patient. When things go awry and actions are not taken, death ensues.
5. To figure out how failure to act on an important lab test resulted in death, consider four stages in the specimen testing process. Errors can occur anywhere along this chain. The first stage begins immediately after the specimen is obtained. It has to be properly labelled so that the right sample is tested. Examining the wrong person's body fluid guarantees an incorrect analysis. Blood and urine must be properly collected, handled and stored to prevent biological changes. Any degeneration will mar test readings. These potential problems occur before testing begins.
6. The second stage is the actual testing. Nowadays the analysis of the patient's tissue specimen is usually performed correctly. Errors are much fewer than in the past because computerization has automated testing over the last 20 years. Machines are not infallible though, and technical problems can lead to improper results.
7. Thirdly, test results must be correctly communicated to the person ordering them in a timely manner. If results take too long to arrive, a window for life-saving therapy may be missed.
8. Finally, the test results need proper interpretation.
9. Unnecessary tests or procedures. All tests or procedures could lead to death in rare instances. Some tests are much more potentially dangerous than others. (Compare the risk of a coronary angiogram to a urinalysis.) The more tests or procedures carried out, the greater the risk of one being fatal.
10. Medication mistakes. In 2006 a patient in an American hospital could expect one medication error every day.[22] Fortunately, most of these mistakes were not lethal. There are several

reasons medication errors occur. When fatal, the person administering the medication often lacks complete information about a patient's drug allergies or other medications being taken. The wrong medication and too much of the right medication can both be fatal.

11. Surgical error. Even though hospitals and operating rooms have procedures to prevent this from happening, surgeons do not always correctly identify their patients. Death can occur when the wrong patient is operated on. The wrong kidney being surgically removed from a patient with only one functioning kidney will cause death. Patients also die during the operation when improperly monitored, for example, when an unnoticed poor connection to an intravenous line allows air entry to cause fatal air emboli.
12. Uncoordinated care. Failure to properly inform a replacement at shift change may lead to inadequate observation of an ill patient or failure to administer a life-supporting medication.
13. Medical device malfunction. A cardiac defibrillator that will not shock or a pacemaker wire that breaks can both lead to death.
14. Hospital acquired infection leading to sepsis and death. This is discussed in detail in Chapter 6.
15. Failure by staff to appreciate symptom significance. For example, missing warning signs of a myocardial infarction's onset may result in a potentially avoidable fatal cardiac arrest.
16. Premature discharge from hospital. This is not really a death in hospital, but when a person dies shortly after returning home when their condition had not become stable, it is considered hospital related.
17. Patient-controlled analgesia (people managing their pain by themselves). People are sometimes sent home with a pump that allows an analgesic to be dispensed whenever pain becomes intolerable. The machine contains a computer that must be correctly set up to deliver the required dose of medication. If a nurse improperly codes the machine, an excessive amount of medication may be delivered. With an opioid, too high a dose can lethally suppress breathing.[23]

Perisurgical Errors

There is always the risk that an anaesthetic will kill a patient during surgery or in the post-operative period in the recovery room. General anaesthetics are much more lethal than local anaesthetics. Fortunately, any type of anaesthesia is rarely fatal in developed countries. One German paper in 2011 suggested that only four healthy people were likely to die in every million administrations of general anaesthetics.[24] Others put the rate higher, considering people in all states of health. Coroners are safe to suppose death is likely once every 10,000 to 20,000 administrations of anaesthetics.

An anaesthetic gas may fatally impair the heart muscle's ability to function. Whether this will happen cannot be predicted in advance of surgery. Similarly, an anaesthetist administering either wrong drugs or wrong doses during the procedure can lethally depress both heart function and breathing capacity.

Lack of oxygen will always kill an intubated person. Inadequate oxygen occurs in two ways. Since the airway tube inserted into the mouth must not be obstructed in any way and properly positioned, a wrongly located or blocked tube can be fatal. Secondly, enough oxygen must steadily flow through the tube to provide adequate ventilation that keeps the blood's oxygen level within normal limits. Should the blood's oxygen level drop too low during anaesthesia, the heart may stop beating.

A cardiac arrest on the operating table may result from an inadequate quantity of blood reaching the heart during surgery. Blood pressure swings up and down quite rapidly during trauma operations. Multiple blood transfusions accompany trauma surgery. An anaesthetist may simply be unable to administer enough blood fast enough to replace the continuing blood loss before it can be finally stopped.

Percentage-wise, more deaths probably occur during trauma surgery than during any other type of surgery. However, cardiac surgery of any sort, thoracic surgery, neurosurgery, and orthopaedic surgery all tend to have more intraoperative deaths than other surgeries. Some deaths are related to the anaesthetic itself, the procedure or the care, but more often dying results from the added stress of surgery upon an underlying disease.

Fatal surgical errors take many different forms. One well-publicized mishap is the failure to remove an instrument or packing from a patient before suturing up the surgical incision. Dying from such a misadventure is relatively uncommon though. A human body usually manages to cope quite well with new internal foreign bodies. Just over 5% of such cases are fatal.

Cutting a blood vessel or duct or accidentally puncturing an organ during a surgical procedure ends in death more than 5% of the time too. Fortunately, the numbers are low — in the period from 2000 to 2002, only 2,419 such deaths occurred in the whole United States. Haemorrhage from loose sutures or clips that come off arteries can occasionally be fatal, but in even lower numbers. In 2004 only 726 American patients bled to death when their clips came loose.[25]

Post-Operative Deaths

The post-operative period is dangerous for any patient. For some patients their metabolism may simply be so dysfunctional that survival is impossible. Careful fluid monitoring after surgery is very important. Intravenous fluid management that goes askew can be lethal. Fluid management error was considered to be fatal 1,327 times in the United States in 2000-2002 constituting about 20% of that year's post-operative metabolic deaths.

The process of wound edges pulling apart is termed dehiscence. A wound opens when sutures fall out or when they are not tight enough in the first place. Both are common occurrences that are rarely lethal. Of those that end up being fatal, only 10% involve any physician error. The rest result from natural processes within the body. The United States reported 615 such fatalities between 2000 and 2002.[26]

Pulmonary emboli develop from leg clots that form after surgery. This expected complication may be minimized, but not eliminated, by using anticoagulant therapy. Sometimes surgeons forget to prescribe it. Any clotting in the absence of an anticoagulant is considered a preventable complication, even though there is no certainty that anticoagulant therapy would have prevented the clot from developing.

Occasionally some people develop a fatal reaction to a blood transfusion. One potentially lethal error is transfusing the wrong type of blood. To ensure compatibility, procedures exist to check that the type of blood administered matches the patient's own. When investigating a transfusion death, a coroner needs to ascertain whether that process has been followed.

It is quite common for breathing failures in the post-operative period, and one third of the time resuscitations are unsuccessful. One fifth of the time some medical error is the cause of deaths arising from post-operative respiratory failure.

In 2016 Harvard investigators published a paper in the *British Medical Journal*.[27] They concluded that hospital errors were the third leading cause of hospital deaths after cancer and heart disease. Since then both hospitals and physicians have begun to pay more attention to the systems within their institutions, looking for flaws that might lead to these errors occurring.

Still, people are going to continue dying in hospital forever. Hospitals will continue to treat the very ill and injured with many fatal outcomes despite the very best of care. Coroners need to recognize that some people have unrealistic expectations of outcomes of their relatives' treatment. They expect miracles, but alas, we live and die in a secular world.

NOTES

1 Smith, V. (2008). *Clean: A history of personal hygiene and purity*. Oxford, UK: Oxford University Press, p 142.

2 Stanford School of Medicine. (n.d.). *Palliative care: Where do Americans die?* https://palliative.stanford.edu/home-hospice-home-care-of-the-dying-patient/where-do-americans-die/

3 Statistics Canada. *Table 13-10-075-01: Deaths by place of death (hospital or non-hospital)*. doi: 10.25318/1310071501-eng

4 United Nations Development Program. (2019). Human development report 2019: Beyond income, beyond averages, beyond today. http://hdr.undp.org/sites/default/files/hdr2019.pdf

5 Kastor, A., & Mohanty, S. K. (2018, January). Disease and age pattern of hospitalisation and associated costs in India: 1995–2014. *BMJ Open 8*(1), e016990. doi: 10.1136/bmjopen-2017-016990

6 Ray, K. (2018, September 10). 4300 Indians die daily, due to poor hospital care. *Deccan Herald*. https://www.deccanherald.com/opinion/panorama/4300-indians-die-daily-due-692128.html

7 See note 2 above.

8 Joshi, R., Lodhe, R., Agrawal, S., & Jain, A. P. (2014). Hospital based infectious disease related proportional mortality study. *Journal of Global Infectious Diseases, 6*(1), 10–16.

9 Berstock, J. R., Beswick, A. D., Lenguerrand, E., Whitehouse, M. R., & Blom, A. W. (2014). Mortality after total hip replacement surgery: A systematic review. *Bone & Joint Research, 3*(6), 175–182.

10 Tsang, C., Boulton, C., Burgon, V., Johansen, A., Wakeman, R., & Cromwell, D. A. (2018, February 21). Predicting 30-day mortality after hip fracture surgery. *Bone & Joint Research, 6*(9). doi: 10.1302/2046-3758.69.BJR-2017-0020.R1

11 Panula, J., Pihlajamaki, H., Mattila, V. M., Jaatinen, P., Vahlberg, T., Aarnio, P., & Kivela, S.-L. (2011, May 20). Mortality and cause of death in hip fracture patients aged 65 or older: A population-based study. *BMC Musculoskeletal Disorders, 12*, 105. https://bmcmusculoskeletdisord.biomedcentral.com/articles/10.1186/1471-2474-12-105#citeas

12 Haque, M., Sartelli, M., McKimm, J., & Abu Bakar, M. (2018). Health care-associated infection: An overview. *Infection and Drug Resistance, 11*, 2321–2333.

13 Koch, A. M., Nilsen, R. M., Eriksen, H. M., Cox, R. J., & Harthug, S. (2015, December 29). Mortality related to hospital-associated infections in a tertiary care hospital: Repeated cross-sectional studies between 2004–2011. *Antimicrobial Resistance and Infection Control, 4*, 57. https://aricjournal.biomedcentral.com/articles/10.1186/s13756-015-0097-9

14 Nicolle, L. E. (2014). Catheter associated urinary tract infections. *Antimicrobial Resistance & Infection Control 3*, 23. doi: 10.1186/2047-2994-3-23

15 Melzer, M., & Welch, C. (2013). Outcomes in UK patients with hospital-acquired bacteraemia and the risk of catheter-associated urinary tract infections. *BMJ Postgraduate Medical Journal, 89*(1052), 329–334.

16 Gahlot, R., Nigam, C., Kumar, V., Yadav, G., & Anupurba, S. (2014). Catheter-related bloodstream infections. *International Journal of Critical Illness & Injury Science, 4*(2), 162–167.

17 Centers for Disease Control and Prevention. (2011). Vital signs: Central line-associated blood stream infections - United States, 2001, 2008, and 2009. *Morbidity and Mortality Weekly Report, 60*(8), 243–248.

18 Charalambous, C., Swoboda, S. M., Dick, J., Perl, T., & Lipsett, P. A. (1998). Risk factors and clinical impact of central line infection in the surgical intensive care unit. *Archives of Surgery, 133(11), 1241–1246.*

19 Joint Commission Center for Transforming Healthcare. (n.d.). Surgical site infections. https://www.centerfortransforminghealthcare.org/improvement-topics/surgical-site-infections/

20 Bouldin, E. D., Andresen, E. M., Dunton, N. E., Simon, M., Waters, T. M., Liu, M., … Shorr, R. I. (2013) Falls among adult patients hospitalized in the United States: Prevalence and trends. *Journal of Patient Safety, 9*(1), 13–17.

21 Makary, M. A., & Daniel, M. (2016). Medical error—the third leading cause of death in the US. *British Medical Journal*, 353:I 2139. doi: 10.1136/bmj.i2139

22 Eastman, P. (2006). IOM report: Medication errors injure millions. *Emergency Medicine News, 28(9), 44–46.*

23 A Train Education. (n.d.). *Types of medical errors.* https://www.atrainceu.com/content/3-types-medical-errors

24 Gottschalk, A., Van Aken, H., Zenz, M., Standl, T. (2011). Is anesthesia dangerous? *Deutsches Arzteblatt International, 108*(27) 449–474.

25 Health Grades. (2004). *Patient safety in American hospitals.* Appendix F. http://www.providersedge.com/ehdocs/ehr_articles/Patient_Safety_in_American_Hospitals-2004.pdf

26 See note 25 above.

27 See note 21 above.

17
Work-Related Deaths

When a person dies on the job, a coroner is always called to investigate because nobody is expected to die at work. Workplace deaths are actually quite common, since adults usually spend a third of their lives working. Most workplace fatalities are natural events that fate has decreed will happen at a worksite. A death at work is investigated in the same way as any other, with one exception. If the spouse or a family member believes that work had anything at all to do with its cause, the coroner should always order an autopsy. Its findings will provide the maximum amount of medical information available to government departments and tribunals that must decide whether to compensate a deceased worker's family.

Since the start of the Industrial Revolution, workplace conditions have improved dramatically throughout the developed world. Safety at work is legislated, and almost nobody has to get up in the morning worrying about being killed at work. Not all of today's jobs are still completely safe though, and some are inherently dangerous. Still, few people die at work in the First World today, but "human factors" — that is, carelessness or some sort of misconduct — mean that accidental deaths will continue in even the safest workplace for years to come.

Most people know which types of work are dangerous. The satirical revue *Beyond the Fringe*, correctly observed that "judgin'" was safer than "minin'" because judges didn't have to worry about falling rocks.* Mining will probably always be one of the world's most dangerous jobs. In most courts, presiding and ruling should always be one of the safest. The bulk of today's most dangerous jobs are found in underdeveloped countries that have lax workplace safety and construction laws. Their safest jobs are usually found in factories or offices, but even

* *Beyond the Fringe* was a theatrical revue written and performed by Alan Bennett, Peter Cook, Jonathan Miller and Dudley Moore. It opened in Edinburgh in 1960, later transferring to London and New York.

working there can be risky. In some factories, faulty machinery leads to fatalities. Buildings also collapse, crushing those working inside.

Work has two ways of killing people. The more common is an accident. Less frequently the work's environment leads to a disease that ultimately kills the worker much later on — often in retirement. Many more First World workers die from work accidents than from work-induced disease. The numbers dying vary between countries and industries.

There are differences within a country too. In 2016 the province of Manitoba was the safest part of Canada to work in; that year, Manitoba had only 0.8 fatal injuries per 100,000 workers.

That same year the far northern Arctic territory of Nunavut appeared to be the most dangerous. Nunavut had a death rate of 4.5 per 100,000 workers, nearly six times as high as Manitoba's. Here it is important to interpret what the statistics mean. There are fewer than 40,000 people in Nunavut. A high proportion are young and do not work. I do not know exactly how this figure was arrived at, but it almost certainly involves a single death. One death in Nunavut drastically changes the death rate. If nobody had died in 2017, it would then have become the safest place in Canada to work (statistically speaking).[1] Please note that more recent figures are available, but the 2017 statistics were chosen to make the point.

Combining all the provincial and territorial statistics adds up to 905 people dying at work in Canada in 2016, which may not seem like a large number. However, each one was thoroughly investigated by multiple agencies. In some cases, inquests were held to allow public access to the death investigation. For example, Ontario holds inquests on any death that occurred while mining or working at a construction site.[2] In addition to reviewing the circumstances surrounding each death, an inquest allows a jury to recommend actions to prevent future similar deaths.

Canada's most dangerous jobs have two things in common: the work is largely outdoors and is very physically demanding. Fishermen and trappers die on the job most often. Miners, quarriers and people working with oil wells have the second-highest number of fatalities. Loggers and others in the forestry industry as a group come in third.

Construction workers are fourth-most likely to die while working, and transport and storage workers are fifth. All these jobs have to be considered inherently dangerous.[3]

The U.S. Bureau of Labor statistics for 2018 tell a similar story. American occupations with the lowest percentage of workplace deaths are computer and mathematical work, legal jobs, teaching and a category called "life, physical and social science occupations." Police and firefighters were in the middle. In the whole of the United States in 2018, 108 police and sheriff's patrol officers and 64 firefighters died when injured on the job.[4]

A lot of people perform inherently dangerous work where few are killed. Soldiers deployed overseas, police officers on the bomb disposal squad, taxi drivers and ice-road truckers recognize that the work they do puts them at risk all the time. When harmed, they are more often injured than killed by their work accidents. Many more emergency department physicians than coroners deal with these workers.

Workers in the Third World have different causes of death. Since those nations' statistical gathering capabilities are poor, it is hard to be certain of the number of deaths. Some lethal occupations are found only in the Third World. One example is breaking up ships, a fatal business for many workers, that is done largely in the Indian subcontinent. At least 90 people died breaking up unneeded tonnage on the shores of Bangladesh alone between 2005 and 2012. The types of accidents that killed them were not unique. Some workers fell to their deaths from higher parts of the vessel. Others were crushed by falling iron plates. Electrical shocks transmitted through the metal remnants of the ship electrocuted a third group. Toxic gases suffocated some more. A final mechanism of death in ship breaking is exploding gases.[5]

Farm workers in informal tropical economies also suffer deaths peculiar to their environment. Some arise from fatal falls out of palm trees while gathering coconuts. A Papua New Guinea physician reported two cases of death of workers who were struck by falling coconuts.[6] In India, elephants and tigers kill rural farm folk when their farming encroaches on the animals' usual habitat. India recorded 1,144 such deaths between April 2014 and May 2017.[7]

Sewing machines are rarely associated with death. However, the Bangladesh government has counted deaths in the ready-made garment industry since 2013. That was the year the Rana Plaza building in Dhaka collapsed and killed 1,134 garment workers when its walls and ceilings fell on them. Bangladeshi building inspectors have a difficult job. Since 2013 another 40 workers in the garment industry have died, mostly from fires. While that number seems high, 500 people died in garment factories from 2006 to 2010, so the 2013 figure actually shows a significant improvement.

Human Factors

Age

Inexperienced workers are considered especially at risk of workplace injury or death. During the 10 years between 1980 and 1989, 670 16- and 17-year-old adolescents died of workplace accidents across the United States. Interestingly though, the ratio of teenage deaths to teens employed was lower than the corresponding ratio for older workers. During the years 2015 to 2019, the rate of deaths per 100,000 workers aged 18 and 19 varied between 1.9 and 2.6, while the rate for deaths of all workers was approximately 3.5 per 100,000 each year.[8]

In Ontario, "young workers" is considered to include anyone up to the age of 25. In the five years from 2011 to 2015, 33 young Ontarian workers died accidentally.[9] Most of Ontario's accidental workplace deaths occurred in those aged between 40 and 60 years. The United States records the highest number of workers' deaths between the ages of 45 and 65.[10] The highest proportion of fatal workplace injuries is found in those over 65 years of age. Figures will vary somewhat, but they should be similar throughout the developed world.

Sex

It is usually men who die from workplace trauma. Women may like to believe this statistic proves that they are more careful than men. But these are just statistics; they have to be interpreted. Again, take Ontario as an example. In the 10 years from 2008 to 2017, 91% of workplace deaths due to injury occurred in males. However, 76% of these deaths occurred in construction, transportation and manufacturing, and in services sectors with an overwhelmingly male workforce. In most developed countries, 90% or more of all workplace deaths are male, and most workers die in male-dominated occupations.[11]

Alcohol and Drug Use

Since alcohol and drug use are enormous problems for society at large, one would suspect that drug and alcohol consumption must be especially dangerous at work. It is. Of the 5,147 American workplace deaths in 2017, unintentional overdoses of alcohol or street drugs while in the workplace accounted for 272 of them. Almost 5% of workplace accidental deaths involve voluntary consumption of a toxic chemical.[12] Many fatal accidents result from physical or mental impairment caused by consuming a less-than-fatal quantity of these chemicals. Epidemiologists are not yet absolutely sure of this, but proof may be forthcoming. A couple of autopsy studies of work accident deaths detected alcohol in the blood 20% of the time. Deaths in motor vehicle accidents, from falls, and when being caught in or under equipment are all associated with recent consumption of alcohol more often than other types of workplace fatalities.

Other Factors

In many cases there may be a relationship between an employee's physical condition, skill and training (or lack of it) and their accidental death at work. Most people would suspect these factors have a role in fatal accidents, yet proof remains elusive. Should a relative raise these as possible factors related to the cause of death, don't disagree, but leave the question to labour ministry investigators. Surviving relatives should be reassured that labour ministry investigators will consider those factors at length before issuing any final report about their relative's death.

How Fatal Accidents Occur

1. Vehicles

By far the greatest number of fatal work accidents involve transportation vehicles. Most happen on highways and involve collisions, usually between vehicles, but occasionally with an animal. Some truck drivers die in a vehicle rollover or when their truck jack-knifes into an immovable object. Occasionally a pedestrian within a work zone is struck by a passing vehicle. These accidents happen both on highways and also in non-road areas such as quarries. In 2017, the United States reported that vehicle accidents accounted for about 40% of all workplace deaths.[13]

2. Crushing

A second large group of deaths results from an object or some piece of equipment striking a person. A similar type of death occurs when a heavy piece of material or equipment falls and lands on a worker. Powered machinery can be lethal for the worker using it too. Workers caught in operating machines may be squashed or bleed to death. Anywhere in the world, falling structures or material may crush or kill anyone beneath them.

3. Falls

Falls at work can be fatal. A trip or slip while standing or when walking sometimes causes death, usually from bleeding or a head injury. More commonly, death results after falling from a height, sometimes due to structural or equipment collapse. More commonly a worker who is not attached to a protective lifeline falls off a building or through an open space.

4. Hazardous Workplaces

Some workplaces that are inherently dangerous can lead to death when a worker is careless or when an unforeseen event occurs. In governmental terms these are described as "hazardous environments." People can drown at work, freeze to death, burn fatally or die from dehydration. More commonly though workers suffocate, quite often while in some sort of confined space.

5. Confined Spaces

A confined space can be found in any place not designed for habitation that is either completely or partially enclosed. Air won't flow freely in it. Though the space may contain normal air before entry, the initially life-supporting atmosphere changes to a lethal one as the worker's lungs consume the air's oxygen and replace it with carbon dioxide. Once a surrounding atmosphere becomes mostly carbon dioxide, anyone within it who is not wearing an oxygen tank to assist breathing loses consciousness and dies.

Confined spaces are not always limited to the interior of a building or some other structure. They can occur outdoors too. For example, farmers' manure pits are confined spaces. These manure pits produce hydrogen sulphide, a foul-smelling heavier-than-air gas that sits in the pit. Anyone staying in a manure pit long enough to breathe in too much hydrogen sulphide loses consciousness and dies of asphyxia. Other historically fatal confined workspaces include silos, vats, hoppers, utility vaults, tanks, water supply towers, sewers, pipes, access shafts, truck or rail tank cars, aircraft wings, boilers, manholes, pump stations, digesters, and storage bins. The possibilities are seemingly endless.

In the United States from 1992 to 1998, there were 523 cases of fatal "occupational inhalation", a mortality rate of 0.56 deaths per 1,000,000 worker-years. Men's rate (1.01 per 1,000,000) was higher than women's (0.03 per 1,000,000). Mining was the industry with the highest mortality rate (6.64 per 1,000,000). The service industry occupation with the highest rate was firefighting (3.54 per 1,000,000). The group including farming, forestry, and fishing occupations experienced a mortality rate of 2.84 per 1,000,000. Nearly half of the inhalation victims were constructing, repairing, cleaning, inspecting, or painting when they died. Carbon monoxide, the gas most frequently fatal, caused one third of all inhalation deaths. Workers die from inhaling carbon monoxide twice as often in the winter as in the summer. These deaths are more common as workers age. Those older than 65 had the highest mortality.[14]

6. Electrocution

People also electrocute themselves at work. Fortunately, that does not happen often. Still, 166 Americans died of electric shock in 2019.[15] In Ontario, whenever an electrical death occurs at a construction site an inquest follows. In those that I have presided over, the electrocuted worker had either removed their protective gloves before moving a piece of metal that inadvertently contacted an electrical current while they were still holding it, or a live wire unexpectedly touched some bare skin.

7. Homicide and Suicide

Finally, people can be killed at work intentionally. Workers commit suicide in the workplace in the same ways that they commit suicide anywhere else. Workplace homicides are a significant worry in the United States. In 2017, 458 Americans were shot to death at work, while 351 died of stabbing.[16] This is less of a problem in other countries. For example, the United Kingdom had only one intentional workplace death occurred in the year 2013/2014.[17] Most other countries' numbers of workplace homicides will fall between these two figures.

The American ratio of male to female workplace homicides is about 4 to 1. Cashiers, supervisors of retail sales workers, and police officers were the occupations with the highest numbers slain at work. Other risky occupations included taxi drivers, gas station attendants, private security guards, stock handlers and baggers, barbers and bartenders.

Occupational Disease

The other way work leads to death is when a fatal disease develops after exposure to some substance in the work environment. Most of these diseases develop slowly and become fatal long after the final exposure occurred. Coroners are not usually involved in these deaths at all. In countries with workers' compensation systems, spouses of deceased workers usually receive a pension when one of these diseases kills their mate.

Financial compensation will only be granted after the disease can be definitely attributed to work. A disease's relationship to work is usually determined by comparing its frequency of occurrence in a workplace to the frequency in the populace at large. The multiple ways statistics can be interpreted leads to considerable political involvement in determining which diseases should be compensable in different industries.

The interpretation of these statistics is continually tested by lawyers, unions, advocacy groups and indeed anyone with a particular interest in attributing death to a toxic workplace exposure. Causative associations between substances found at work and disease slowly change over time. They vary in different legal jurisdictions because governments respond differently to pressure groups. One of the most active such groups in any country is the firefighter's union. Their work will likely be never-ending because firefighters are exposed to so many noxious chemicals in their line of work. Firefighters receive compensation for only a few diseases attributed to smoke exposure; their unions believe that many more diseases should be compensable.

Cancer

There are some groups of diseases that are generally accepted as being work related. One such group consists of cancers. Mesothelioma, a particularly aggressive form of lung cancer, is now 80% of the time found in workers exposed to asbestos fibres. Working with talc may produce mesothelioma too. If a worker has any past history of exposure to asbestos and develops mesothelioma, work will be considered the cause of the disease. Exactly how the fibres of asbestos trigger the development of cancer in the mesothelium, a body tissue, is not yet known. However, the disease is almost always fatal within five years of its discovery.

Other deaths from lung cancer occur in people who work with arsenic, cadmium, chromium compounds, or silica, and those who work in nickel refining. Fatal lung cancer can also develop among workers who are exposed to a lot of carbon, be it from coke oven fumes, soot, tars, oils or in coke gasification. Lots of substances in foundries cause lung cancer, as can high levels of radon gas exposure while on the job.

Another substance that causes fatal tumours is vinyl chloride. This chemical becomes part of polyvinyl chloride, a substance now primarily used in the manufacture of plastic pipes and bottles. Workers at plants where there is a high level of exposure to the chemical develop angiosarcoma of the liver. Vinyl chloride can probably also cause another type of fatal liver tumour, hepatocellular carcinoma. Any relationship between vinyl chloride and fatal cancers is decided by a battle of the epidemiologists. Outcomes vary in different jurisdictions around the world. Vinyl chloride can only kill people manufacturing this component of plastic, not the public using the final plastic products. Though liver cancer is very common, only a small percentage of fatal cases are caused by exposure to vinyl chloride.

Lethal nasopharyngeal and sinus cancers occur in woodworkers exposed to a lot of sawdust. They may also prove fatal for workers involved in manufacturing formaldehyde or isopropyl alcohol, people refining nickel, and those exposed to a lot of leather dust or mustard gas. Not everybody who is afflicted with these cancers at work dies from them, but some of these tumours are fatal. Formaldehyde and mustard gas also cause cancers of the mouth, and asbestos, mustard gas and isopropyl alcohol are associated with larynx cancer. All these malignancies can end workers' lives.

Skin cancers come with jobs exposing workers to arsenic, coal tars or mineral oils in industrial processes. Not all skin cancers are lethal. The most fatal type of skin cancer is malignant melanoma. It often occurs on body parts – such as lips and arms – that are exposed to the sun among people working outdoors unprotected. Melanomas kill farm labourers, construction workers and even ski lift operators. Their death is not really due to their job as much as the environment in which they work.

More lethal for workers is exposure to a lot of carbon. Carbon has been known to cause cancer since at least 1775, when Sir Percivall Pott first realized that climbing in sooty chimneys caused chimney sweeps to develop scrotal tumours. Carbon continually applied to other parts of the body will trigger cancer too. This commonly happens in the lungs and the stomach. In heavy smokers it is always tricky to attribute lung cancer solely to work. It is similarly difficult to blame the work environment for stomach cancer when the person ate a lot of smoked foods.

Bladder cancer can often arise in manufacturing workers who use dyes, textiles, rubbers, paints, plastics, aluminium or leather-tanning chemicals. Taxi drivers and bus drivers who are exposed to chemicals in diesel fumes regularly have more bladder cancer than the general public. To develop cancer requires a very long exposure, perhaps up to 30 years. The best-known causes of bladder cancer are aniline dyes. However, 2-naphthylamine, 4-aminobiphenyl, xenylamine, benzidine and o-toluidine are equally carcinogenic.

It is always a concern that people working with X-rays, such as radiologists and X-ray technicians, might develop leukaemia and other blood cell tumours. That was probably more likely before 1950, when dosages used were higher and safety precautions less stringent. Nowadays there is not considered to be any significant relationship between that sort of work and cancer. Blood cancers are now more frequently found in workers exposed to benzene, ethylene oxide or herbicides.

Establishing the relationship between work and death from cancer is left to a government or a tribunal. A coroner need only take note of the possible relationship. In the coroner's world a cancer death is a natural one. Whether it was solely, primarily or even slightly related to work exposure is decided by a different process. The numbers of work-related cancer deaths are never certain. In Ontario from 2003 to 2011, there were 136 construction workers, 7 electrical and utility workers, and 6 transportation workers who had their fatal lung cancer attributed to work.

Infection

Infectious diseases are inherent risks of the job in health care. Doctors and nurses who cut their skin with a needle or scalpel may find their patient's blood intermingled with their own. A patient with hepatitis B, hepatitis C or AIDS may transmit that disease to the health-care worker. The risk of transmission is low, and the risk of death is lower still, yet workplace deaths do occur from all three of these infections.

Agricultural workers are continually exposed to pests while outdoors. They may be bitten by mosquitoes that may spread malaria, West Nile virus or Zika virus. Ticks may carry Rocky Mountain spotted fever or Lyme disease. Most of the time these infections are not fatal, but some deaths occur every year. Over 400,000 people around the world die every year from malaria.[18] Many are workers, and it is reasonable to assume that at least some were bitten while they were working.

Circulatory Disease

Since cardiac disease especially is extremely prevalent, people die of heart attacks at work all the time. Some work features, like extreme heat or cold, may increase the likelihood of a heart attack. Miners and foundry workers have a higher than average risk of developing heart attacks. Ski instructors and freezer workers, particularly women, find themselves in a similar situation. It is always hard to attribute fatal heart disease to the workplace since it is so common.

Academics discuss the association of noise, electromagnetic radiation and vibration with an increased risk of cardiovascular disease too. No definitive conclusions have been reached, and the debate continues. Lots of modern jobs are very sedentary, and desk work makes a person twice as likely to develop a heart attack as a person who moves around and exercises at work every day. When a person does irregular heavy work, or when it is hectic, there is also an increased risk of cardiac death.

Some chemicals are associated with an increased risk of cardiovascular problems. Carbon disulphide, which is used as a solvent in viscose rayon, is an example. A more widespread chemical is carbon monoxide, a gas to which firefighters and diesel mechanics working in enclosed areas are exposed. When one of these people has coronary artery disease, the decrease in the concentration of oxygen transported to the heart can lead to angina, heart attack or even sudden death.

A chemical used in paint or varnish remover is methylene chloride. People who work with this all the time risk chest pain and death if they have underlying coronary arteriosclerosis. Other solvents, particularly bromofluorocarbons and trichloroethylene, may cause fatal cardiac arrhythmias. These chemicals are used in dry cleaning, degreasing, painting, and chemical manufacturing. Since most individuals are not exposed to high enough levels, workplace fatalities are few. Deaths occur much more commonly when sniffing the solvents recreationally.

Cobalt was suspected of causing an epidemic of death from cardiomyopathy in the 1960s, when it was used to stabilize the foam in beer. As soon as the mineral was removed from the beer these deaths stopped. Though cobalt is used in the production of metal alloys and drill bits, no similar death effect is seen in the workplace. Arsenic is used in smelters and in vineyard pesticides, and has also been known to contaminate beer. At the start of the twentieth century, an "arsenic epidemic'" among Manchester beer drinkers caused 6,000 people to develop cardiac problems and 70 to die.[19] Arsenic can cause ventricular fibrillation, so this may have been the mechanism of death, though it is not officially known to have caused the Manchester deaths.

One initially puzzling epidemic of chest pain and cardiac deaths at work occurred in 1950s munitions workers. Eventually physicians figured out its cause. While at work these people were exposed to nitrates.

The nitrate esters in the air dilated their blood vessels. Employees going home for the weekend started to suffer nitrate withdrawal. This led to coronary artery spasm, angina, myocardial infarction and even sudden death. This often occurred on Mondays, before they had a chance to inhale nitroglycerine again.

Most cardiac deaths are considered natural events, and only rarely is any attempt made to link them to a job. Statisticians have looked for an increase in cardiac deaths in various occupations, such as police officers, firefighters and players of American-style football. Right now, it has not been shown that these jobs cause an increased number of cardiac deaths.

Stress

A lot of people believe that people can work themselves to death, especially if they are workaholics. Over the past half century researchers have discovered that to be probably correct. One situation that is hard on the heart is described in Karasek's job strain model.[20] It deals with the common situation in which an employee's work is psychologically demanding but allows little ability to make any decision at all. When a worker is socially isolated this is more stressful. The Whitehall Study[21] concluded that exposure to jobs with high effort and low reward doubled the risk of heart disease. Jobs requiring constant vigilance, such as air traffic controllers, sea pilots and professional drivers, are also associated with cardiovascular disease. The more cardiovascular disease, the more deaths.

While the overwork problem has been little investigated in the Western world, governments in Asia, particularly in Japan, have been quite concerned about it for some time. In Japan 25% of the average "salarymen" work more than 60 hours a week. Their deaths at work are called *karoshi*. The cause of these deaths is usually a stroke or a heart attack. However, a number also commit suicide. Stress-induced workplace suicides also have a name — *karojisatsu*.

The International Labour Organization (ILO) has looked at Japan's *karoshi* problem and attributes the deaths to several factors.[22] One is long and excessive hours of work; a second is the failure to meet corporate goals. In Japan the social contract is that lifetime employment is provided in return for loyalty to the company. This social norm forms the basis for the country's rampant workaholism. When staff cutbacks are needed, long-term employees may be dismissed or forced to resign. Often, prior to their departure there is a period during which they are bullied. Being unemployed means a loss of face and, for men, even a lethal loss of masculinity. Japanese middle managers also commit suicide during corporate restructurings when torn between protecting their staff and laying off workers.

South Korea and China have a similar problem. In South Korea death by overwork is called *gwarosa.* Koreans used to work longer than did the Japanese — 68 hours per week. The resultant high number of deaths made the government decrease the maximum number of work hours per week to 52. The government apparently only enacted this decrease after discovering that it was losing many of its own employees to *gwarosa.*[23] In China, overwork death is called *gualosi.* Chinese businesspeople (usually men) need to develop networks and connections called *guanxi.* Networks include not only fellow businessmen but also powerful regional politicians and members of the Communist party. Forming these connections usually involves drinking in nightclubs every night. A lot of businessmen become alcoholics. While running a company, these men feel obligated not only to their own families, but also to their employees and their families. Sometimes when problems at work occur this becomes overwhelming. An overworked and alcoholic death may follow.[24]

Shift work also makes cardiovascular disease develop faster. In this context, *shift* usually means night work, but studies use varying definitions. Three possible links to disease and death have been put forward:

- The natural circadian rhythm is disrupted, and as a result the worker tends to eat more at night. This may lead to higher blood cholesterol levels than would otherwise be the case. Anginal pain and heart attacks are common in the early morning. Inadequate oxygen supply to the cardiac musculature triggers angina. When a job requires great cardiac effort in the middle of the night, angina may occur in a person with arteriosclerotic heart disease. Automobile workers used to call night shifts at the plant "widow makers."

- Shift work decreases the availability of social support. Most people are asleep while the shift worker is up and toiling. They perform their own jobs while the shift worker sleeps. This lifestyle risks developing coronary artery disease.
- Shift work also leads to unhealthy behaviours. Common ones are smoking and missing meals. Shift workers tend to develop excessive centrally deposited adipose tissue.

All three of the above are risk factors for coronary artery disease that can cause a cardiac death.

Neurological Disease

Neurological conditions caused by exposure to toxins at work are not usually fatal. Occasionally death does result from toxic encephalopathy that developed from exposure to a very high dose of pretty well any organic solvent. A toxic encephalopathy may start with a slight euphoria. In fatal cases it rapidly progresses to stupor, then coma, perhaps seizures, and finally death. The circumstance in which death occurs is usually an acute exposure to a toxin. Exposure is easily determined by speaking to coworkers and, in most countries, a very concerned ministry of labour inspector. Gases such as those used for anaesthetics, carbon monoxide, hydrogen sulphide and cyanide can also cause a fatal toxic encephalopathy when a person is exposed to them in high enough doses.

Kidney Disease

In the United States, 8.2% to 14.5% of deaths from chronic kidney disease was thought to be due to occupational exposure to agents that damaged the kidneys.[25] Silica, solvent and metal exposures were the most common causes. Family members of a person who worked in an industry where exposure to these products is common may raise work as a possible contributing factor to death. When they do, acknowledge it to be possible.

However, many other diseases end up in kidney failure. Particularly when one of these (such as diabetes) is present, a coroner should not report a possible workplace contribution to the death. Determining the precise cause of any workplace disease is the job of a Workers' Compensation tribunal. The coroner must describe and classify the cause of death. For example, if a man died of a mesothelioma, the coroner should give that as the cause of death and classify it as a natural occurrence. A Workers' Compensation Board or tribunal may attribute the origin of the disease the man's exposure to asbestos, given that he spent five years working at removing insulation 30 years before his death. The tribunal may further attribute responsibility for this to whoever was his employer at that time. Secondly, a coroner needs to look at the circumstances of the death to see whether anything done differently might have prevented it. When death is accidental and there are steps that could be taken to prevent future similar deaths, a coroner should highlight them in the report of the investigation.

However, if the cause of death is a disease rather than injuries from an accident, a coroner should be careful when reporting investigation findings. Any association known to exist between disease development and the work environment can be noted, but nothing more. Leave determination of any cause and effect relationship between the work environment and the fatal condition to the appropriate government labour ministry and adjudicative tribunal to deal with. That determination is not the coroner's to make.

NOTES

1 Tucker, S., & Keefe, A. (2018). *2018 Report on work fatality and injury rates in Canada.* https://www.uregina.ca/business/faculty-staff/faculty/file_download/2018-Report-on-Workplace-Fatalities-and-Injuries.pdf

2 Coroners Act R.S.O. 1990, CHAPTER C.37 Sec. 10(5).

3 Barton, A. (2014, January 15). And the top 10 most dangerous jobs are ....*The Globe and Mail.* https://www.theglobeandmail.com/life/the-hot-button/and-the-top-10-most-dangerous-jobs-are/article16352517/

4 U.S. Bureau of Labor Statistics. (2019, December 17). *Census of fatal occupational injuries news release. https://www.bls.gov/news.release/archives/cfoi_12172019.htm*

5 Young Power in Social Action. (n.d.). *Death trap!* http://www.shipbreakingbd.info/death_trap.html

6 Barss, P. (1984). Injuries due to falling coconuts. *Journal of Trauma: Injury, Infection, and Critical Care, 24*(11), 990–991.

7 Associated Press in New Delhi. (2017, August 1). More than 1,000 people killed in India as human and wildlife habitats collide. *The Guardian.* https://www.theguardian.com/environment/2017/aug/01/over-1000-people-killed-india-humans-wildlife-territories-meet

8 U.S. Bureau of Labor Statistics. (n.d.). *Rate of fatal injuries per 100,000 full-time equivalent workers by age group. https://www.bls.gov/charts/census-of-fatal-occupational-injuries/rate-of-fatal-work-injuries-per-100000-fte-by-age.htm*

9 Ontario Ministry of Labour, Training, and Skills Development. (2016, July 21). *New and young workers.* http:www.labour.gov.on.ca/english/hs/sawo/pubs/fs_youngworkers.php

10 U.S. Bureau of Labor Statistics. (2018, December 18). *Census of fatal occupational injuries news release. https://www.bls.gov/news.release/archives/cfoi_12182018.htm*

11 Workplace Safety and Insurance Board (WSIB) Ontario. *By the numbers: 2019 WSIB statistical report.* http://www.wsibstatistics.ca/

12 Gonzalez, G. (2019, January 9). Safety experts sound alarm on addiction-related workplace deaths. https://www.businessinsurance.com/article/20190109/NEWS08/912326038/Safety-experts-sound-alarm-on-addiction-related-workplace-deaths

13 See note 10 above.

14 Valent, F., McGwin, G., Bovenzi, M., & Barbone, F. (2002). Fatal work-related inhalation of harmful substances in the United States. *Chest, 121*(3), 969–975.

15 Electrical Safety Foundation International. (n.d.). *Workplace injury & fatality statistics. https://www.esfi.org/workplace-injury-and-fatality-statistics*

16 See note 10 above.

17 Health and Safety Executive. (2014). *Health and safety statistics: Annual report for Great Britain 2013/14.* https://www.hse.gov.uk/statistics/overall/hssh1314.pdf

18 World Health Organization (WHO). (n.d.). World malaria report 2020. https://www.who.int/teams/global-malaria-programme/reports/world-malaria-report-2020

19 Dyer, P. (2009). The 1900 arsenic poisoning epidemic. *Brewery History, 130,* 65–85.

20 Karasek, R. A., Jr. (1979). Job demands, job decision latitude, and mental strain: Implications for job redesign. *Administrative Science Quarterly, 24(2), 285–308.*

21 Marmot, M. G., Rose, G., Shipley, M., & Hamilton, P. J. (1978). Employment grade and coronary heart disease in British civil servants. *Journal of Epidemiology & Community Health, 32(4), 244–249. https://jech.bmj.com/content/32/4/244.short*

22 International Labour Organization. (2013, April 23). *Case study: Karoshi: Death from overwork.* https://www.ilo.org/global/topics/safety-and-health-at-work/resources-library/publications/WCMS_211571/lang--en/index.htm#:~:text=Karoshi%20is%20a%20Japanese%20word,been%20used%20since%20the%201970s.&text=The%20media%20have%20frequently%20used,important%20social%20problem%20in%20Japan

23 Haas, B. (2018, March 1). South Korea cuts "inhumanely long" 68-hour working week. *The Guardian.* https://www.theguardian.com/world/2018/mar/01/south-korea-cuts-inhumanely-long-68-hour-working-week

24 Osburg, J. (2013). *Anxious wealth: Money and mortality among China's new rich.* Stanford, CA: Stanford University Press, 141.

25 Sponholtz, T. R., Sandler, D. P., Parks, C. G., & Applebaum, K. M. (2015). Occupational exposures and chronic kidney disease: Possible associations with endotoxin and ultrafine particles. *American Journal of Industrial Medicine, 59*(1), 1–11.

18

Poisoning Deaths

There are too many poisons to talk about all of them. In fact, a large enough quantity of virtually any chemical will be poisonous. Most poisoning deaths that coroners investigate arise from street drugs, prescribed medications or chemicals manufactured for household or industrial use. These poisonous compounds have usually been taken to elicit a pleasurable sensation or to commit suicide. Russia and North Korea still poison people nowadays, but the use of poisoning as a political tool has declined dramatically since the days of the Borgias. Few coroners are ever involved with such a state-sanctioned death.

Prescription medications used in suicides have changed with time. Fifty years ago, barbiturates were widely prescribed sedatives. They soon became the most popular drug used by people to kill themselves. Nowadays barbiturates are so infrequently prescribed that they are generally unavailable and rarely cause any deaths.

Poisons can be swallowed, inhaled or absorbed through the skin. People using illicit drugs smoke them, sniff them, stuff them into their anuses (a process called buffing), or inject them. The poison usually finds its intended way into their veins but occasionally ends up in fat or muscle tissue instead. A poison becomes lethal when the amount in a person's bloodstream leads to some physiological change that stops an essential organ from working any more.

The amount required for a compound to become lethal is lower when a person consumes multiple drugs with similar effects on the body over a short period of time. The effect of a relatively small amount of a potentially life-threatening drug becomes fatal once amplified by others previously consumed or taken at the same time.

Opioids

Currently, fatal opioid overdoses are the most publicized type of poisonings. At one time, opioids were natural compounds derived from opium poppies. Nowadays many others are manufactured for recreational use by chemists working in underground laboratories throughout the world, especially in China. Commonly used medical opioids include opium, heroin, morphine, codeine, oxycodone, methadone, Dilaudid (hydromorphone or dihydromorphone), tramadol, buprenorphine (Suboxone in Canada) and fentanyl. Fentanyl in one of its many forms is currently responsible for most poisoning deaths.

Many, if not most, opioid poisoning deaths are accidental. Users purchase all sorts of illicit drugs from their local dealers. Since these compounds can also be bought online, sales competition is fierce. The illicit drug world lacks quality control. Users do not really know what they are consuming. Many vendors don't know what they are selling either, but dealers invariably assure purchasers that any drug they sell is pure. That is often untrue because a fentanyl compound has been added to the expected chemical being purchased. Its purpose is to deliver a more profound high. Fentanyl can be added to any drug. Alprazolam (Xanax) bought on the street nowadays has commonly been topped up with fentanyl.

Oxycodone

Opioids have long been used to treat severe pain caused by injuries and cancer. Oxycodone, which its maker Purdue Pharma branded as Percodan, worked quite well. However, it became a very popular drug and was heavily over-prescribed by physicians until it finally fell out of favour. Purdue's aggressive marketing strategy to doctors was extremely successful. While past generations of physicians had been taught to use the weakest strength of analgesic necessary to manage pain, Purdue emphasized the use of high doses of strong opioids to ensure the pain completely disappeared. Their marketing convinced the medical profession for a while that this practice was completely safe.

That message led to Percodan, its sister drug Percocet (with added acetaminophen or paracetamol), and its long-acting version Oxycontin becoming the drug of choice to manage virtually any type of pain. Tolerance to the effect of oxycodone as a pain reliever developed fairly rapidly. Higher doses became necessary to relieve pain, and more and more of the drug had to be prescribed. Some physicians turned into oxycodone or Oxycontin "mills" — they prescribed the drug in large quantities to people who resold it for recreational use. Abusers on the street crushed Oxycontin and injected or snorted the drug until the company produced a type of pill that prevented such abuse.

That change worked. Oxycodone deaths occur less frequently today than was the case a couple of decades ago, but the new formulation of oxycontin is not the only reason. Fentanyl has now replaced oxycodone as the most lethal opioid seen by North American coroners.

Methadone and buprenorphine (Suboxone) are dispensed to people to manage their opioid addiction, but these drugs can be abused too. Many of the opioid drugs that cause an opioid toxicity death are dispensed by a pharmacist filling a legitimate prescription. Some drug purchasers, even addicts, do not take their prescribed medications — they sell them instead. If asked where the opioid came from, do not speculate on its source unless you have located a prescription. Just explain the alternatives.

Opioids kill by depressing respiratory centres in the brain. High doses often kill very quickly, but at other times dying lasts for hours. Respiration slows. The user loses consciousness, possibly chokes, gurgles or snores, and then stops breathing. Death follows about five minutes later. Even when death comes slowly, users are unconscious most of the time. The one nice thing that can be said about an opioid overdose death is that it is painless.

Some first-time users die immediately, even though taking a "normal" dose of the drug. This is presumably due to individual sensitivity, but their deaths could be caused by an acute allergic reaction to the compound. Exactly why this happens will always remain a mystery. No ethics board would ever approve an experiment to study the matter.

Fentanyl

Fentanyl, widely used for pain relief in hospitals, is now the most common cause of fatal acute drug toxicity deaths that coroners investigate. It is a manufactured rather than a natural opioid, and it comes in many forms. The multiplicity of varieties makes testing for its presence in blood complicated. Innovative chemists who manufacture opioids in "underground" laboratories constantly change their structures, in fentanyl especially. The reason why is unclear. It may simply be to give the user a better high, for novelty, or perhaps to produce the drug more cheaply.

Two societal problems arise when the fentanyl structure changes. First of all, the drug's potency changes. Carfentanil is a type of fentanyl so powerful that veterinarians use it to manage pain in elephants. However, carfentanil is so toxic to humans that a small amount absorbed through the skin can make people very sick, if not kill them. Police officers tend to be very aware of this problem. New varieties of fentanyl can be more lethal than their predecessors.

The second problem is that the constant modifications of illicit drugs pose great challenges to forensic laboratories. A technique that successfully identifies and quantifies one type of fentanyl frequently cannot even detect a novel compound with a minor modification. Deaths from the consumption of a suspected fentanyl that is undetectable by testing lead toxicology chemists to search for some new chemical structure. Once the new drug is finally recognized, toxicologists set to work to develop a test for the compound. This is not always a rapid process. Perfecting a new test usually takes quite a bit of time.

To give an example of the problem's complexity, consider what Ontario faced in January 2018. The Centre for Forensic Science in Toronto notified Ontario coroners that it was looking at 44 opioid compounds. The Centre could detect 33 of these by screening methods. Chemists were able to quantify how much was in the body in 21 of these cases, but in 6 cases there was not even a name for the drug the Centre was trying to assess. These six drugs were simply described by letters and numbers.

If a person dies after consuming a type of fentanyl for which no test has yet been devised, the coroner will receive an inaccurate toxicology report. The coroner will still strongly suspect a drug toxicity death but be unable to prove it by toxicological testing. This situation leaves the coroner no alternative but to tell the relatives three things:

- A drug toxicity death is likely.
- Given the current limitations to toxicological testing, it is impossible to prove it.
- Therefore, the means of death will to have to be classified as "undetermined."

Rapid death happens in habituated drug users too once they develop pulmonary oedema. The fluid that builds up in their lungs in these sudden deaths causes dried froth to collect on the drug user's lip. This froth is visible whenever the body is discovered shortly after death. Why pulmonary oedema occurs is currently inexplicable.* All one can tell inquiring relatives is that pathologists do not yet know why pulmonary oedema occurs in habitual drug users, but they are working on it.

Anaesthetists and attendants at drug injection sites deal with another problem with fentanyl. Suddenly chest and jaw muscles become rigid — usually seconds or minutes after the drug enters the body but occasionally hours later. Spasm of the vocal cords prevents air from entering the chest. A minute later these people lose consciousness and five minutes later they die from what is referred to as "wooden chest syndrome."[1]

Heroin

Heroin is the strongest opiate the opium poppy (*Papaver somniferum*) produces. It can be smoked, snorted, swallowed, buffed and mainlined, but most deaths occur by intravenous injection. Most overdose deaths are found in experienced users rather than people trying the drug for the first time. People inject heroin in jail, but opportunities to do so

* Its failure to occur in first-time users suggests some sort of allergic response to repeated drug stimulus.

are sporadic; this makes heroin injection for the incarcerated a less than regular event. Most jailed heroin users' ability to tolerate the drug decreases while imprisoned.

This makes the days after their release very dangerous. Often the first thing on the mind of a newly released prisoner is to locate a source of heroin supply. The new-found freedom is celebrated by shooting up, an action that often has fatal consequences. A heroin dose that might have been easily tolerated before the person went to jail often becomes lethal upon the person's release.

Heroin is frequently only one of many drugs that have been taken either together or sequentially just before death. Heroin depresses the central nervous system quite quickly. Alcohol does too, but more slowly. Consuming both first slows breathing and then stops it completely. Heroin use with alcohol kills. Equally lethal is combining heroin with a benzodiazepine like Xanax.

People die of a heroin overdose relatively soon after taking the drug. Through that short dying period consciousness turns into coma where breathing slows gradually until it finally stops. The coroner can assure the relatives death was quite painless. People using heroin likely have no idea that they are dying.

Cocaine

Cocaine is another drug that has medical value but that users purchase "on the street" for recreational purposes. It causes death differently from opioid drugs. Cocaine triggers anxiety-producing cardiac arrhythmias that can be uncomfortable and sometimes fatal. Even when optimally managed in an emergency department, cocaine-induced arrhythmias do not always respond to either medical treatment or defibrillation.

Cocaine also stimulates the autonomic nervous system and raises blood pressure. Once the person is high, a cerebral artery aneurysm may rupture and cause a fatal stroke. Cocaine can end more lives than just that of the user. When a pregnant woman ingests cocaine, it may cause foetal death by tearing the placenta from the uterine wall. Without any more blood from the mother the foetus dies, aborting the pregnancy.

Cocaine can be taken in many forms. Chronic users sniff it so often that long-term users develop a hole in their nasal septa (the tissues separating nostrils). A popular rock form in which cocaine is abused is called *crack*, which can be sniffed, taken by mouth or injected. In India cocaine has been absorbed by urethral instillation, and Indian prostitutes insert cocaine vaginally.[2]

Rectal cocaine use has produced fatalities. Drug smugglers (also called *mules*) who have inserted condoms full of cocaine up their rectums to transport the drug across international boundaries sometimes have one rupture. This can be fatal for the drug mules, who are suddenly exposed to a high dose of cocaine speedily absorbed through their large intestines.

Doctors use cocaine to stop nose bleeds and occasionally as a local anaesthetic. People who die from cocaine toxicity rarely get the drug from a physician, though. Almost always it is purchased from an illicit street vendor.

Amphetamines

For years physicians have safely used amphetamines, in low doses, to treat attention deficit hyperactivity disorder (ADHD), narcolepsy, obesity, depression and chronic pain. As a result, much is known about this drug family's workings. Those interested and able to understand chemistry and physiology should read Wikipedia's thorough discourse on amphetamine's pharmacokinetics. It has everything anyone could want to know about how these drugs work.

That amphetamines enhance performance was a Second World War discovery. Since then people have repeatedly experimented with them. Students take amphetamines to stay awake so they can study late into the night. Truck drivers use amphetamines to improve their reaction times and stay awake when driving on long trips. Athletes find they increase muscle strength and endurance when competing. Males take amphetamines to improve penile erections and increase their desire for sexual intercourse. All these uses require dosages much higher than those doctors prescribe.

The effects of amphetamines vary with a person's state of health. A user who has heart disease risks death from myocardial infarction, cardiogenic shock and haemorrhagic strokes. Amphetamine overdose can result in suffocation from pulmonary oedema. Sometimes amphetamines trigger a psychosis. A person might jump off a cliff while under the delusion that it is possible to fly. Amphetamine-induced behaviours include virtually any imaginable dangerous act. Amphetamine toxicity can also lead to death from kidney failure when the drug stops urine production.[3] A coroner can only consider death arose from an amphetamine overdose upon receipt of a toxicologist's report finding an elevated blood level of the drug.

Ecstasy

For a couple of decades police have been aware of a type of amphetamine commonly used at "raves" that can be fatal. It is colloquially called ecstasy and currently has no medical use whatsoever. The drug may become useful if future experiments assessing its value in treating severe post-traumatic stress disorder pan out. Still, it will be some time before ecstasy can be sold by pharmacists, so the need for users to purchase the drug illicitly from a dealer will continue.

Ecstasy is a chemical named 3,4-methylenedioxymethamphetamine, which is usually shortened to MDMA. While this drug has been known about since 1912, and for a time was used in psychiatry, nowadays MDMA is always purchased illicitly.[4]

Street acquisition means that any drug purchased may not be pure MDMA. Manufacturers add some other compound, like ephedrine, to augment the hoped-for pleasurable sensations. These can be many, and include a generalized sense of well-being, happiness, self-confidence, empathy, closeness to others, relaxation, inner peace, enhanced sensory perceptions, boosted sexuality and an altered sense of time.[5] Sensations usually begin 30 to 60 minutes after taking the drug, peak at 75 to 120 minutes, and then plateau for 3.5 hours before fading in 4 to 6 hours.[6] MDMA is usually swallowed in pill form or snorted in powder form.

Exactly how death occurs in any case of MDMA use varies. Fatal vascular effects of MDMA arise from both intracranial bleeding from severe hypertension and from clotting throughout the body (disseminated intravascular coagulation) associated with low blood pressure.[7]

Death may also result from convulsions or cerebral oedema. These neurological causes of death can be accompanied by respiratory distress syndrome and a very high body temperature. Hallucinations caused by overdoses sometimes lead to accidental death. When an MDMA user's dead body is discovered without any information about what happened, an autopsy may fail to clearly explain how the drug killed the user. In that case all one can say is that death was due to drug use.

Ecstasy is popular, but few actually die from using the drug. The best estimate is that worldwide 21.3 million people took MDMA in 2017.[8] In England and Wales in 2019, only 78 people died from its abuse.[9] One can calculate the approximate number of ecstasy deaths expected in any country by dividing its population by that of England and Wales and multiplying by 78. Users believe that the drug is quite safe while coroners conclude the opposite. Coroners will undoubtedly be asked to investigate every death involving MDMA.

Other Street Drugs

LSD, lysergic acid diethylamide, may cause hallucinations leading to an accidental death. A person might die falling off a cliff while running from a large imaginary vampire bat. LSD will not kill by itself. Nor do "magic mushrooms" that contain the hallucinogenics psilocybin and pseiocin. Similarly, mescaline, a chemical that comes from a cactus, sometimes used to achieve similar sensations, will not kill people who ingest it.

Nor is marijuana or any cannabis-containing product, when simply taken by itself, lethal. "Angel dust", also known by PCP, the initials of its chemical constituent,* is another matter. It is often used in combination with other drugs, but PCP by itself has been reported to cause death when it raises the body temperature extremely high, causes heart failure or triggers an intracranial haemorrhage.

* 1-phenylcyclohexyl piperidine hydrochloride

Acetaminophen / Paracetamol

This ubiquitous drug, usually referred to in Canada by its brand name, Tylenol, has two different generic names – paracetamol or acetaminophen. Small amounts are safely used to relieve pain and diminish fevers. At recommended dosages Tylenol has virtually no side effects and is one of the blandest medications available. However, large quantities can be lethal.

Until governments recommended children stop taking aspirin because of its association with Reye's syndrome, most households treated pain and fevers with aspirin. In those days, many died from aspirin poisoning. Today death from aspirin overdose is so rare that most coroners will never investigate one. Paracetamol (or acetaminophen) overdose deaths are much more common.

Canada averaged only 68 fatal acetaminophen (Tylenol) poisonings each year between 2000 and 2011.[10] One wonders if Canadian Tylenol deaths are under-reported. Australia had 170 people die of paracetamol overdose in 2016 and it has little more than half Canada's population.[11] It is tricky to find good numbers of acetaminophen deaths for the United States (one FDA estimate was 458 deaths per year[12] averaged over a decade, which seems low) or the United Kingdom. A coroner will investigate all Tylenol poisoning deaths to determine whether they were accidental or suicides.

People die from acetaminophen poisoning by simply taking lots of Tylenol pills. Since it takes about 20 g of acetaminophen to kill someone, 40 or more extra strength (500 mg) tablets or at least 60 regular strength (325 mg) tablets have to be swallowed at once. Large people require more Tylenol than those who are smaller to achieve similar fatal effects. Far fewer pills may prove to be lethal when they are taken in combination with any other drug that affects the body in the same way.

Ingesting a lethal quantity of acetaminophen does not kill quickly. For a day or so after taking an overdose of Tylenol a person may feel nothing at all. Once the acetaminophen starts to damage the liver, fatigue, nausea, vomiting and abdominal pains start. Appetite disappears, and people start to feel generally unwell as their liver gradually stops functioning. Tylenol poisoning does not cause a loss of consciousness, though eventually mental confusion may occur when the liver failure gets bad enough. Death is slow — anywhere from three days to six weeks.[13]

Insulin

Death from insulin toxicity can happen accidentally, but insulin suicides and homicides are becoming increasingly common. Nurses seem to have chosen insulin as a painless way to kill patients or residents they have been looking after. The multiple deaths caused by Elizabeth Wettlaufer[14] in Canada and by Beverley Allitt[15] in Britain are well-publicized examples of this phenomenon.

Self-injected, therapeutic insulin usually only enters muscle or fat. With suicidal or homicidal intent, insulin is injected intravenously. Diabetics all know that if they begin to feel dizzy, confused, irritable, jittery, anxious, depressed; perspire profusely; or note their heart beating rapidly, they have taken too much insulin and need to quickly consume sugar to counteract it.

These symptoms probably occur in fatal insulin overdoses too. If the fatal dose of insulin is administered intravenously in a high enough amount, these sensations probably do not last very long. Someone who is not diabetic will not understand the significance of what is going on. Consciousness quickly disappears, and death is painless.

A coroner can also tell relatives that pathologists and toxicologists have their work cut out for them in these cases because while it is possible to detect insulin derived from animals, it is not possible to detect human insulin. Pathologists derive most valuable glucose levels from the vitreous humour, the jelly-like liquid behind the lens in the eye. Rapid tissue decomposition after death makes blood and other tissues valueless for determining whether death was due to insulin toxicity.

Ethylene Glycol

Another common method of poisoning in countries that experience cold winters comes from the ingestion of ethylene glycol, an antifreeze solution for automobiles. The chemical is also used in some solvents, so ethylene glycol is easily available all around the world, even in the tropics. Alcoholics who have got to the stage of drinking anything they can get their hands on sometimes consume ethylene glycol and die.

Quite often the chemical is used to commit suicide. It does not take much. Perhaps 225 mL may be enough for an 80 kg (176 lbs.) adult.[16] Anyone drinking ethylene glycol feels the same symptoms of drunkenness that ethyl alcohol produces. However, the drunk feeling disappears quite rapidly. Convulsions may precede the stupor that sets in and finally turns into a terminal coma lasting less than a day.

A coroner speaking to relatives can analogize the symptoms of an ethylene glycol death to simple drunkenness. Relatives will then interpret the coroner's comments in that light. Most will decide that, all things considered, their deceased relative did not suffer too much.

Corrosive Poisons

Hundreds of years ago in developed countries, many poisoning deaths — usually suicides — occurred from people swallowing strong acid or alkali solutions. Now that there are many less painful lethal compounds easily available, fewer people die such horrible deaths. Third World coroners still investigate these deaths though. In India in 2012, for example, 200,000 people died from ingesting corrosives.[17] Corrosive liquids in the home and factories include battery acid, descalers, metal cleaners, rust removers, bleach, lye, toilet bowl cleaners and drain cleaners. All are potentially lethal when swallowed.

Drinking acid or alkali causes severe pain along the length of the gastrointestinal tract. Ingested chemicals react with any tissue they touch, initially causing a chemical burn and terminally perforating the gastrointestinal tract, usually in the oesophagus or stomach. When aspirated the chemical makes tracheal or bronchial tissues bleed. Lung irritation develops into pulmonary oedema and suffocation. Survival for more than a day often leads to a fatal pneumonia ending the pain. Without hospitalization and sedation, life may continue for several very painful days.

A perforated oesophagus allows the contents of the gastrointestinal tract to flow into the surrounding area of the chest. A painful inflammatory condition called mediastinitis develops and makes breathing increasingly difficult until death finally stops it.

Whatever is in a perforated stomach flows into the abdomen's cavity, inflaming its lining, the peritoneum, and causing severe abdominal pain. Untreated, death follows in a couple of days.

Agricultural Chemicals

Farmers around the world have benefited from chemicals that kill insects and weeds to produce better harvests. Developed countries carefully control these chemicals. Developing countries have less strict rules, which results in many fatal ingestions of these chemicals. In Sri Lanka from 1975 to 1980, 1,000 people a year died from acute pesticide poisoning. In 2011 there were 1,757 pesticide deaths comprising 46.6% of all Sri Lankan suicides that year.[18]

Sri Lanka is not the only place where people choose to kill themselves with pesticides. Many Asians use them to commit suicide. From 2002 to 2009, pesticide ingestion was the third most common method of Taiwanese suicide. In Samoa and southern Trinidad, some 70% of suicides are reportedly due to ingesting paraquat.[19]

Paraquat is an excellent herbicide that kills weeds throughout the world. Only about 5% of it is absorbed when drunk orally, but the chemical is so toxic that a mouthful, perhaps 10 mL, will be lethal.[20] Unsuspecting people have been known to die after mistakenly drinking paraquat decanted into a bottle. Paraquat irritates any tissue it touches. The mouth mucous membranes and tongue burn the moment any enters the mouth. Any paraquat aspirated into the lungs causes bleeding, pulmonary oedema and death within a couple of weeks.

Paraquat absorbed through the gastrointestinal tract leads to liver necrosis and death from progressive renal failure. These slow painful deaths usually occur in hospital in most developed countries. European, North American and Australasian coroners are unlikely to ever investigate a paraquat death, however.

Organophosphorus pesticides are also widely used around the world. Parathion is the most toxic chemical among them, but malathion and dichlorvos are lethal too. These chemicals all kill insects by interfering with their ability to produce the enzyme cholinesterase.

Humans need cholinesterase to break up an essential neurotransmitter called acetylcholine. Once a person ingests a product that causes serum cholinesterase to decrease by more than 70%, acetylcholine builds up in nerves' neurotransmitter sites. At this point the person starts to feel depressed, lacks motivation, has difficulty concentrating, and becomes tired, confused and forgetful.

The chemicals make people feel hopeless and irritable. They cause rumination, trigger headaches and cause blurry vision. After chemical ingestion people belch, fart, feel nauseated, have diarrhoea; alternatively, they become constipated and their bellies bloat. Muscles become sore, weaken or twitch. Nerves tingle. Hands or feet may become cold. Bladder control disappears. Death can occur within an hour of swallowing paraquat, but usually it takes several hours to days.

Sarin

Another synthetic organophosphorus compound is sarin, a colourless, odourless liquid that all coroners hope to avoid. Sarin is not a pesticide but a highly volatile gas that is used as a weapon. The 1993 Chemical Weapons Convention[21] banned sarin production and stockpiling. Since then the world learned that Iraq definitely had it, and several other governments probably have covert supplies of the gas stashed away somewhere. Sarin is a tool for terrorists too. The most famous recent terrorist use of sarin in gaseous form was the Japanese subway attack in 1995.[22]

Sarin kills the same way parathion does but much more quickly. Death can follow just 10 minutes of inhalation. The nose of a person inhaling it starts to run. The chest tightens. Pupils constrict. Vision blurs. Drawing a breath becomes hard. Drooling starts. Waves of nausea are followed by vomiting, defecation and finally loss of control of all bodily functions. Muscles start to twitch and jerk before turning into terminal convulsive body spasms.*

A coroner unlucky enough to be involved in a sarin poisoning shortly after it happens must be very careful. Any clothing on the bodies will have absorbed some of the gas, so it can continue to expose people to sarin for another half an hour. Protective gear must be worn

* Death results from a combination of two processes: increased mucus production in the bronchial tree blocks air entry into the lungs, and airway spasm narrows the diameter of the bronchial tubes through which air flows. The decreased air flow leads to a period of unconsciousness before breathing finally stops.

when coming near the body of a person who died from sarin poisoning. The gas can penetrate the skin, so every bit of the coroner's body has to be completely covered.

Historic Poisons

History and literature are full of poisons that still exist but have fallen so much out of use for suicides that they cause death rarely nowadays. The hemlock Socrates poisoned himself with two and a half millennia ago is an example. Since nobody appears to have recorded Socrates's death agonies, we can all hope the sage died quite quickly from respiratory paralysis after his muscle tissues broke down and his kidneys failed. These unpleasant effects only occasionally arise from hemlock poisonings nowadays. The average coroner will never investigate one.

Strychnine was a popular poison in the nineteenth and twentieth centuries, when it was easily obtainable for the purpose of killing rats. Now strychnine has become generally unavailable to prevent its use as a poison. A fatal strychnine poisoning was quite horrible. Shortly after ingestion severe convulsive spasms of all the muscles in the body would begin. Eventually strychnine paralysed the nerves supplying the lungs. Death eventually arose from asphyxia. Strychnine is still made, but the difficulty in obtaining any makes it unlikely a coroner will investigate a strychnine poisoning death.

In the 1940s, arsenic poisoning came to the attention of the moviegoing public in the film *Arsenic and Old Lace.* Arsenic was indeed a type of poisoning once used by criminals. A death from arsenic is unlikely nowadays. Arsenic poisoning usually was the result of repeated ingestion of small amounts of the chemical. Swallowing a large amount of arsenic would have been foul. People usually spit any liquid containing arsenic out of their mouths, but not always. There is quite an extensive history of women successfully poisoning food and drink they offered to their husbands, members of their families and others in order to achieve some financial benefit. One of the earliest arsenic poisoners on record was Giulia Tofana, who died in Rome in 1659.

Repeated arsenic ingestion causes people to lose hair, become nauseated, have recurrent diarrhoea, develop headaches and feel drowsy.

At the end they become comatose and may terminally convulse while dying. Arsenic is found in water in many areas of the world. An accidental accumulation of large amounts of water-borne arsenic could theoretically cause accidental death. Most arsenic deaths investigated by coroners are due to deliberate poisoning.

Cyanide

Cyanide has long been known to be poisonous. It is found in the smoke of burning polymers that are fatal in a high enough concentration. The Zyklon B gas used in Nazi death camp extermination chambers during the Second World War was cyanide. However, the chemical was used on both sides. Allied commandos sent to destroy the Vemork heavy water plant in 1943 were given cyanide pills with rubber coating. Their instructions were to bite into them if captured. Death was then expected to occur within three minutes.

People inhaling cyanide experience headaches, dizziness, convulsions and shortness of breath when pulmonary oedema develops during the minute or less before they lose consciousness. Cyanide poisoning is always a possibility for coroners to consider, but the odds of any coroner ever investigating a cyanide poisoning death are very low.

Russian Poisons

Russians have a history of poisoning that goes back at least as far as Rasputin. In the past century the Russian state has deployed several poisons to kill suspected turncoats. Coroners in jurisdictions where Russian exiles live may become involved with deaths due to Russian state-sponsored poisoning. Otherwise these deaths will simply be items of professional interest. The Russian armamentarium of poisons seems vast, so there is no certainty that a new poisoning will look anything like its predecessors.

Since the Second World War, Soviet and subsequent Russian governments have imaginatively killed people using several different poisons. One case that fascinated the public in 1978 involved an agent killing Georgi Markov, a Bulgarian playwright and defector, while waiting for a bus on Waterloo Bridge in London.[23] A projectile from an umbrella that had been laced with ricin penetrated the skin of one of his legs; he died four days later.

Ricin

Ricin is a poison made from the castor bean. It is usually only fatal when inhaled or if the poison enters the bloodstream. Eating or drinking ricin irritates the gut. About 10 hours after ingestion, the person vomits and has bloody diarrhoea. A drop in blood pressure and fainting follows. Seizures start. Death follows one or two days later. Ricin is said to be fatal as early as four hours after inhalation, but (supposedly) always by 24.* However, Georgi Markov managed to continue living for four days after the chemical entered his bloodstream.

Gelsemium

Russian and Chinese contract killers as well as the Russian government have often used gelsemium, the chemical extracted from "heartbreak grass", an Asian plant, to assassinate their victims. After eating or drinking the chemical a person becomes weak, dizzy, nauseated and may convulse before dying. Gelsemium blocks transmission at the neuromuscular junctions that cause respiratory failure and death in as few as 30 minutes.

Polonium

Polonium-210 is a radioactive element extracted from uranium ore. Aleksander Litvinenko was offered tea poisoned with polonium in 2006. Litvinenko developed the symptoms of acute radiation sickness. He died three weeks after exposure to the element.[24] He may be the only person (or at least one of very few) ever assassinated by polonium. A coroner investigating another polonium poisoning death is unlikely, but possible.

Novichok

In one of their latest assassination attempts, Russians tried to kill a double agent and his daughter at Amesbury in the United Kingdom[25] using Novichok, a chemical that is an acetylcholinesterase inhibitor

* Ricin prevents cells from making proteins. Death occurs cell by cell. Life usually ends with congestive heart failure and shock.

like the organophosphates previously mentioned. Novichok causes headaches, nausea, vomiting, dizziness and confusion before it renders a person unconscious. Death results when transmission blockage at neuromuscular junctions causes asphyxia or heart failure.

The Russian agents were unsuccessful in killing their intended targets, but they did kill a woman who had picked up and sprayed herself with a discarded perfume bottle containing the agent. Novichok may be the most powerful nerve gas developed so far. Coroners need to be aware that it exists. Novichok may be deployed again in future.*

Thallium

Thallium is a metal derived from ores. It has been known to be poisonous for more than a century, and it is thought to be on Russia's current list of useful poisons. If a Russian dissident's death is the subject of investigation a coroner must consider thallium poisoning a possible cause. Russia is not the only state historically to have used thallium this way. France, Rhodesia (now Zimbabwe), East Germany and Iraq are all known to have poisoned people with thallium. Though very toxic in high doses, thallium has medical value in small doses. As a poison it acts slowly and mimics many other illnesses. Fatal doses of thallium can be ingested, inhaled and even absorbed through the skin.

The drug affects many organs, which causes many different symptoms. First come indigestion, nausea, vomiting and burning sensations in the hands or feet. Thallium's pathway to death progresses through delirium, hallucinations and convulsions, ending in a terminal comatose state. Low non-lethal doses of thallium cause hair loss. This takes two to three weeks to occur, so quick thallium death will not be accompanied by baldness.

As thallium toxicity worsens people develop nausea and diarrhoea. Their mouths become sore, their legs and skin burn, lines develop on their nails, and their skin atrophies. Since the chemical affects the heart, liver, kidneys and bone marrow, and has been associated with subarachnoid haemorrhages in the brain, practically any painful symptom that one could imagine has been associated with thallium poisoning.

---

* A loose translation of *Novichok* is "new kid on the block."

Thallium used to be a very effective rat poison but, in most places, it is no longer available. Any thallium poisoning cases a coroner might investigate nowadays will probably be intentional. The person poisoned will likely have received a high dose and have died quickly.

NOTES

1 Torralva, R., & Janowsky, A. (2019). Noradrenergic mechanisms in fentanyl-mediated rapid death explain failure of naloxone in the opioid crisis. *Journal of Pharmacology and Experimental Therapeutics 371*(2), 453–475.

2 Chopra, I. C., & Chopra, Sir R. N. (1958). *The cocaine problem in India.* https://www.unodc.org/unodc/en/data-and-analysis/bulletin/bulletin_1958-01-01_2_page005.html

3 Vasan, S., & Olango, G. (2017). *Amphetamine toxicity.* Treasure Island (FL): StatPearls.

4 Freudenmann, R. W., Oxler, F., & Bernschneider-Reif, S. (2006). The origin of MDMA (ecstasy) revisited: The true story reconstructed from the original documents. *Addiction, 101*(9), 1241–1245.

5 Merle Gordon, S. (2001, July 5). What are the effects of the drug ecstasy? *Scientific American.*

6 Liechti, M. E., Gamma, A., & Vollenweider, F. X. (2001). Gender differences in the subjective effects of MDMA. *Psychopharmacology, 154, 161–168.*

7 DrugWise. (2017). *Why do people die after taking ecstasy?* https://www.drugwise.org.uk/why-do-people-die-after-taking-ecstasy/

8 United Nations Office on Drugs and Crime. (n.d.). *Annual prevalence of the use of drugs by region and globally. https://dataunodc.un.org/drugs/prevalence_regional-2017#ecstasy*

9 Stewart, Conor. (2020). Death from use of MDMA/ecstasy in England and Wales 1993–2019. *Statista.* https://www.statista.com/statistics/470824/drug-poisoning-deaths-mdma-ecstasy-in-england-and-wales/

10 Yang, J., & Cribb, R. (2015, September 17). What you haven't been told about acetaminophen. *Toronto Star.* https://www.thestar.com/life/health_wellness/2015/09/17/up-to-68-canadians-on-average-die-from-acetaminophen-annually.html

11 Australian Bureau of Statistics. (2016). *Drug induced deaths in Australia: A changing story.* https://www.abs.gov.au/ausstats/abs@.nsf/Lookup/by%20Subject/3303.0~2016~Main%20Features~Drug%20Induced%20Deaths%20in%20Australia~6

12 Lee, W. M. (2004). Acetaminophen and the US acute liver failure study group: Lowering the risks of hepatic failure. *Hepatology, 40*(1), 6–9.

13 Proudfoot, A. T., & Wright, N. (1970). Acute paracetamol poisoning. *British Medical Journal, 3*(5722), 557.

14 Ferguson, R. (2017, June 26). Case of killer nurse Elizabeth Wettlaufer to be subject of public inquiry. *Toronto Star.* https://www.thestar.com/news/queenspark/2017/06/26/case-of-killer-nurse-elizabeth-wettlaufer-to-be-subject-of-public-inquiry.html

15 Batty, D. (2007, December 6). "Serial killer nurse Allitt must serve 30 years. The Guardian. https://www.theguardian.com/uk/2007/dec/06/ukcrime.health

16 Brent, J. (2001). Current management of ethylene glycol poisoning. *Drugs, 61*(7): 979–988.

17 Anthony, L., & Kulkarni, C. (2012). Patterns of poisoning and drug overdosage and their outcome among in-patients admitted to the emergency medicine department of a tertiary care hospital. *Indian Journal of Critical Care Medicine, 16*(3), 130–135.

18 Knipe, D. W., Padmanathan, P., Muthuwatta, L. Metcalfe, C., & Gunnell, D. (2017). Regional variation in suicide rates in Sri Lanka between 1955 and 2011: A spatial and temporal analysis. *BMC Public Health, 17*, 193. https://bmcpublichealth.biomedcentral.com/articles/10.1186/s12889-016-3961-5

19 Pestizid Aktions-Netzwerk e.V. (PAN Germany). (2003). *Paraquat and suicide.* http://www.pan-germany.org/download/fact_paraquat2.pdf

20 Krieger, R. (Ed.). (2010). *Hayes' handbook of pesticide toxicology* (3rd ed.). Elsevier.

21 Organisation for the Prohibition of Chemical Weapons (OPCW). (1997, April 29.) *Convention on the prohibition of the development, production, stockpiling and use of chemical weapons and on their destruction.*

22 Pangi, R. (2002). Consequence management in the 1995 sarin attacks on the Japanese subway system. *Studies in Conflict and Terrorism, 25*(6), 421–448.

23 Mackie, L., & Andrews, J. (1978, September 12). Defector's mystery death. *The Guardian.* https://www.theguardian.com/world/from-the-archive-blog/2020/sep/09/georgi-markov-killed-poisoned-umbrella-london-1978

24 Nathwani, A. C., Down, J. F., Goldstone, J., Yassin, J., Dargan, P., Virchis, A., . . . Harrison, J. D. (2016). Polonium-210 poisoning: A first-hand account. *The Lancet, 388*(10049), 1075–1080.

25 Dodd, V., Harding, L., & MacAskill, E. (2018, March 8). Sergei Skripal: Former Russian spy poisoned with nerve agent, say police. *The Guardian.* https://www.theguardian.com/uk-news/2018/mar/07/russian-spy-police-appeal-for-witnesses-as-cobra-meeting-takes-place

19

Deaths in Custody

Taking people into custody does not occupy much of the average police officer's day. Detectives on television always seem to arrest at least one person every hour. That is far from reality. One police officer described herself to me as an armed social worker who spent most of her time typing reports on her cruiser's computer. On the site of a death investigation, coroners frequently arrive to find police officers, jointly investigating the death, doing their best to console one or more of the dead person's relatives. This type of work and bureaucratic tasks in both car and office occupy a far greater part of a police officer's day than does making arrests.

The responsibility of police who arrive at a death scene is to determine whether it resulted from a crime. Most deaths do not. Once a doctor appears to formally pronounce the person dead and sign a death certificate the police can leave. If no doctor is coming, or if the death seems unnatural, even though not the result of criminal activity, police roles and responsibilities vary in differing jurisdictions. Many will operate in a fashion similar to Ontario, where investigating officers switch their figurative hats (Ontario police usually don't wear hats anymore except at funerals) after they have determined that no crime has been committed. One officer then assumes the role of coroner's constable to assist the coroner to complete the ongoing coronial investigation. This is the common way coroners interact with police officers.

Less commonly, arrests trigger interaction between a coroner and the police. Any death that occurs throughout the legal process following an arrest needs to be investigated by a coroner. This chapter reviews the different types of death occurring in the various venues in which arrested people find themselves as the legal process unfolds.

During Arrest

Most arrests go smoothly. Some suspects even voluntarily surrender themselves at the police station. Police chiefs and police officers all hope for uneventful arrests but understand that many will be anything but. People commonly resist arresting officers, and this resistance is sometimes fatal. Coroners investigate deaths that occur during an arrest. It's arguable those people die while not yet in police custody because they die while still fighting arrest.

Custody requires that a person be brought under police control. Some agencies keep a single count of the number of people who die during or shortly after arrest. That makes it very difficult to determine at what stage of the arrest process a death occurred. To thoroughly deal with death while in custody, consider custody to include the process of being arrested or detained before control over the suspect is actually achieved.

Arresting an unwilling person is dangerous for both police officer and the person being arrested. This danger takes different forms. Strong males unwilling to submit to arrest probably constitute the largest group likely to hurt or kill a police officer. These men only occasionally die during the course of an arrest. Armed resisters, also usually men, form a second group who die while being arrested. Their deaths commonly result from pointing a gun at the arresting officer, firing it, or lunging at the officer with a knife. Two other groups of people whose deaths during arrests coroners commonly investigate are the mentally ill and addicts who are high on drugs.

All these groups of people have something in common. They act violently and frighten, if not terrify, police officers. Nowadays police are usually armed. Their weapons include batons, stun guns that shock (like Tasers) and, of course, guns loaded with metal, or sometimes rubber, bullets. From media reports one might conclude that shooting suspects during arrests is common, and the police see it as simply part of the job. In most parts of the developed world these shootings are so unusual that none go unreported. Perhaps an occasional cop considers these shootings are just part of the job, but that's really "fake news." Most police officers never even fire their guns in the line of duty let alone actually shoot someone. Every firearm discharge makes the officer with the smoking gun anxious.

Obviously, the relatives of anyone killed during an arrest will be terribly upset and angry. The police are almost equally disturbed. Coroners who speak to police officers shortly after someone has been killed during an attempted arrest find them all stunned and upset. Shootings are traumatic for the police officers as well as for the victim's family. Officers are all aware of the paperwork, questioning and stress that will accompany their force's ensuing internal investigation.

But that's not the real reason these officers feel terrible. First, they never intended to kill the suspect — they just wanted to arrest him. Death was totally unexpected. Secondly, just like everybody else, police officers feel remorseful when they kill somebody. Deaths during an arrest are uncommon, but they do happen. The death upsets all police officers involved in the arrest, but the most remorseful is the one who killed the suspect.

Police are repeatedly reminded about the proper use of escalating levels of force needed to make an arrest. Every police department has a variation of the wheel of escalating force (see Figure 19.1) to depict what police officers are taught about how to arrest a person. The arrest process starts by instructing a suspect to submit. Most people do. Deaths rarely occur when no force is required to make an arrest. A person with severe heart disease might experience a fatal ventricular

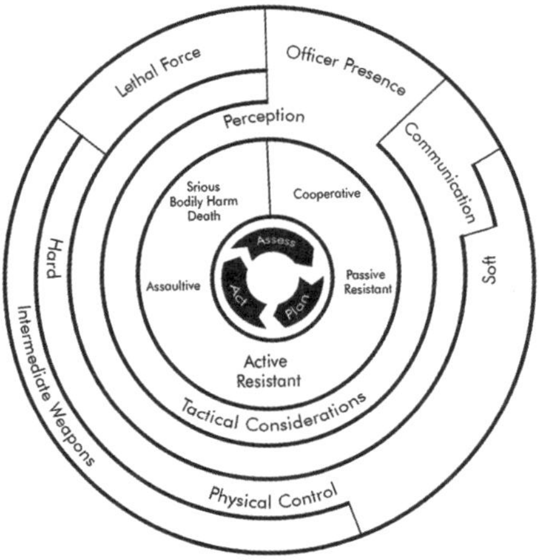

Figure 19.1: The wheel of escalating force

fibrillation if overstressed by an unexpected arrest. Otherwise, it is hard to see how the simple request to submit to arrest could be lethal.

Physical force is another matter. A police officer's appropriate application of physical force sometimes results in death during especially combative arrests. The person being arrested may simply be obnoxious and pugnacious. Many are also intoxicated by alcohol. "Fighting drunks" have been known to die while being arrested. The mentally ill are always at danger of dying during an arrest when arresting officers perceive them (quite often correctly) to be irrational and dangerous. A final group of people who die resisting arrest are high on drugs.

Force can be fatal when it causes head injuries. Police batons, fists and feet have all delivered lethal blows to the skull while trying to bring an unwilling suspect into custody. Sometimes death results from a head striking a wall, floor or any hard object during the process of being subdued. People have also been suffocated when arresting officers sit on their chests or kneel on their necks. When violent people — psychotic or high on drugs — flail around, throwing furniture off apartment balconies or destroying interior furnishings, multiple police officers may need to lie across their bodies or sit on them to subdue their frenzy enough to gain control. In North America these people are said to be in the grips of "excited delirium."[1]

The widely publicized death of George Floyd in the United States in 2020 made the world aware of the danger of a police officer kneeling on a suspect's neck. This is not the only way application of force to the neck during an arrest can be lethal. Two types of chokeholds, improperly applied, can be fatal. Side-of-neck pressure can compress the carotid arteries. Front-of-neck pressure compresses the windpipe and, when fatal, often breaks the larynx. Martial arts practitioners are taught how to use these holds safely. To avoid possible deaths, many police forces simply instruct their officers not to apply any pressure to the neck during an arrest.[2]

To bring people in the throes of excited delirium under control, police officers have to sit or lie on them. Police only dismount a suspect's body once they are finally able to handcuff both of the person's hands together. When this can't be done quickly, the officer's weight on the suspect's chest and abdomen makes breathing increasingly difficult. The man (almost always) is usually lying face down, so his breathing is not easily visible to the arresting officer. Should it stop, if not immediately noticed, asphyxiation follows. Pathologists attribute this type of death to asphyxia caused by compression, a subject dealt with more thoroughly in Chapter 3, Respiratory Deaths.

The third level of force available to a police officer attempting to make an arrest is the stun gun. Its use always carries the risk of death. When the Taser was first invented it seemed quite safe. The weapon simply delivered enough shock that police could quickly subdue a suspect. However, the passage of time has shown that, in some unlucky people, the Taser induces a fatal cardiac arrhythmia. Though Taser deaths are infrequent, they do happen and often are videotaped.

When Tasers won't work to subdue a suspect, police can fire projectiles, some of which are lethal. Police load pistols with real ammunition for their own protection. Rubber or plastic bullets that are not meant to be lethal are usually issued only for riot control. Rubber bullets are not used to make an arrest – just to disperse an unruly crowd. Real bullets are the usual way a police officer uses lethal force. A bullet is only supposed to be fired when a police officer is frightened for his/her own life or needs to protect somebody else's.

Recent widely shared American videos show police officers shooting suspects walking or running away who pose no danger to the officers firing the guns. These actions seem blameworthy, but the reasons for them do not concern a coroner. Blame is a subject for a police force's senior officers and the courts. Whenever an officer kills a person during an arrest, the coroner simply categorizes the death as a homicide. The question of whether the homicide is justifiable or culpable is a decision that will be made by others.

One other way people commonly die during the arrest process results from the police chasing them. A chase involving cars can end in a fatal crash. The suspect's death occurs in the same way as it would in any other fatal collision. Should the car leave the road to end up in a body of water, death occurs in the same way as any drowning. When cars, or even people, being chased on foot end up falling over a cliff or off a raised highway, the mechanism of dying resembles that experienced by anyone falling from a similar height.

Custody really only starts when a person is physically controlled by a police officer or when handcuffs have been snapped onto a suspect's wrists. Nothing fatal usually happens in the next few stages of the arrest process. Once arrested, people are usually safely transported to the police station to be photographed, fingerprinted and then charged before being led off to the cells. During this time, it is possible for a person to die naturally from a heart attack. It is also possible for a suspect to die unnaturally from a bag of illicit drugs they swallowed, or when a condom full of an opiate they stuffed up their anus bursts in the colon, but this is very unusual. Only once jailed are deaths more likely to happen.

In the Police Cells

There are three ways people die in police cells. Most commonly it's from some natural cause, like a heart attack. Not everybody arrested is a fit, healthy 18 year old. Many much older, unhealthy people are detained for all sorts of criminal misbehaviour. It is simply their lot to die in a jail cell rather than somewhere else of no medico-legal concern at all.

A second group is people who consumed alcohol or used an illicit drug before being arrested and jailed. Arresting officers are trained to take anyone they suspect might be impaired by alcohol or drugs to be checked out at a hospital to ensure safe incarceration. This process is not flawless. Sometimes the person may have abused some substance and yet does not seem impaired in any way. That means jail without medical assessment. At other times, a physician clears a suspect as safe to be jailed, but this turns out not to be the case.

In either situation, after being lodged behind bars, a lethal event happens. An intoxicated person may lie down on a bed in the cell and go to sleep. At some point breathing ceases. Most modern cells have some form of electronic surveillance. In older jails the jailer regularly checks all inmates at predetermined times, both during the day and at night. The state an inmate inflicted on himself by ingesting drugs or alcohol is always the prime reason for his death in a police cell. But there is a contributing factor — the boredom of a jailer's job.

Some jailers sit in an office and periodically leave to check on inmates, say every 15 to 30 minutes. Others sit hour after hour staring at an array of monitor screens looking at people who show very little movement much of the time. Either way, this is very boring work. At night especially, tired jailers sometimes fall asleep. Even during the day, it is quite easy for a jailer to drift off when there is nothing to look at beyond grey pictures of the inside of a cell with a person lying on a bunk. The video allows anyone watching to try to ascertain that an inmate is still breathing, but the officer needs to be wide awake to do so.

Exactly when a sleeping person stops breathing is not that easy to discern even when the observer is alert. Only five minutes or so without respirations will be lethal. It may take longer than five minutes for a jailer to realize that breathing has stopped. Ontario requires that an inquest be held into every cell death, and in inquests over which I have presided, the inmate has always been discovered to be dead when checked up on.

People jailed in police cells also hang themselves. Nobody ever knows the reason why. Undoubtedly, distress occasioned by finding themselves in jail plays a role. To hang themselves, potential suicides usually shred their clothes or bedsheets to be used as ligatures. They always seem able to find some point in any cell from which they can suspend themselves. It only takes a few minutes for them to fatally asphyxiate themselves.

These are the most common means by which people die in police cells, but other, very unusual, ways are possible. One cell occupant might assault and kill another. This must happen occasionally, and when it does criminal charges are laid. The coroner's role in its investigation is likely minor. In older jails where opportunities to escape exist, a prisoner might die in an attempt to get out. That death would be accidental, and the coroner's role in the death investigation would probably be significant. Similarly, if an explosion produces fatal toxic gases or cause part of a cell to fatally crush a prisoner, the coroner will be very much involved.

In Prisons

Most people convicted of a serious crime are sent to prison. In many jurisdictions, the type of jail differs depending on the length of the sentence. In Canada, incarceration facilities change when a sentence is two years or more. Inmates jailed for a sentence lasting two years or less are the responsibility of a province. Incarcerations for longer than that take place in federal institutions, which are referred to as penitentiaries. Both short- and long-term institutional inmates die in the same ways. Penitentiaries have more natural deaths than do provincial prisons because there are many more elderly penitentiary inmates. Prisoners incarcerated for life terms age and die within their prison walls in the same manner as if living outside.

Because the United States has such a huge prison population, its statistics probably provide the best understanding of the ways people die in jail. Roughly 90% of all deaths in American jails arise from natural causes. The five most common conditions that killed American prisoners, in descending order of importance, were cancer, heart disease, liver disease, AIDS–related illness, and respiratory disease. Suicide accounted for 6% of prison deaths, homicide accounted for 2% of deaths, and drug and alcohol intoxication and accidents resulted in 1% each.[3]

Far fewer people are jailed in Canada. The Canadian Correctional Investigator issues an annual report reviewing the operations of federal penitentiaries. In the 2016–17, the investigator looked at the 47 deaths that occurred in penitentiaries across the country. Thirty-seven inmates died of natural causes, three committed suicide, one accidentally died of a drug overdose and there was one homicide. The ratio of causes was quite similar to that in the United States.[4]

My experience refutes the current judicial view that prisons are educational and rehabilitation institutions. The many Ontario coroners' inquests into penitentiary deaths over which I have presided led juries to understand that prisons are violent places, rife with drugs and illicitly manufactured alcohol. Ontario's jails are spartan and unattractive. Inmates' next-door neighbours are not very nice people.

An inmate's daily routine is tedious and stultifying. Inmates routinely ignore the well-intentioned educational programs correctional staff provide in the hope of bettering the inmates' lives once they are released. As a result, expectations from these programs are very low. Success is considered to be getting an inmate to attend all classes rather than having the course change some aspect of his behaviour. Jails in other jurisdictions may differ, but probably not very much.

This unpleasant environment explains some prison deaths. First there is homicide. A penitentiary population contains a higher percentage of killers than any similar-sized group in society. Most prison homicides are culpable and arise from situations that are not unique to jail.

Jails are full of gangs. Some penitentiary killings are gang revenge against members of a different gang. At other times a slight to a powerful inmate offends the "prisoner's code" and mandates death at the hands of another inmate. Some, typically sex offenders, are killed by fellow prisoners who dislike the nature of their crime. Coroners simply investigate the facts surrounding the death. The culpability of the homicide is a matter for a judge.

Killings in jails happens in many ways, but two are common. Inmates fashion knives, called shivs or shanks out of pieces of metal or hard plastic (see Figure 19.2). Either a single convict or a group of prisoners corners the intended victim in an area where they cannot be easily seen. That location makes it hard for any watching correctional officer to see who stabs the inmate to death. The other option inmates use to kill fellow prisoners is brute force. Convicts are punched, strangled or kicked to death.

A prisoner's killing is often planned to occur in the penitentiary's exercise yard. However, the outcome is not always what the plotters expect. To ensure the designated victim cannot escape his death

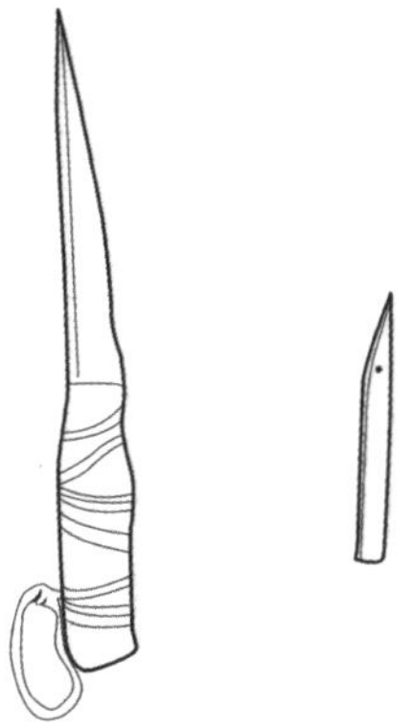

Figure 19.2: Inmates make weapons out of metal or hard plastic, often using eating utensils.

in the yard, prisoners form a circle around both the victim and his designated hitman. If the victim is killed quickly, the group can then disperse leaving the dead inmate's body on the ground without anyone being held responsible. However, guards on the parapet above often realize what is going on. They order the attempted killing to stop immediately. Should it continue in spite of the warning, a guard will shoot the hitman. When a guard sees that one inmate is in immediate danger of being killed by another, the aggressor can be shot to save the victim's life.

In Ontario, where all prison deaths require inquests, I have presided over dozens, if not hundreds, of these fatalities. Most juries investigated deaths by stabbings and physical force; only one considered a death caused by a guard having to shoot a prisoner who was trying to kill another inmate. Most penitentiaries in the province are in my region, so it is probably safe to assume that Ontario correctional officers very infrequently kill prisoners. That will also likely be the case throughout the developed world.

In prison, death by suicide is three times as common as death by homicide. Suicides are invariably by hanging. Many Ontario prisons have bunk beds to house two prisoners in a cell. The upper bunk provides the beam from which a suicide-intent inmate can suspend himself by a piece of torn clothing or bedsheet wrapped around his neck. Guards make rounds regularly. When a guard discovers a prisoner hanging, he simply sounds an alarm and waits for other guards to arrive. Only then can a guard safely enter the cell. This delay for help to arrive and permit safe entry always extends the time before resuscitation can start by minutes.

When there were two people in the cell, juries thought that the cellmate might provide some evidence about the hanging. That never happened in any inquest where I presided. Police investigators always advised the jury that the cellmate claimed to be asleep and to hear nothing. An inmate planning to commit suicide while alone in a cell always seemed to be able to hang himself just after the guard made a round to look in on his cell. That ensured an adequate suspension time for death to occur before the guard discovered his hanging body on his next round.

Hanged inmates are cut down by the guards as soon as possible after discovery. Resuscitation in the cell is vigorous and continues for quite a while. Eventually the inmate is moved to the prison's nursing station, where the body is finally declared dead. Occasionally a lengthy resuscitation period returns circulation but leaves the inmate with cerebral anoxia. In those cases, the prisoner is transferred to a hospital, supported by a ventilator for some period of time before being declared dead minutes after disconnection from the ventilator. There are probably other methods for committing suicide in jail, particularly if drugs can be obtained for the purpose, but none ever came to my attention.

Another type of jail death is the accident. Some convicts do actually die from head injuries when slipping in the shower. More accidental deaths arise from poisoning. Common penitentiary poisons are homebrew alcohol, manufactured somewhere in the prison, or illicit drugs smuggled in. Homebrew alcohol can kill in two ways. An inmate can drink so much that breathing stops when his brain's respiratory centre can no longer trigger another breath. Less commonly, the homemade hooch contains *Clostridium botulinum*, which can cause fatal botulism.[5]

Drugs are available in most penal institutions despite never-ending efforts to keep them out. Drug overdoses kills prisoners in exactly the same way as does an illicit drug overdose taken outside the prison walls. Drug users in the outside community often consume opiate drugs in the presence of friends who can administer Narcan in case they start to become stuporous. That does not happen in jail. Isolation makes the use of drugs in prison even more dangerous than their use would be in the outside world. Most drug users in prison do their illicit drugs safely though. There were only 595 prison drug deaths in the United States during the years from 2001 to 2014.[6]

In Halfway Houses

Halfway houses are the least secure form of penal custody. In Canada they are called community correction facilities. Deaths in these institutions are rare. They can be natural, but their residents are probably more likely than the population at large to die of a drug overdose, be killed by a gang member, or even to commit suicide. However, it is hard to find statistics on this to back up this suspicion.

Every death that occurs in such a halfway house is likely to be widely reported, so anyone interested can probably learn about all deaths occurring in his or her community simply by going to the Internet. If the deaths are unnatural, they are investigated by coroners. At some point, these deaths will be separately counted, but in the jurisdictions I looked at, that time does not yet seem to have arrived.

NOTES

1 Takeuchi, A., Ahern, T. L., & Henderson, S. O. (2011). Excited delirium. " *Western Journal of Emergency Medicine, 12*(1), 77–83.

2 O'Reilly, N. (2020, June 13). Why police chokeholds were banned in Ontario nearly 30 years ago. *The Hamilton Spectator.* https://www.thespec.com/news/hamilton-region/2020/06/13/why-police-chokeholds-were-banned-in-ontario-nearly-30-years-ago.html

3 Noonan, M. E. (2016). *Mortality in state prisons, 2001–2014: Statistical tables.* https://www.ojp.gov/ncjrs/virtual-library/abstracts/mortality-state-prisons-2001-2014-statistical-tables

4 Office of the Correctional Investigator. (2017). Annual report of the office of the correctional investigator 2016–2017. https://www.oci-bec.gc.ca/cnt/rpt/annrpt/annrpt20162017-eng.aspx

5 Centers for Disease Control and Prevention. (2018). *Pruno: A recipe for botulism.* https://www.cdc.gov/botulism/pruno-a-recipe-for-botulism.html

6 Noonan, M. E. (2016.). Mortality in state prisons, 2001–2014: Statistical tables. (Table 1, p. 4). https://www.bjs.gov/content/pub/pdf/msp0114st.pdf

20

Deaths by Suicide

Humans have long chosen suicide as a means to end life. The earliest recorded reference to suicide may be the Debate between a Man and his Ba (Soul) in which an ancient Egyptian in the Middle Kingdom period debates with his soul whether or not to commit suicide.[1] While in that era the choice of suicide was a philosophical exercise, the act was considered a sin by the early Christian church[2] and receives disapproval in the Quran to the present day.[3]

It is certain suicide was common in times gone by. Physicians in ancient Greece were concerned about suicide in women, the young and the elderly. However, most Greeks were stoics. They viewed committing suicide as generally undesirable, but it became permissible when their gods gave people a sign to kill themselves.

The possibility of being made a slave after capture or losing a battle were the sorts of signs from a god that might lead an ancient Greek to suicide. In possibly the most famous example in ancient Athens, Socrates drank hemlock when his failure to acknowledge Athenian gods and his introducing of new gods led to his conviction for impiety and corruption of youth. His death was the result of a judicial execution by suicide, with Socrates his own executioner.[4]

In imperial times Romans saw suicide a reasonable alternative to dishonour. It was common practice for a person, facing trial, to "fall on his sword" rather than face the dishonour of a guilty judgement. Romans were not the only people of the time to use suicide in this way. Hannibal, a Carthaginian, also committed suicide to atone for his failure to conquer the Romans.[5]

In most Christian countries people who committed suicide were not allowed to be buried in church graveyards from at least the Middle Ages until recent decades. Christian and Muslim countries frowned on suicide generally. Nowadays, in most countries with a Christian or

Muslim heritage, suicide is generally considered to result from depression or some other mental illness.

Considering suicide to be an act of desperation that would not be contemplated by a sane person is possibly a cultural construct. Japanese culture has long had an honourable history of suicide. Samurai facing defeat in battle used their swords to disembowel themselves in an act called *seppuku*. Japanese who were of lesser status tried to achieve an honourable death when they committed *hara-kiri*. In the Second World War, Japanese fighter pilots sacrificed their lives dive-bombing enemy ships. These pilots were known as kamikazis. Some hara-kiri still continues in the present day.

Japan currently has a high rate of suicide. Both males and females favour suicide by hanging, jumping or suffocation. These suicide choices are common in most other countries where firearms are not easily accessible. Japanese suicides are often committed by students who fail to pass examinations, youths unable to find work and isolated elderly males.

Japan has a very high rate of suicides, but Koreans, Lithuanians and Greenlanders kill themselves even more frequently. Depending on which statistics you look at, any one of these three countries can be said to have the world's highest rate of suicides. Japan has no history of Islam at all and little of Christianity. High rates of suicide are also found in central and northern Europe and Sri Lanka.

In France 12.1 per 100,000 people commit suicide each year. Rates vary a lot in other countries, with Africa having the world's lowest (although admittedly the statistics on Africa are poor). This paucity of African suicides may also be cultural though. In the United States, whites commit suicide more frequently than do African-Americans. The male to female ratio of Americans who died from suicide in 2018 was 3.56:1. Men prefer to commit suicide with firearms, women with drugs. Over 50% of U.S. suicides in 2019 involved the use of a firearm.[6] (In the United Kingdom, both sexes prefer suicide using drugs and, in the past, gassing themselves).

Most countries with coroners accept Western medical theories of diseases and their treatment. These include the general view that people who commit suicide must be suffering from some sort of mental illness, usually depression. The public at large generally agrees with this position.

A coroner discussing suicide with a physician will find both usually share this view. Few medical practitioners consider suicide possible in the mentally healthy. However, in this multicultural world that may not always be a relative's view. Some will perceive that the suicide's life was so intolerable that death was the best, or only, way to escape its problems. This philosophical view won't pop up often in discussions with coroners, but it does sometimes. When it does listen and make no comments. More often a relative did not see the suicide coming and simply asks, "Why?"

Of course, the coroner cannot answer that question. Nor can anyone else for that matter. In some deaths people try to perform a "psychological autopsy." This process simply reimagines a mental state. The examination may isolate a tipping point that triggered suicide. However, it can never explain why suicide was the chosen option to solve the problem. The answer to "Why?" has to be "Nobody can answer that question."

One other stock phrase to remember is "You are not to blame for the suicide." It can't be emphasized too strongly that suicide is an act of free will. There are always other options to deal with an unhappy situation. The choice to commit suicide is made only by the person committing it. It is never anyone else's fault. Nobody derives any benefit from feeling guilty about someone else's suicide.

Coroners should point out that guilt is destructive. The dead relative gains no benefit when a surviving family member tries to take responsibility for the suicide. It is equally important to reassure an employer that disciplinary action does not make an employer responsible for an employee's subsequent suicide. It is not a coroner's job to be a psychotherapist, but it is a kindness to grieving relatives or upset employers to say something like this while talking to them at the time of, or shortly after, viewing the body.

A coroner can hope that these words will help to prevent future mental distress in a living person. A coroner's timely remarks give any therapist who might later become involved helpful impartial comments to work with. The coroner's words at the death scene are rarely forgotten and often ruminated upon.

Relatives also benefit from hearing that death was speedy and painless when that was the case. Usually, nobody knows what actually happened when a person committed suicide. The act is most often undertaken alone and unobserved. In the infrequent cases where a suicide is videoed, police seize the film. They usually do not provide it to the family since it would be too upsetting.

People generally don't want to inflict pain on themselves. Using whatever tools are available suicides kill themselves in the speediest and least painful way they can find. Some methods of committing suicide are more common than others. Types vary country by country.

One other question that is often asked is "Was there a suicide note?" Suicide notes are commonly, but not always, written. Investigating police and coroners always look for one. When a note has been drafted it is frequently left out in an obvious place for ease of discovery. Suicide notes were once almost always written on paper. Nowadays, a computer or a cellphone is a common location, though notes may be found almost anywhere. Occasionally, and hopefully not very often, a pathologist's assistant discovers a suicide note in a trouser pocket while undressing a body in preparation for the autopsy.

Coroners frequently read suicide notes before turning them over to investigating police officers. Some notes contain an apology. Others simply explain why the suicide was necessary. Another group of notes assesses blame. The content is irrelevant to a coroner's investigation unless the note is likely to cause great harm to a reader. A coroner is simply looking for evidence of suicidal intent. The existence of the note, regardless of its content, actually establishes this. Once perused, the coroner has no continuing need for the document. Nor do the police, once certain that no crime was involved.

Family requests for a suicide note should be referred to the police who will initially have custody of the document. Usually, a police service eventually accedes to persistent family requests for the note. When its content assigns a lot of blame police tend to push back against the request before reluctantly agreeing to release the note. They want to prevent any misery the words will cause a surviving family member who reads it. Experienced police officers are quite skilled at stifling a family's request to minimize this hurt. However, when the family is persistent even though warned about its contents, police will yield possession of any suicide note.

Remember that the police seized the suicide note under the coroner's authority, though. If you think the suicide note will be particularly harmful to some future reader, get it back from the police. Take the suicide note to a knowledgeable lawyer to see whether there is some legal way you can avoid giving it to whichever person is entitled to it. There may be some law in your jurisdiction that will permit a coroner to refuse to release it on the basis that it is likely to cause harm to someone.

Poisoning

Suicide using an overdose of drugs was known in antiquity and is common today. Socrates drank hemlock to end his life. In the twentieth century, while awaiting judgement at Nuremberg, Hermann Goering committed suicide with a cyanide pill. In the ensuing decades, when barbiturates were widely prescribed to induce sleep, many suicides involved their use. Two of the most famous Hollywood stars who died of barbiturate overdoses were Marilyn Monroe and Judy Garland.

Nowadays barbiturates are less commonly available and are used in fewer poisoning suicides. Taking the world as a whole, 30% of poisoning suicides involve pesticide ingestion.[7] Most pesticide suicides take place in heavily populated Asian countries. Their lethal effects are discussed in Chapter 18. In the United States, the most commonly used poison for suicide varies. In all states sedatives and antidepressants generally rank among the chemicals most frequently used.

Narcotics are used for suicide too. However, many people ingest them seeking pleasurable sensations. Consequently, without a suicide note it is difficult to tell the difference between an accidental death and a suicide when someone dies from a narcotic overdose.

Benzodiazepines are a family of drugs commonly prescribed to manage anxiety. While they are very relaxing, benzodiazepines overdoses by themselves are not often lethal. Three of the best-known drugs in this family are sold as Valium, Xanax and Ativan. It is unlikely that a coroner will ever investigate a suicide solely caused by a high dose of benzodiazepines. Most of these pure benzodiazepine overdoses simply result in a long stay in bed, on the floor, on a couch or in a hospital intensive care unit. In coroners' cases, death usually resulted from the combined effects of benzodiazepines with some other drugs.

In past decades, tricyclic antidepressants were the drug of choice to treat depression. Amitryptyline (brand name Elavil) was one such drug. Excessive amounts caused fatal cardiac arrhythmias, making them a popular vehicle for suicide. Tricyclics have to be prescribed by a physician. Newer antidepressants have made tricyclics less frequently prescribed, though they are still used to treat chronic pain. Decreased prescribing has lessened their use for suicide nowadays.

After Prozac became widely used in the 1980s, its family of selective serotonin uptake inhibitors (SSRIs) became favoured drugs to treat both anxious and depressed patients. The numbers of antidepressant suicides declined. Then someone reported an increase in suicides in people under 25 years of age and this received wide publicity.[8] A movement blaming SSRIs for teenaged suicides arose.

The argument for blaming teenage deaths on SSRIs was epidemiological (based on statistical analysis). Statistical interpretation varies depending on who does it. The role of an SSRI in a death might become an issue for coroners if toxicological testing reports SSRIs in the blood of a teenager who committed suicide. Many depressed teenagers will have taken an SSRI without any problem. Only in suspected suicides by drug ingestion do coroners order toxicological testing. Coroners need a very good reason to deviate from that practice.

While SSRIs might induce suicidal thoughts in children or young adults, informed opinions differ on whether they actually do. A coroner should stay out of that debate. Even with proof that a teen has been taking a prescribed SSRI, a coroner should only attribute death to the drug when a toxicologist detects a fatal blood level. Refer any further inquiry from parents (usually) about the drug to either a government website or any psychiatrist who has been involved in the child's care.

Opiates are another class of drugs often used in suicide. Since a person planning to use them to commit suicide often finds it difficult to ascertain the lethal dose, prior attempts might have failed when too little was taken. Relatives readily tell coroners about past failed attempts. The more opiate regularly used in the past, the higher the dose needed to relieve pain or simply get high. Long-time recreational opiate users require a much higher dose to kill themselves than do the opiate naive.

Morphine was once the opiate coroners most commonly found in suicide investigations. It is now less frequently prescribed to control severe pain. Oxycodone (brand names Percodan or Percocet) or hydromorphone (brand name Dilaudid) have now become frequently used for pain control, even when the pain is only of moderate intensity. Some suicides arise from overdoses of prescribed opioids, but most current opiate overdose deaths are recreational accidents.

Opiate overdose deaths are virtually painless. Sleep, or loss of consciousness follows ingestion. The time till death varies with the drug taken and its dose. Barbiturates and opiates affect the brain's respiratory centre to slow breathing and induce sleep. When these medications are swallowed in a suicide, the gap between each breath gradually widens until, terminally, Cheyne–Stokes gasping respirations herald death.

Acetaminophen or paracetamol (Tylenol) is an easily accessible drug that can be lethal when a large number of pills are taken. A large enough overdose puts a person to sleep with few other symptoms felt. The lethal amount varies with a person's size. People using acetaminophen to commit suicide sometimes do not take this into account. Taking an inadequate number of pills results in misery.

Tylenol poisoning damages the liver, causing nausea and vomiting, abdominal pain, jaundice, confusion and fatigue. Blood stops clotting properly, and bleeding starts. Kidney failure and body swelling follow. When pancreatitis accompanies liver failure, abdominal pain tends to be much more severe.

Liver failure stops the destruction of by-products of the body's metabolism. These compounds collect in the blood and cause hepatic encephalopathy. While dying, a person becomes drowsy and forgetful, experiences personality changes, and may even convulse at times before finally entering a period of calm that precedes death. Paracetamol suicides are common in the United Kingdom, but less so in most other countries.

Suicide due to salicylate poisoning from an Aspirin overdose was quite common until the last quarter of the twentieth century, when the use of Aspirin to relieve pain or to lower temperatures became less common. Nowadays the United States probably sees fewer than 50 cases of suicide per year from any sort of salicylate poisoning.[9] Most new coroners will probably never investigate one.

Previous paragraphs have described deaths due to a single drug overdose. Quite often more than one drug is taken to commit suicide. Pills may be washed down with beer, wine or spirits. Some of these drugs may affect the heart, but many more stop breathing. Alcohol depresses respiration too. The toxicological explanation for many deaths is that while the action of a single drug might not be enough to cause breathing to cease, the cumulative effect of two or more drugs does so and is lethal.

Particularly when alcohol accompanied a fatal mixed-drug overdose, a coroner can safely say that dying was unlikely to have been accompanied by any pain. Sleep would have come on fairly rapidly — perhaps in half an hour to an hour. Death would then have followed minutes or hours later, but who can say how long? That time will always remain a puzzle because people metabolize drugs differently depending on their body size, sex, race, and so on. A coroner should not hazard a guess.

Hanging

Suicide by hanging is common worldwide. Almost everyone knows how hanging works. Houses contain ample material with which to hang oneself. Ropes or wires for normal household use are stored in every home and can be easily hidden when someone plans to use them for suicide. Hanging frequently takes place when everyone else is out of the house.

But not always. People intent on suicide sometimes use a pretext to go to the basement or leave the house to go to a garage or barn. That ensures nobody will follow very quickly or start to wonder about something being wrong very quickly. This allows adequate undisturbed time for people intent on suicide to hang themselves. Most suicidal hangings occur at home.

There are many ways to hang oneself in a house. Basement and garage overhead beams, both wooden and metal, are strong enough to support the weight of a hanging body. With a rope already looped around a person's neck, its other end is easily tied around a beam. Since most basement ceilings are low this is often done while standing on a plastic basket, box or chair. The rope is typically tied around garage beams by standing on a stepladder, box or chair. Garages and basements are probably the most common sites, but hangings can occur throughout the house. When a beam is used, hanging occurs once the box, chair or stepladder is kicked away to leave the suspended body dangling in the air, feet unable to touch the ground.

Rods securely attached to or embedded in the walls of a closet are the upstairs crossbeam of choice for hangings. The rod's height above the floor allows easy attachment of the other end of a rope looped around the neck. Hanging is then accomplished by voluntarily flexing the knees to let the body drop. The rope then pulls tight around the neck, either cutting off blood flow to the brain or causing death by suffocation.

Another household method of hanging uses a doorknob. These doorknob hangings start in a kneeling position. The rope, wire or cord is looped in a noose around the neck with the other end tied to the doorknob. Completion of the hanging requires a lunge forward so that the rope jerks tightly around the neck to cause death.

Household doors become gallows when a rope is wedged securely between the top of the door shut tightly into its frame. Inside the room at its other end is a noose, slipped around the neck of a person standing on an object, like a chair, that can be easily kicked away. Without the chair's support the body drops and the rope tightens, killing the person whose dead body remains hanging against the door until it is discovered.

Bannisters provide another type of beam for suicidal hangings. This type of suicide is not uncommon in two-storey houses and avoids any need for a chair. With a noose around a person's neck when the rope is secured around the bannister a jump over the railing completes the suicide.

In the best-case scenario, the tightened noose suddenly stops blood flow to the brain. Loss of consciousness is almost instant. At other times the noose only compresses the trachea. This stops air from entering the lungs leading to death by suffocation. Rarely does suicide by self-hanging produce the type of neck fracture a hangman aims for. The so-called hangman's fracture is discussed in Chapter 22.

Fortunately for the police, relatively few people hang themselves outdoors. Locating a body hanging in a pine tree in a forest is very difficult. This is true even in wintertime, when footprints in the snow lead toward the tree's location. Bodies hanging in deciduous trees are more easily seen than in conifers, provided the body hangs from a lower limb. In the case of a tree being heavily leafed, a body hanging high up toward the tree's crown may not be discovered until the leaves are shed in the fall.

Even when searchers know that a body likely hangs somewhere in the woods, hours or days may still pass before anybody sees clothing among the foliage. Urban hangings are discovered more quickly. Hangings in public parks usually happen at night. The body is then usually discovered the next morning or at most a day or two later by a jogger or someone out walking a dog.

Gunshot

People who own firearms commit suicide by shooting themselves. Farmers and hunters usually have long guns at home, but almost nobody in Canada owns pistols. Consequently, a rifle or shotgun is the suicide weapon of choice. Most people who use guns for suicide tend to be very knowledgeable. They calculate a fatal shot that will cause death speedily with minimal pain.

Most people seeking to commit suicide with a firearm figure that a gunshot wound to either the head or heart should cause immediate loss of consciousness and aim their guns accordingly. Sometimes the shots miss though, for a couple of reasons. The first is inadequate anatomical knowledge. A misdirected aim will miss a vital organ, occasioning a much slower and more painful death.

The second reason is that the gun may move when fired. Guns recoil after their triggers are pulled. To prevent its barrel from moving, a successful suicide needs the firearm so tightly wedged that the bullet cannot deviate from its intended path. A common technique is to place a barrel's tip into the mouth. Usually this works as planned. The person's loss of consciousness is then instant. Improperly positioned guns may simply blow off the jaw or part of the face. Dying then lasts quite a bit longer, during which time the pain is exquisite.

Rifle shots make a small entry hole in the skin. If an exit wound exists, its size is often larger. How one dies depends on the shot's trajectory through the body. A bullet through the brain stem immediately disrupts breathing, heartbeat and consciousness. Death follows within five minutes. Shots in other parts of the body kill differently.

Death results from bleeding, whether inside the skull or from a wound to another part of the body. The larger calibre the bullet, the more bleeding and the speedier the death.

Some people shoot themselves in the heart by pulling the trigger of a rifle with its barrel tip pressed against their chest walls. Others choose to securely position a rifle at a distance from a chair in which they sit with a gun's barrel pointed at the heart. A long wire or string mechanism is set up to pull the trigger. Once pulled, a bullet pierces the heart, immediately disorganizing its electrical activity and stopping its beating. No more blood is pumped to the brain. The shooter instantly loses consciousness.

Shotgun suicides are far messier than those caused by rifle shots. This is especially true when a shotgun barrel tip discharges into the mouth. Much, if not most, of the head is blown away. The fewest possible family members (preferably none) should view such a body.

A shotgun blast into the mouth causes instant death. Bits of brain and skull get blown all over the house. The force of the skull's explosion usually embeds some bits of bone in the walls and in the ceiling. Relatives need to be warned when this happens. The family will have to clean up the mess after police and the coroner leave. Some companies specialize in this type of cleaning. Where it appears relatives can afford it, the coroner should recommend the family hire one of these cleaning companies and not re-enter the room until it has been returned to its former state.

Suffocation

One unanticipated consequence of the automobile's invention was the use of its tailpipe exhaust to commit suicide. Only toward the end of the twentieth century did the number of people dying from this type of carbon monoxide poisoning start to decrease. Concern about pollution led to better catalytic converters. Newer automobiles started producing up to 99% less carbon monoxide in their exhausts. Since carbon monoxide was the killer, people could run some car motors for a long time without asphyxiating themselves.

The most common form of carbon monoxide poisoning required simply closing a garage door with a car inside and the motor running.

Carbon monoxide is a product of incomplete combustion that attaches itself to haemoglobin in the blood instead of oxygen. These red blood cells with carbon monoxide attached circulate without carrying any oxygen to the body's tissues. This leads to loss of consciousness and a painless death. The garage will have been full of carbon monoxide when police arrived. By the time the coroner gets to the scene, the garage will have been aired out so that it is safe to enter and view the body.

This twentieth century method of suicide is relatively less common today. Its replacement is death by incomplete combustion from burning charcoal in a closed area.

The automobile is still one of two popular venues for this type of suicide. The other is a small room with its windows and doors duct-taped shut. A lighted cooking implement using coal, oil, kerosene or naphtha produces a lethal amount of carbon monoxide in this enclosed space. This type of suicide is nicknamed "death by Hibachi."

People have long committed suicide by tying airtight material around their heads. As soon as they were invented, plastic bags replaced textiles for this purpose. A plastic bag covering one's head, tied tightly around the neck, prevents any new oxygen from being delivered to the lungs. Instead, exhaled carbon dioxide increasingly becomes the only gas within the bag. Rebreathing it induces first loss of consciousness and then death. In recent years this time-honoured method of suicide has been augmented by the addition of helium to the dying process, and the bag over the head has been called a suicide bag.

Suicide societies promote death by helium pumped into a bag tied around the neck. Helium is an inert gas that causes the oxygen level in the blood to drop very quickly without triggering the breathing reflex. As a result, consciousness is lost within 5 to 10 seconds.[10] A number of videos of these suicides have been made showing apparently peaceful deaths. No feeling of suffocation is thought to occur. Suicide kits using this mechanism are available online. Helium inhalation may be the most painless method of dying.

Since death by helium administration requires a lot of apparatus to carry it out, there is never any question about whether such a death is a suicide. Frequently relatives know that helium causes a relatively painless death. Most family members also understand the circumstances that may have triggered this type of suicide. Helium deaths don't seem to involve the question "why" as often as do other types of suicides.

Death by gassing oneself was a popular method of suicide in the latter half of the twentieth century in the United Kingdom. The American writer Sylvia Plath famously ended her life this way. This form of suicide relied on the fact that coal gas combustion, occurring in most British houses of the era, produced a large amount of carbon monoxide as its by-product. When natural gas, which burns much more efficiently, replaced coal gas, this type of suicide virtually stopped.

Jumping

Jumping off an urban apartment balcony, off a cliff in the country, or off a bridge spanning a waterway is a worldwide method of suicide, more common in some countries than others. Coroners investigate all lethal falls from great heights. A suicidal jump is invariably fatal when the take-off spot is high enough above the landing site.

People whose business is climbing poles or trees for a living use 9 metres (30 feet) as the height at which a fall becomes fatal. A jump from that height might indeed be lethal, but that is not certain. A jump from four or five storeys above the ground is usually, but not always, fatal. Children who fall between 12 and 15 metres (40 to 50 feet) only die 50% of the time.[11] Jumps from a point 46 metres (150 feet) above land or 76 metres (250 feet) above water are fatal 95% to 98% of the time.[12] Which body part first strikes the ground is a major factor affecting the likelihood and speed of death. When the jumper lands head first, death is certain. Massive brain damage causes instant loss of consciousness. The skull fractures; the brain is crushed and lacerated, tearing multiple blood vessels. Death can be considered instant.

Dying after a flat landing results from multiple injuries and blood loss. Many bones break, chest injuries impair breathing, and any head injury involves brain damage too. Lucky jumpers who land flat on the ground die from massive bleeding when their aorta tears. This leads to almost immediate loss of consciousness and a rapid death.

Circles scratched in dust on the ground means fingers moved and death did not occur instantly. If noted, don't mention this to family members. Instead, discuss falling deaths in generalities. Explain how great force to the head renders one immediately unconscious. Avoid suggesting that the jumper suffered at all before death. Family members are upset enough about the suicide that they do not want to think that their relative's death was accompanied by any type of pain at all.

Drowning

Suicide by drowning is relatively uncommon, but most coroners investigate at least one case every few years. Non-swimmers sometimes simply wade out into deep water until it is over their heads. Others take a fatal leap from a structure such as a bridge, pier, dock, or building at the water's edge. Some jump from natural features on the water's edge, such as the winter's ice or a cliff. Suicides that occur by falling from a boat are the hardest to be certain about.

Once sunk in the water, whatever the temperature, it only takes a few minutes to die from drowning. People who can swim know they will have to overcome a natural reflex to start swimming in an effort to stay afloat. This is often managed by tying a stone, an anchor, or some other type of weight to their legs to ensure their bodies stay submerged so that drowning is quick. These attached weights make it easy to differentiate a suicide from an accidental drowning.

Drowning is only uncomfortable for seconds. From the moment of initial submersion to unconsciousness usually takes less than a minute. Death follows a few minutes later. The last three to five minutes of life are painless. Relatives of those drowned rarely ask about pain while dying. Chapter 12 describes the process of dying when drowning in more detail.

Bleeding

Suicide from blood loss, after cutting one's body, is relatively uncommon in Ontario, where I work. Some people commit suicide by cutting their wrists, less commonly by cutting their necks or femoral arteries (in the thigh), and in most societies (except perhaps Japan) still less commonly by lacerating abdominal blood vessels. I suspect the reason for the relative rarity of the latter is that deeply lacerating oneself hurts a lot. There are nerve endings in the skin, muscles, arteries and bones. Cutting nerves is extremely uncomfortable.

A large lacerated artery pumps blood out of the body quite rapidly. (Rates of flow in some large arteries can be found in Chapter 5). Blood loss itself is not painful. Bleeding just weakens and fatigues. Dizziness follows until terminal coma sets in to end it. Then all body systems start to shut down. Death finally arrives when too little blood remains in the circulatory system to deliver adequate oxygen for the survival of vital organs. This happens after the loss of a half to two thirds of the body's blood.

The bigger the artery lacerated, the quicker one bleeds to death. If two blood vessels are completely severed, death will occur doubly fast – but the cutting will cause twice the pain.

Electrocution

Electrocution is an uncommon method of committing suicide. Most coroners never investigate such a case. Usually only electricians or others with great familiarity with electrical currents choose to commit suicide by electrocution. They attach coins or copper strips to their bodies to act as the anode and cathode points between which the lethal electricity will flow. Another way to create similar electrodes is to tie copper wire around wrists (or other body parts). Suicide by electricity is then completed by touching a live wire.

Most people intent on an electrical death know that the normal household current is sufficient to electrocute a person. Their deaths start with a muscle spasm that is not very painful, because the current almost immediately reaches the heart, disrupting its normal rhythm and causing pumping to cease. The electrocuted person passes out, and minutes later death follows.

The bathtub often plays a role in electrocution. Water surrounding a body easily transmits electricity. A hair dryer is one common power source of electrical bathtub deaths. A radio is another. To cause fatalities these devices must be operating when they enter the bathtub water. Nowadays some have circuit breaking technology that stops electrical flow. Only appliances lacking a circuit breaking feature are lethal.

Most bathtub electrocution deaths are accidental, but one German forensic paper reported 30 probable bathtub suicides, 11 of which left notes. In Germany, at least, people are both aware that bathtub electrocution is a feasible suicide option and also practise it.[13]

It is also possible to climb up some types of high voltage pylons carrying electricity. Loss of consciousness from electrocution results immediately when a bare hand touches one of these high voltage wires. Climbing such a pylon is tricky though. Usually only people very savvy about electricity commit suicide in this manner.

A similar suicide can be committed by touching the electrical rail in electric subway (underground train) systems. These rails carry high voltage, often 1500 volts, electrocuting in a fashion analogous to the electric chair. The immediate result of touching the rail line is loss of consciousness. Muscle spasms occur, but the person immediately loses consciousness before dying a few minutes later. Death is relatively painless.

There is more to read about electrical deaths in Chapters 14 and 22.

Exposure

The Inuit (formerly known as Eskimos) have lived in the Arctic for centuries. Their survival has always been very difficult. Food could only be obtained periodically. Families and whole communities shared (and still do) everything among all members to ensure survival. When supplies were running short, elderly Inuit sometimes concluded that their food consumption imperiled the rest of their clan. They offered to die in order to allow the rest a better chance of survival on the rations that remained. The elder might be taken out and placed on an iceberg, or simply left behind, outdoors, to die alone after everyone else moved on.

In Canada this is not known to have happened since the Second World War.[14] The Inuit have now moved into small permanent villages, and no longer travel from place to place living in temporary igloos. Nowadays, residents of northern countries commit suicide by exposure to the elements, particularly during the winter, by simply staying out of doors too long. As their body temperature drops, drowsiness turns into unconsciousness and then death from hypothermia. The speed of dying varies with the temperature, weather, and clothing worn.

More information is on this is available in Chapter 11.

Vehicular Impact

Ever since the Rocket started rail travel in 1829, people have thrown themselves in front of a train's engine in order to commit suicide. In England in the 1860s, the number of such suicides jumped following a newspaper report revealing the ease of killing oneself using the new-fangled train as a tool. The London Tube opened in the same decade. It proved to be an equally effective instrument of suicide.[15]

A train's high speeds and long braking time for stopping makes it impossible for its engineer to avoid striking a person who is intent on suicide. American trains are only involved in 300 to 500 suicides per year, but in Europe the figure is much higher. Over 10% of all Dutch suicides involve trains.[16] The figure is similar in the Flanders section of Belgium, though it drops to only 6% if the entire country is considered. In Germany, suicide by train is slightly higher at about 7% of their total.[17] Japan has a lot of train suicides too.

How the train kills a person depends on the body's position on the tracks. If the person intent on suicide places his or her neck over one rail, the wheels will decapitate the body as the heavy engine and cars repeatedly pass over the neck. Death is very speedy. If the person is sitting, standing or walking on the tracks at the time of impact, death arises from multiple injuries.

The force with which the train strikes the person or the force with which a body lands on the ground makes immediate loss of consciousness very likely even if the body remains intact, which is not always the case. Quite often a human body's tissue cannot withstand the force of an onrushing train and tears apart into little bits. That type of death is certainly instant.

Where the body remains relatively intact death is usually swift. There can be many injuries, but death commonly arises from rapid blood loss from multiple lacerated arteries. Death comes rapidly, particularly when the aorta is torn or the head severely injured.

Roughly 90% of suicide attempts involving above-ground trains succeed, but as few as 59% (66% in New York City[18]) of people who jump from a station platform in front of a subway train die. The reason is straightforward. Above-ground trains are usually travelling at high speed when they hit a person, whereas subway cars are slowing as they come into a station. However, when the subway runs on electricity, electrocution can also occur should the jumper's skin touch the electric rail. If the death is not caused by electrocution, it is traumatic.

People who dive from the sidewalk under the slowly turning wheels of a bus don't always die, but they usually do. When wheels crush the head or chest, consciousness is lost immediately and death follows soon after. If other parts of the body are injured enough to eventually cause death, the person may initially be both alert and conscious. Broken bones, crushed nerves and bleeding muscles hurt a lot while dying this way. Death usually arises either from exsanguination or a head injury.

Automobiles are used in suicides too. Police frequently suspect a suicide when a car driven by a lone healthy occupant crashes into an abutment or other solid object. Their suspicions increase if the driving conditions are good, and the relatively new car is in excellent condition. Police suspicion is not enough though. Coroners cannot deem an automobile fatality to be a suicide simply because they suspect that might be the case.

The law has a presumption against suicide based on the commonly held, reasonable belief that most people do not want to kill themselves. Without clear evidence that the collision was due to more than just a driver daydreaming at the wrong time or some sort of automobile malfunction, a coroner has to determine the death to be accidental. Statistics on the frequency of suicide-induced vehicle deaths vary. It happens more than one would think. Researchers estimate suicides account for 1.6% to 5.0% of automobile fatalities.[19]

Airplane suicides are not common, but one cannot say they are rare either. Between 1983 and 2003, 36 pilots in the United States killed themselves this way. Most flew their own planes. When the only person who dies is the pilot in a single plane, that is a sad suicidal event. It is much worse when a suicidal commercial pilot crashes a plane. The pilot's death is a suicide, but the passengers' deaths are all murders.

Commercial airline pilots' suicides have received worldwide attention a couple of times in recent years. One probable suicide that took place in 2014 resulted in 239 passenger deaths when the pilot of Malaysian Airlines flight 370 downed his plane somewhere in the Indian Ocean. A more certain suicide led to another 150 passengers deaths when the pilot crashed Germanwings Flight 925 into the Alps in 2015.

Those reconstructing the Malaysian Airlines flight and crash concluded that the passengers and crew probably slowly asphyxiated long before the plane hit the water. If so, their deaths would have been relatively painless. However, the Germanwings flight deaths would have all been traumatic and potentially painful, even if only momentarily. Since these types of deaths are so unexpected, most family members of passengers killed this way are uniformly irate and inconsolable. A coroner's role in these deaths is primarily to order autopsies on bodies that are found; few coroners will ever be required to do this.

Unusual Methods of Suicide

No coroner is likely to investigate deaths where people set themselves aflame, but this does happen. This millennium's single most famous fiery suicide was probably that of Mohamed Bouazizi. His was probably also the most consequential since it triggered the 2011 Tunisian revolution and ultimately led to the Arab Spring throughout the Middle East.

In India's rural areas it is still possible that a widow might throw herself on her husband's funeral pyre in the ritual of *suttee* or *sati*. Though officially banned since 1829,[20] the ritual suicide still occurs occasionally — one did in 2008.[21] This type of suicide seems specific to India even though Hindus now live in many other countries. In Japan, people have committed suicide by jumping into volcanoes.

Tropical suicides include being eaten by crocodiles. A South African man jumped into a crocodile infested river. The beasts immediately attacked, and his death was speedy if indescribably painful.[22] A Thai woman achieved the same result by jumping into a crocodile pond at a zoo.[23] Long ago Cleopatra was supposed to have caused an asp to bite her after hearing of Mark Antony's death. In 2016 in Michigan a suicidal young woman, high on drugs and hoping to be torn apart, died of multiple injuries after entering a yard inhabited by two pit bull dogs.[24]

In Northern Ireland during the Troubles, Bobby Sands became an IRA saint when he starved himself to death over a period of 66 days. Nine other IRA prisoners did the same.[25] An even slower suicidal path comes from infecting oneself with a fatal disease such as HIV. Death comes after the disease has followed its normal course, however long that may be.

Suicidal attacks are sometimes carried out with the intention of somebody killing the assailant. "Suicide by police" is one such method that has been much discussed in the media. When initially looked into, it may not be obvious that suicide was the person's intent. It often takes detailed investigation before that truth becomes apparent. This form of suicide distresses not only the deceased's family but also the families of the police officers involved — especially the officer responsible for the killing.

When a person commits suicide by inhaling a poisonous gas, the investigation may endanger an investigator. Common poisonous gas deaths are generally discussed in Chapter 18. Hydrogen sulphide needs to be thought of when undertaking suicide investigations, so it is discussed here.

To commit suicide some people create hydrogen sulphide by mixing a detergent or toilet bowl cleaner with a sulphide-containing product like a pesticide. Hydrogen sulphide gas is rapidly produced by this mixture, so quite often the containers used to create the gas can be found near the body. The skin of a person killed by inhaling hydrogen sulphide is cherry red in colour; the skin areas exposed to the gas have a greenish overtone.

Hydrogen sulphide affects humans differently depending on its concentration in the air. The low concentrations of hydrogen sulphide found in the air surrounding a pulp and paper mill creates a rotten egg smell and may irritate some people's eyes. A decomposing body only produces enough hydrogen sulphide to produce a foul smell. At a high concentration hydrogen sulphide becomes a "knock-down gas" that will cause immediate loss of consciousness followed by death after only a few inhalations.

A more moderate concentration of hydrogen sulphide causes fatigue, coughing and shortness of breath that may end up as bloody pumonary oedema. The smell of rotten eggs has to be a warning signal. For police and coroners, hydrogen sulphide's odour usually arises from a very decomposed body. Occasionally it is the result of a suicide, in which case the death scene is potentially hazardous.

Sometimes a note is left outside the room where such a suicide occurred. In that case whoever discovers the note should turn around, leave the building and call whatever organization in that munipality deals with toxic gases. Their staff need to come to the site to ensure that the scene is safe for humans to enter before police, a coroner or any other investigator goes in to look at the suicide scene. Fortunately for everone involved, this type of suicide is uncommon.

NOTES

1 The dispute between a man and his Ba. Papyrus Berlin 3024. See discussion at https://en.wikipedia.org/wiki/Dispute_between_a_man_and_his_Ba

2 Cholbi, M. (2017). Suicide: The Christian prohibition. In *Stanford encyclopedia of philosophy*. https://plato.stanford.edu/entries/suicide/#ChrPro

3 *The Noble Quran. M. Khattab (Trans.), Chapter 4, Verse 29. "...And do not kill 'each other or' yourselves. Surely Allah is ever Merciful to you."*

4 Laios, K., Tsoukalas, G., Kontaxaki, M. I., Karamanou, M., & Androutsos, G. (2014). Suicide in ancient Greece. *Psychiatriki, 25*(3), 200–207.

5 van Hooff, A. J. L. (2002). *From autothanasia to suicide: Self-killing in classical antiquity*. Routledge.

6 American Foundation for Suicide Prevention. (n.d.). *Suicide statistics*. https://afsp.org/suicide-statistics

7 Gunnell, D., Eddleston, M., Phillips, M. R., & Konradsen, F. (2007). The global distribution of fatal pesticide self-poisoning: Systematic review. *BMC Public Health, 7*, Article 357. https://doi.org/10.1186/1471-2458-7-357

8 McLean, J., & Bruser, D. (2012, October 29). Health Canada brushes off reports of serious side effects. *Toronto Star*. https://www.thestar.com/news/canada/2012/10/29/health_canada_brushes_off_reports_of_serious_side_effects.html

9 Runde, T.J., & Nappe, T. M. (2020). *Salicylates toxicity*. StatPearls (Internet). Treasure Island: FL. https://www.ncbi.nlm.nih.gov/books/NBK499879/

10 Clayton, G. D., & Clayton, F. E. (Eds.). (1994). *Patty's industrial hygiene and toxicology* (Vol 2, Part F). 4th ed.). New York: Wiley-Interscience.

11 Barlow, B., Niemirska, M., Gandhi, R. P., & Leblanc, W. (1983). Ten years of experience with falls from a height in children. *Journal of Pediatric Surgery, 18*(4), 509–511.

12 Stone, G. (1999). *Suicide and attempted suicide*. Da Capo Lifelong Books.

13 Bockholdt, B., & Schneider, V. (2003). Death by electrocution in the bathtub (translated from a Russian journal). http://www.medline.ru/public/art/tom4/art97.html

14 Leighton, A. H., & Hughes, C. C. (1955). Notes on Eskimo patterns of suicide. *Southwestern Journal of Anthropology, 11*(4).

15 O'Donnell, I., & Farmer, E. D. T. (1994). The epidemiology of suicide on the London underground. *Social Sciences and Medicine, 38*(3), 409–418.

16 van Houwelingen, Kerkhof, J. F. M., & Beersma, D. G. M. (2010). Train suicides in The Netherlands. *Journal of Affective Disorders, 127*(1-3), 281–286.

17 Lukaschek, K., Baumert, J., Erazo, N., & Ladwig, K.-H. (2014). Stable time patterns of railway suicides in Germany: Comparative analysis of 7,187 cases across two observation periods (1995–1998; 2005–2008). *BMC Public Health, 14*, Article 124. https://doi.org/10.1186/1471-2458-14-124

18 Buiso, G. (2013, June 2). Suicide is leading cause of subway passenger deaths: MTA data. *New York Post.* https://nypost.com/2013/06/02/suicide-is-leading-cause-of-subway-passenger-deaths-mta-data/

19 Schmidt, C. W., Shaffer, J. W., Zlotowitz, H. I., & Fisher, R. S. (1977). Suicide by vehicular crash. *The American Journal of Psychiatry, 134*(2), 175–178. https://doi.org/10.1176/ajp.134.2.175

20 *Bengal sati regulation, 1829.* http://www.bareactslive.com/WB/WB615.HTM

21 The Times of India. (2008, October 13). Woman jumps into husband's funeral pyre. https://timesofindia.indiatimes.com/india/woman-jumps-into-husbands-funeral-pyre/articleshow/3587874.cms

22 Maclean, S. (2011, April 18). Suicide by crocodile: Missing farmhand, 44, "waded into croc-infested river after row with girlfriend." *Daily Mail.* https://www.dailymail.co.uk/news/article-1378046/David-Lubisi-40-commits-suicide-crocodile-fight-girlfriend.html

23 Moran, L. (2014, September 16). Depressed Thai woman killed herself by leaping into zoo's crocodile pit: Report. *New York Daily News.* https://www.nydailynews.com/news/world/thai-woman-killed-leaping-crocodile-pit-report-article-1.1941136

24 Blakeley, K., & Towner, M. (2015, December 10). Death of mother, 22, who was mauled in pit bull attack is bizarrely ruled a suicide as medical examiner says she climbed into their enclosure on purpose to get mauled. *Daily Mail.* https://www.dailymail.co.uk/news/article-3354472/Death-mother-22-mauled-pit-bull-attack-bizarrely-ruled-SUICIDE-grieving-fiance-sticks-breed.html

25 O'Keeffe, T. M. (1984) Suicide and self-starvation. *Philosophy, 59*(229), 349–363.

21

Deaths by Homicide

For those who enjoy films (and who doesn't?), the word *homicide* frequently pops up in police dramas. An intrepid team of investigators track down a man (usually) who is believed to have committed a homicide. When eventually cornered, he is either shot and killed or, more often, arrested and charged with murder. This type of homicide is always culpable and therefore a crime. Police and prosecuting attorneys are very interested in criminal homicide, but homicide occurs in non-culpable ways much more often than criminal ones. Homicide is simply the act of one person killing another.

Society permits people to kill one another in circumstances that vary from country to country. In wartime, killing enemy combatants is accepted by people throughout the world as an expected consequence of their nation's entry into military conflict. Coroners do not investigate deaths of combatants in warfare. Armed forces throughout the world record and investigate wartime deaths in their own differing ways.

Judicial execution is another form of homicide that is much less common today than in the past. Nowadays many countries have abolished the death penalty, and even in those countries that still retain the death penalty, fewer are executed than in the past. China and Iran, the countries that probably carry out the highest number of executions right now, have questionable statistics and no coroners. A few common law jurisdictions around the world continue to have the death penalty, and in those places, coroners are still called upon to investigate them.

Euthanasia is a type of homicide that is gradually being accepted in more and more countries. The Netherlands and Switzerland pioneered the practice of allowing physicians to assist the incurably ill to a painless death. Now some American states and all of Canada, since a Supreme Court decision in 2015,[1] allow euthanasia. In Canada the process is called medical assistance in dying (MAID), and in some provinces, coroners scrutinize each death.

Nowadays, police in many countries bear arms. They are permitted to kill armed and threatening people in order to protect themselves or anyone else at risk of being killed by an assailant. The coroner's investigation that follows provides a public review and certifies exactly how a person was killed under those circumstances. Many jurisdictions also have any death involving the police reviewed by a supervisory body. In Ontario this organization is called the Special Investigations Unit, commonly referred to by its initials: SIU.

Correctional officers in jails are also authorized to kill inmates under certain circumstances. People in jail, particularly those in maximum security institutions, are all potentially very dangerous. A guard attacked by a prisoner is permitted to kill the attacking inmate in the course of defending himself. That action is considered a justifiable homicide. The other circumstance in which a guard may kill a prisoner is to prevent one prisoner from killing another. In this circumstance the correctional officer may shoot and kill the attacking inmate to prevent him from killing his intended victim.

All these types of homicides mentioned so far have been intentional. People kill each other by accident too, of course. The number of ways that accidental killings can happen would mystify an Einstein. Each of these deaths is unexpected. Police investigate these fatal accidents to determine whether the death resulted from a crime. A parallel coroner's investigation determines and categorizes the cause of death. Whenever a homicide is not criminal, the coroner's role includes examining its circumstances to look for anything that could have been done differently in an effort to prevent future similar deaths.

Some homicides that were initially considered non-culpable in the past have included state sanctioned or "winked at" killings carried out by government employees or an approved third party. In the twentieth century, enormous numbers died in Nazi and Cambodian death camps. After wars ended and governments changed, a number of the murderers who considered that they were only doing their job were brought to justice. Some were executed.

Smaller numbers of drug dealers have been killed with impunity by South American, Central American and Philippine death squads.

These countries do not have coroners, so none of these deaths will ever be the subject of a coroner's investigation. Jamaica has both death squads and coroners though. That is the one country where coroners might investigate such deaths.

Homicides do not account for a great portion of a coroner's work. The world is much less dangerous nowadays than it used to be. In Canada, prior to European colonization, Indigenous nations were in a recurring state of combat with one another. Deaths in these skirmishes was common and occurred repeatedly throughout North America. There are no Canadian or American statistics for that period, but European records have allowed scholars to speculate on mediaeval death rates on that continent. The estimated homicide rate in fifteenth-century Amsterdam has been calculated at 47 per 1,000 people.*[2] Today, the European homicide rate has dropped to about 3.0, which is less than 7% of that number.[3]

Ottawa, a city of one million where I work as a coroner, has about 15 criminal homicides each year. The city has 15 coroners. This means that each coroner is only likely to become involved with one or two murders per year in an average year. That is probably the case for any coroner across the English-speaking world, with the exception of the United States or Jamaica. Only the most common causes of homicides are addressed in this chapter.

Shooting

People are usually shot with guns, though arrows from bows or bolts from crossbows are also still occasionally used as lethal projectiles. Many other devices fire some form of potentially lethal missile, but the coroner's focus on firearms reflects the statistical reality of shootings nowadays.

Today's typical urbanites, including coroners, have little knowledge about guns. Fortunately, coroners only need to understand a little about the three types most used for killing people — shotguns, pistols and rifles. Pistols and rifles usually fire only one bullet at a time. Shotguns can fire a single slug, but more often they fire many small

* However, scholars question the accuracy of this and all other mediaeval homicide figures because the population statistics of the time are unreliable.

balls of shot that spray over a wide area. Forensic pathologists need a bit more familiarity with gun types than do coroners, but the police are the death investigators who really need to understand everything about firearms.

Shotguns have a smooth-bored barrel and come in several different gauges (called *bores* in the United Kingdom). Only two are common — 12 gauge and 410. The 12 gauge is the larger of the two and is the type usually involved in deaths. Both gauges kill in the same way. Shotguns fire shells (see Figure 21.1). Shotgun shells have a metal base, have walls made of plastic (sometimes made of cardboard instead), and contain gunpowder, wadding and round lead shot of varying but uniform size. The individual balls of shot may also be separated with plastic pellets so that shot, separators and wadding can all be fired from the gun when a firing pin strikes the base of the shell.

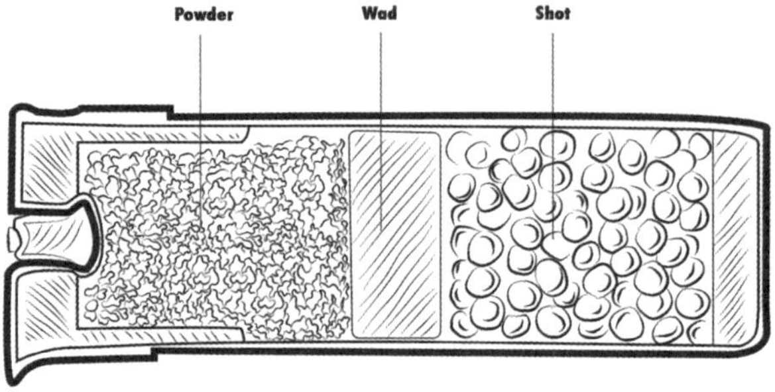

Figure 21.1: Shotgun shells contain gunpowder, wadding and round lead shot.

Rifles have a spirally grooved barrel that allows a single bullet to fly out with accuracy. Pistols, the weapons used in about half of all fatal shootings in the United States, are rifled too. Civilian rifles require the operator to pull the trigger to produce each shot. Military weapons continue firing as long as a trigger is held down.

In countries that have coroners, other than the United States, virtually all shooting deaths involve pistols, hunting rifles or shotguns. In the United States some military weapons are available to the general public. Pistol or rifle ammunition (shown in Figure 21.2) usually consists of a metal cylinder with a percussion detonator at the base, an explosive propellant and a bullet tightly packed within the cylinder's walls.

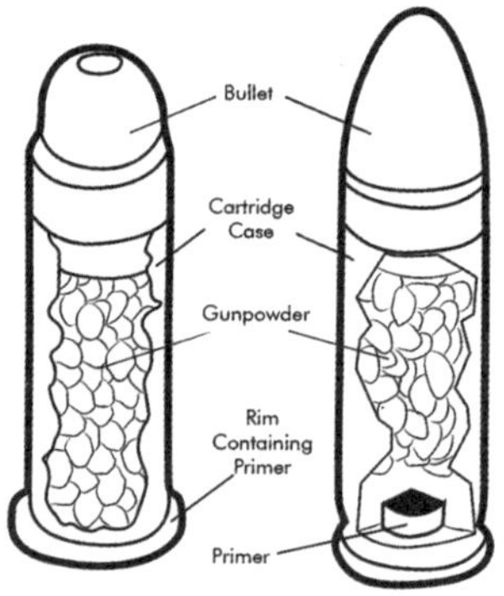

Figure 21.2: Rifle cartridges have different shapes of bullets.

Both shotgun shells and rifle cartridges work the same way. When a hammer triggers firing, the explosive propellant creates a hot gas that hurtles the bullet or shot forward at a high speed. Hunting rifles and pistols fire their bullets at a lower velocity than do military rifles. Pathologists and police investigators spend a lot of time determining exactly how far away from the body the gun was at the time it was fired in a crime. This is important information for any homicide trial, which invariably follows long after the coroner's investigation has been completed.

The occasional coroner may investigate an accidental shotgun death, but much more often it is a suicide or a homicide. As stated in the previous chapter, a shooter frequently places the tip of the shotgun's barrel into his mouth (usually) and then pulls the trigger. This causes an explosion within the skull that often blows away the face and most of the rest of the head. Only the posterior part of the skull remains attached to the neck. A quick look above the body usually reveals parts of the skull or brain embedded in the ceiling. Relatives need to be told this has happened to minimize their distress when they re-enter the room after the body has been removed.

After firing, a shotgun muzzle that was pressed against a chest or abdomen leaves a round wound, sometimes surrounded by the muzzle's imprint, on the skin. The wound's edge should be a bit black. When a shotgun is discharged a short distance from the skin there may be soot around the wound and small punctate spots around the wound; both are caused by particles of gunpowder. When the gun is fired farther away from the body, the shot begins to spread out. In that case pellet holes are visible around the central gunshot wound. Forensic pathologists and police firearms experts who look at these wounds can roughly estimate the distance of a shotgun muzzle from the skin at the time it was fired.

Rifled bullets come in different types and do different degrees of tissue damage depending on their design, but they all cause death the same way. A bullet entering body tissue leaves a trailing tunnel or cavity as it lacerates or crushes all the tissue it passes through. The space created is short-lived. The edges of the damaged tissue quickly press against each other to make the cavity disappear, but the damage is done. Depending on the density of the tissues passed though, the bullet can leave a larger exit wound than an entrance wound.

The single bullet from a discharged rifle or pistol pressed against the skin often leaves a muzzle imprint and black powder marks around the wound. But when the bullet is fired at any distance from the body no blackening around the bullet hole is visible. Bullets from rifles sometimes go right through the body leaving an exit wound, but that is rarely the case in fatal shotgun wounds.

Death from gunshots can be quite rapid. Bleeding from a perforated artery is a frequent mechanism of death. Neurological functions rapidly cease when a shot destroys tissue in many vital parts of the brain. Bleeding from a ruptured artery within the skull will also quickly stop the brain from working anymore.

A shot into the lungs that ruptures a pulmonary artery causes rapid death. Alternatively, the lungs may collapse and allow air to collect in the pleural cavities between the lungs and chest walls. This air collection is called a pneumothorax or, when both pleural spaces fill with air, two pneumothoraces. Both lungs and pleural cavities can also become packed with blood, leading to suffocation. A blood collection in the pleural cavities (the spaces created by the lungs collapsing) is called a haemothorax. (See Figure 21.3.) After being shot, when one dies will vary from a few minutes to very long time. Dying is painless when the shot produces instant loss of consciousness. The longer a wounded person stays awake, the more painful the process.

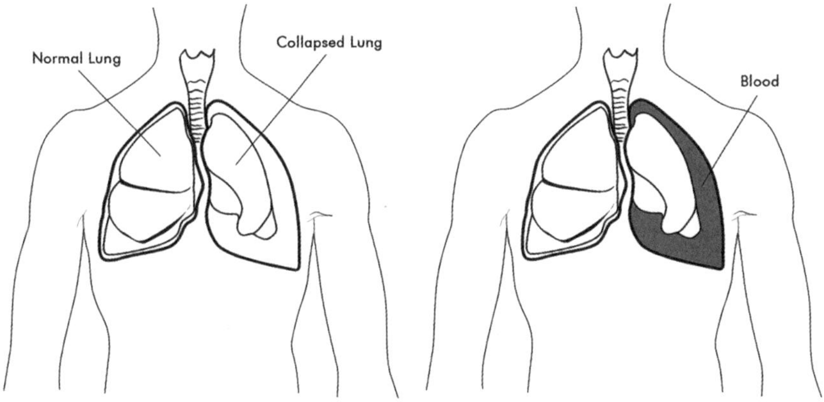

Figure 21.3: Pneumothorax and haemothorax

Some people survive a shooting initially but die later of its complications. Even with the best trauma care future fatal bleeding can happen. Lethal air and fat embolisms can follow too. People also frequently die from an infection that develops in their abdomen, lungs, brain or even bone (osteomyelitis). Death commonly follows an infection's spread into the bloodstream (bacteraemia), leading to sepsis and terminal septic shock. Depending on the region where a coroner works, fatal shootings may almost never happen, be quite frequent or occur regularly.

In 2016 there were 195,000 intentional firearm deaths around the world. Of them 64% were homicides, 27% were suicides and 9% were unintentional. Six countries — Brazil, the United States, Mexico, Colombia, Venezuela and Guatemala accounted for more than half of them.[4] Singapore, Japan and South Korea had the lowest rates of shooting deaths per 100,000 residents. That year, on a per capita basis the United States came in twentieth from the top.

Incised Wounds

A laceration results when a person's skin is torn apart by force. Traction from a blunt instrument can rip the skin's surface, but most fatal lacerations occur when something sharp severs one or more blood vessels. In coroners' cases bleeding continues until a lethal volume of blood exsanguinates. Such wounds are termed "incised", and the action producing them is called an incision.

Incised wounds come in two types. One is a slash, the other a stab; see Figure 21.4. The names are self-explanatory. People know the difference. For a slash wound to cause a rapid death, it must be deep and cut an artery. Death from slashing certainly happens, but coroners see many more fatal stab wounds.

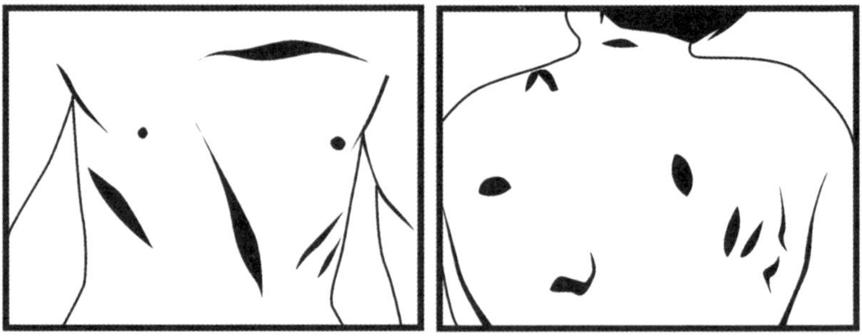

Figure 21.4: Slash wounds are shown on the left; stab wounds are shown on the right.

Domestic disputes sometimes end up with one person fatally stabbed by a kitchen knife or a pair of scissors. Fatal stabbings have also occurred with household tools such as screwdrivers, different types of spikes, such as an ice pick, and even a pitchfork. Prisoners in jail frequently die after fellow inmates impale them with shivs or shanks. (See Chapter 19.)

People have been killed by other common homemade assault weapons, including pieces of razor blade and surgical scalpels attached to a handle. Others have been stabbed to death in drunken brawls with a broken glass bottle, a chisel or even a poker. Street gangs kill with sharp knives of all sorts including switchblades (which are prohibited in Canada). Tools available for lethal stabbings are myriad.

A single wound may be fatal, but in some deaths that coroners investigate stab wounds are numerous. It is not always possible to attribute death to any single laceration. To the untrained eye, including most coroners, a stab wound may look like an innocuous cut. A forensic pathologist can tell a lot about it by simply looking closely at the wound margins. Knife blades have either one or two sharp sides.

Pathologists can often tell whether or not the knife had one blunt side just by looking at the wound margins. Coroners usually can't.

The sharpness of the knife's point is key to its ability to penetrate the skin. The sharpness of the length of the blade matters less. A strong person can drive a knife with a sharp point through a rib or the breastbone. Muscle between the ribs or cartilage is penetrated much more easily. Forensic pathologists and police blood-spatter experts can provide opinions about the amount of force used in a stabbing. Coroners are not expected to know how to calculate it.

Pathologists also form opinions about the direction of thrust, and they can measure the depth of the wound. With this information, they can tie the injury to, or rule out, a weapon that police suspect may have caused the death. Forensic pathologists can also draw on a body of literature that helps them estimate how long before death a wound occurred. Biology being what it is, any opinion has to be imprecise because of wide individual variation. The pathologist interprets the microscopic appearance of white cells in the wound and signs of healing to come up with a range of times.

When a coroner suspects a wound to be the probable cause of death, there is no need to tell the police to look for and seize any weapon that might possibly have been used. The police will immediately declare the area a crime scene. The coroner will be politely (usually) asked to vacate it as quickly as possible without disturbing any evidence. The coroner should point out any possible lethal implement noticed, without touching it, before departure. Police investigators will eventually form their own opinions about the weapon used.

Tying the suspected instrument of death to wounds is the job of a forensic pathologist, not a coroner. Wounding deaths usually have both civil and criminal legal consequences that play out over a period of years. The coroner's role in these cases is minor. After ordering an autopsy the coroner bows out, leaving all further investigation to the police and the pathologist.

One other help that a coroner might be able to provide the police at the death scene is to point out any injuries seen on the backs of hands or forearms. Wrists and knuckles especially may be cut or damaged while the now-deceased victim attempted to save himself. These are called defence wounds and are not usually the cause of death. These cuts simply show that the victim fought back before succumbing to other wounds that were fatal. Defensive wounds help the police recognize that they are dealing with a criminal homicide.

Shooting and stabbing are two of the most common ways people kill one another, but they are far from the only ones. People die when lynched, decapitated, strangled, smothered, poisoned, or clubbed to death, or when shoved off a building or in front of a train. All these other methods of death could also be either suicides or accidental deaths. They are discussed in other chapters.

Serial Killers

It is unusual for coroners to be asked about serial killers while investigating a death. However, when deaths of a similar type occur repeatedly, jurisdictions use whatever means are at their disposal to try to determine whether there is a recurring pattern. Recently an Ontario serial killer became headline news: a nurse, Elizabeth Wettlaufer, was discovered to have killed many elderly people in nursing homes where she worked.[5]

To keep the possibility of a serial killer top of mind it is wise to know something about them. First, very few murderers kill several people. Nowadays every newly discovered serial killer of this magnitude gets global news coverage. This makes it seem as though multiple killings are common, but they are not. Occasional cases of serial killings have been identified throughout recorded history, but the first widely reported were those committed by Jack the Ripper, who killed a number of women in London's East End at the end of the nineteenth century.

For someone to be designated as a serial killer, most people who study the topic consider three murders to be necessary.* Roughly 85% of serial killers are men.[6] That statistic is not much different from killers in general, however. Women serial killers tend to continue their murderous sprees over longer periods than men. The probable reason is that women are not initially suspected of being capable of being serial killers.

* Not the FBI though. At a 2005 symposium in San Antonio, they defined serial killing as "The unlawful killing of two or more victims by the same offender(s), in separate events."

Serial killers have been grouped as sexual killers, team killers, family killers and institutional killers. They have also been categorized by mobility. Some travel and kill, others only kill locally, and some only kill in the same spot every time. There is no single way to explain serial killers. The one thing most have in common though is that, as children, they were often abused by a family member.[7]

Euthanasia

Euthanasia has been practised surreptitiously by family members and physicians for a very long time. Soldiers have traditionally delivered a *coup de grace* as they walked past fatally wounded comrades in arms who were in pain while dying on the battlefield. For millennia, death was delivered by a stab to the soldier's heart using a sword or dagger. In the last couple of centuries, a shot to the heart or head replaced it. In its strictest definition, euthanasia need only be a mercy killing, so consent of the recipient is not a factor. Euthanasia is illegal in most countries.

Since the Second World War, in some countries euthanasia with consent has become permissible. Before such a death can take place the recipient's mandatory consent has to be carefully evaluated. Switzerland was the first country to legalize euthanasia in 1942. The Netherlands joined them in 2002, and now Canada and a number of American states have followed suit. Processes differ from jurisdiction to jurisdiction, but all are similar. The Canadian province of Ontario's system offers an example of how medical euthanasia works.

In Canada euthanasia is only available to the incurably ill suffering pain from a physical ailment. Psychological suffering does not qualify, though this is being revaluated at the time of writing. The legalization of euthanasia in Canada arose from a court decision in 2015. Since then, Canadian legal euthanasia has been termed medical assistance in dying (MAID) in dying, and a federal government webpage has been developed to explain it.[8] To obtain MAID, potential recipients, in the presence of two non-medical and unrelated witnesses, request a doctor's assistance to end their lives. After that a physician needs to discuss the request to ensure MAID is truly the dying person's wish.

This is not an informal conversation. The interrogating physician has to be satisfied with answers to a long checklist of questions. Two determinations are essential. On the one hand, the condition must be both serious and incurable. Secondly, the physician must be satisfied the person requesting MAID fully understands its consequences. To make these determinations properly, the assessing physician must also be sure that the person seeking MAID is experiencing intolerable suffering and, further, is aware of, but rejects, alternative measures to manage the distress.

A ten-day period for reflection follows to ensure there will be no change of mind when confronted with the reality of imminent death. After that ten-day period, a physician who is trained in MAID carries out the procedure. Death can take place in a hospital, home or at some other appropriate site. Quite often the family arranges a death ceremony. Often, many people show up on the day MAID is scheduled to be administered to say their last goodbyes.

Death comes from a cocktail of drugs injected intravenously. The mixtures vary, but most include midazolam, a short-acting benzodiazepine drug that sedates rapidly. Midazolam is often used in initiating anaesthesia before endoscopies or to relax muscles prior to reducing dislocated shoulders. In experienced hands, the drug has been used safely for decades. Midazolam is familiar to many physicians.

A second drug is used to depress respiration. Opioids like morphine, hydromorphone, Percodan or fentanyl serve this purpose well. Following drug administration, the MAID recipient simply goes to sleep. Breathing slows. Death normally occurs within minutes. Family members say their last farewell and leave. When the death occurs in hospital, the body is taken to the morgue. Quite often, when the death takes place at home, funeral home employees have been waiting nearby. They enter the death scene, remove the body from its bed and deliver it to the undertaker's.

Ontario coroners do not attend such a death. The number of people using MAID since its legalization has increased steadily, and the practice is now becoming quite common. Any doctor who administers a MAID cocktail must report the death to the chief coroner's office to ensure that legal requirements have been observed and that the death occurred properly. If MAID becomes a more standard practice, the coroner's role may disappear. Euthanasia will then become a routine part of end of life care. For now, in Canada at least, euthanasia is still novel; in Ontario, the coroner's office still monitors its use.

War

Wars result in a large number of deaths of both troops and civilians. Society accepts that soldiers, sailors and air force members put their lives at risk in theatres of combat. Some death is an expected, inevitable consequence of armed conflict. Investigating deaths on battlefields at the time they occur would be dangerous and impractical.

The deaths of the hundreds or thousands fallen combatants in massive battles in years gone by were never investigated. At best, a senior officer recorded how these men died in some military record. Fewer members of armed forces die nowadays. Their deaths are always investigated. When these deaths happen while at war or while on duty overseas, their investigation remains solely in the hands of the military.

Troops dying on their home turf in peacetime have their deaths investigated by a coroner. Most soldiers are quite young and in relatively good health. Their deaths are not expected unless in combat, so a coroner has to be notified whenever their death occurs suddenly. Coroners' investigations do conclude that some peacetime soldiers die of natural causes, but often their deaths are accidental.

In either case, the focus of the coroner's investigation is to determine whether anything could be done to prevent a similar death in future. The military conducts a parallel investigation of its own as well. If the coroner has ordered an autopsy, a military official will try to obtain its report for its investigation too.

The military investigating body looks at any findings or recommendations that a coroner may have formulated, provided the coroner's conclusions are available before commencement of the military tribunal's deliberations. Both the coroner's report and a final printed autopsy report are frequently unavailable when the tribunal is convened. In my experience, the Canadian armed forces review the death of one of its members very quickly, long before any autopsy report can be completed. The absence of autopsy findings probably detracts little from the value of the armed forces' review. The circumstances surrounding a military death are usually much more important than exactly defining the fatal injury. Military investigations always reach their own conclusions, independent of anything a coroner may find.

Today trauma is the leading killer of wartime combatants. That wasn't always the case though. In years gone by, malaria was one of the biggest killers in the history of war. Alexander the Great probably died of malaria at the age of 33.[9] Alaric, king of the Goths, sacked Rome in the fourth century AD, but malaria killed him soon afterwards.[10] A century later in 452 AD, malaria robbed the army of Attila the Hun of its effective fighting force by the time it reached Rome.

It was not just millennia ago that soldiers died from malaria. More than a thousand years later malaria killed whole British garrisons in North America too. In Canada, during the War of 1812, Lieutenant-Colonel John By, of the Royal Engineers, built a canal along the Rideau River from Bytown (now Ottawa) to Kingston. Its purpose was to transport troops to defend British North America against an invasion by the newly formed United States.

The Rideau Canal was never used in times of war, but during its construction thousands of Irish labourers and British troops died from malaria. The numbers of malarial dead were especially high while dredging a stretch of the Rideau near Kingston. That part of the river was covered by so many malarial mosquitos that the labourers called it "the River Styx" because its environment was so hellish. Nowadays a soldier's death from malaria is very unusual. Most troops take drugs to prevent getting the disease before deployment to malarial areas.

Another common, fatal wartime disease was sepsis. That condition arose when wounds became infected and no antibiotics were available to cure them. At least 620,000 troops died during the American Civil War.[11] In all, 800,000 or more people, including two thirds of the troops,[12] died of infectious disease. Only 34,833 of those died of malaria.[13] Tuberculosis killed many more — it spread easily in crowded military conditions, jails, barracks, and so on. Dysentery took its toll too because of that era's generally poor sanitation. Typhoid fever, rheumatic fever (caused by the now easily treated *Streptococcus*), pneumonia and even measles also killed many Civil War combatants on both sides of the conflict.

Death from many types of infectious diseases continued throughout the First World War, the last major military conflict before the discovery of antibiotics. The Great War killed roughly 10 million civilians and 9.7 million military combatants.[14] Two million of the civilians and over three million troops are thought to have died from disease, most of which was infectious. The Spanish flu started in the last 11 months of the war, adding to the number of both civilian and military deaths. At war's end both troops and the general populace lived in squalid conditions in close contact with others, many of whom were sick. Death from infectious disease remained high for months afterwards.

Twenty years later an even larger war, the Second World War, convulsed the world. At its end, somewhere between 70 and 85 million people had died. The war itself caused 50 to 56 million to die, while another 19 and 28 million more died of infectious disease and famine.* Military deaths from infection declined significantly after the arrival of penicillin. As more and better antibiotics have been developed in the ensuing years, the number of military deaths from infections has declined dramatically. By the time of the 2003 war in Iraq more American soldiers committed suicide than died of infectious disease.

There will always be non-combatant deaths in wars, but in the world's most recent war zones, civilian deaths have greatly exceeded those of soldiers. Civilians don't usually die from infections. During the civil war that started in Syria in 2011, many Syrian non-combatants died when crushed by collapsing buildings. Some were also killed by exploding barrel bombs spraying them with shrapnel. Others died from exposure to chemical weapons.

So, traumatic wartime deaths continue. The difference is that now, more often it is civilians rather than soldiers who are war's victims. Still, these deaths are highly unlikely to ever be investigated by coroners even when the countries where conflict happen have coroners. Society will likely continue to see them as wartime's expected "collateral damage."

Enumeration of deaths and collection of statistics about both military and civilian deaths in wartime has been difficult in the past and remains problematic today. Coroners will not help provide them because they are unlikely to be involved with investigating any of these deaths. Gathering wartime death statistics will always remain the province of armed forces, governments and historians.

---

* These numbers were selected out of a potpourri of different estimates.

NOTES

1 Carter v Canada (Attorney General). (2015). SCC 5. https://scc-csc.lexum.com/scc-csc/scc-csc/en/item/14637/index.do

2 Butterfield, F. (1994, October 23). Historical study of homicide and cities surprises the experts. *New York Times.*

3 United Nations Office on Drugs and Crime (n.d.). Global study on homicide: 2019 edition. https://www.unodc.org/unodc/en/data-and-analysis/global-study-on-homicide.html

4 Global Burden of Disease 2016 Injury Collaborators. (2018). Global mortality from firearms, 1990–2016. *JAMA, 320*(8), 792–814.

5 Gillese, E. E. (2019). *Public inquiry into the safety and security of residents in the long-term care homes system* (Vol. 2). https://www.attorneygeneral.jus.gov.on.ca/english/about/pubs/ltc-review/

6 Hickey, E. W. (1997). *Serial murderers and their victims.* Belmont, CA: Wadsworth.

7 Marono, A. J., Reid, S., Yaksic, E., & Keatley, D. A. (2020). A behaviour sequence analysis of serial killers' lives: From childhood abuse to methods of murder. *Psychiatry, Psychology and Law, 27*(1). https://doi.org/10.1080/13218719.2019.1695517

8 Government of Canada. (2021). Medical assistance in dying. https://www.canada.ca/en/health-canada/services/medical-assistance-dying.html

9 Cunha, B. A. (2004). The death of Alexander the Great: Malaria or typhoid fever? *Infectious Disease Clinics of North America, 18*(1), 53–63.

10 Galassi, F. M., Bianucci, R., Gorini, G., Paganotti, G. M., Habicht, M. E., & Ruhli, F. J. (2016). The sudden death of Alaric I (c. 370–410 AD), the vanquisher of Rome: A tale of malaria and lacking immunity. *European Journal of Internal Medicine, 31*, 84–87.

11 American Battlefield Trust. (n.d.). *Civil War casualties: The cost of war: Killed, wounded, captured, and missing.* https://www.battlefields.org/learn/articles/civil-war-casualties

12 Sartin, J. S. (1993). Infectious diseases during the Civil War: The triumph of the "Third Army." *Clinical Infectious Diseases, 16*(4), 580–584.

13 Otis, G. A., & Huntington, D. L. (1883). *The medical and surgical history of the war of rebellion* (Vol. 2). https://archive.org/details/medicalsurgical32barnrich/page/n5/mode/2up

14 Mougel, N. (2011). World War I casualties. (J. Gratz, trans.). http://www.centre-robert-schuman.org/userfiles/files/REPERES%20%E2%80%93%20module%201-1-1%20-%20explanatory%20notes%20%E2%80%93%20World%20War%20I%20casualties%20%E2%80%93%20EN.pdf

22

Execution Deaths

Most countries that use coroners have abolished the death penalty, making the investigation of deaths resulting from judicial execution relatively uncommon events nowadays. Still, a few jurisdictions remain where judges periodically sentence people to death. That means some coroners will continue to investigate deaths of people executed by their governments.

Any coroner's investigation of an execution is straightforward. There will be no mystery about events that happened up to and including the time of death. An execution is typically the end result of a years-long legal process that included multiple appeals to the sentence. What has happened is clear to every interested person, but, in these cases, coroners are still required to formally investigate the death after the execution is carried out.

Death occurs in different ways depending on the means of execution. A historically common method of execution still in use is hanging.

Hanging

Nearly every country in the world has hanged people, at least since the time of the ancient Greeks.[1] Hanging is an inexpensive, convenient and simple method of execution. Little special equipment is required. It can be carried out essentially anywhere. The training for a hangman is minimal. No certification is required. Most skills in hanging are acquired on the job.

In bygone times when executions were frequent, the position of hangman brought with it a certain amount of public recognition, even if some considered it notoriety. During the career of Albert Pierrepoint (which ended in 1956), the long-time (and one of the last) British hangmen, his name was known worldwide.*

Many countries that have coroners, including the United States, still execute people by hanging. So, some coroners will investigate judicial hangings. In almost all countries hangings are quite rare now. That makes the odds of any individual coroner attending a hanging very low for many and nil for most.

A judicially sanctioned hanging still requires the use of a gallows. As shown in Figure 22.1, this device is formed by a wooden bar atop a post from which is suspended a rope that ends in a noose. The noose dangles above a trapdoor that can be opened using a lever. The hangman ties the noose at the end of the rope around the neck of a condemned person who stands on a trapdoor.

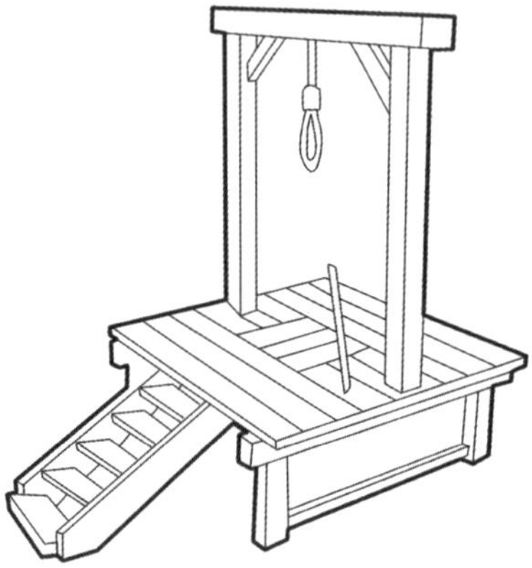

Figure 22.1: Gallows

When the hangman pulls a lever, the trapdoor opens and the condemned person drops through the newly created hole on the gallows' floor. The rope attached to the noose becomes taut. The noose also tightens around the neck as the person drops. At this point the hangman's skill and experience plays a role in what happens next.

---

* Another executioner left his name embedded in the English language. Thomas Derrick, a Tyburn hangman in sixteenth-century England, invented a pulley system for the gallows. It improved on the prior practice of simply tossing a rope over a beam. The mechanism was the basis for the modern-day lifting device called a derrick. Derrick invented his pulley to facilitate his work because he bore a much heavier load than does any modern-day hangman. It is estimated Derrick hanged 3,000 people!

A hangman must consider a couple of factors when planning a hanging. The first is the weight of the condemned person's body. The second is the length of the rope needed. The longer the rope, the longer the "drop" and the more effect gravity will have. If the hangman miscalculates badly, the drop may be too long, and the weight of the body can actually tear the head off. This has been reported to have happened frequently in the past.

Tearing the head off is followed by an instant loss of consciousness of course. Decapitation may produce a sudden but momentary jolt of exquisite pain that will be instantly forgotten because the brain is immediately deprived of blood. Decapitation by hanging is a very bloody but essentially painless death. However, it is considered a bad hanging.

Bad hangings may happen because today's hangmen work infrequently. They lack practice in properly calculating the length of rope that a weight will require for a perfect hanging. Such mathematics will always be problematic at a hangman's first execution. One of the last two people executed by hanging in Canada in 1962 died almost decapitated when the executioner miscalculated the required drop length. The weight of the man's body led to a speedy but messy death from an unplanned partial beheading.[2]

The hangman aims for an optimum combination of gravity and body weight to provide exactly the right amount of force on the spines of the neck. When the noose tightens and the body drops, correct calculations result in the body's weight fracturing a neck vertebra. Ideally this broken bone also severs the spinal cord, causing an instant loss of consciousness followed by death shortly afterwards. Such a successful hanging would produce a momentary sudden sharp pain in the neck instantly forgotten because of an immediate loss of consciousness.

In such a case, knowledgeable observers, of whom there were many in Dickens' day and in the centuries of public hangings preceding Victoria's reign, recognized death when a hanged man "filled his pants." Death relaxes muscles of the anal sphincter and gravity pulls stool downward. A dead body cannot expel stool from its anus by way of muscular contraction. Gravity forces stool, previously contained by the anal sphincter, to fall out of the anus and rectum into the trousers' seat causing a visible bulge. At that point, in the days of public executions, some in the crowd cheered. Others just went home.

The construction and placement of the knot forming the noose varies. The United Kingdom and former British colonies where hanging once occurred (it still does in some) commonly used simple slip knots (see Figure 22.2), or looped one end of a rope around the neck and the other end through a metal eye.[3] In the United States, as moviegoers know from westerns, the hangman's rope is often coiled several times above the knot. The number of coils in the rope varies from six to thirteen.[4]

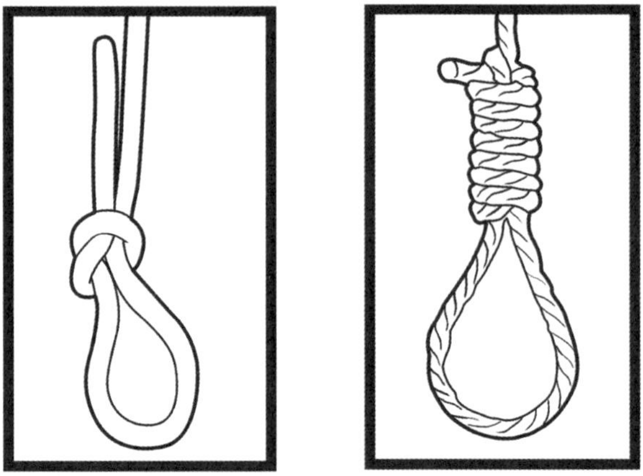

Figure 22.2: A single slip knot (left), and a noose tied using a sequence of slip knots (right).

Such a knot works best when placed in front of the left ear beneath the angle of the jaw. When the body falls and the rope becomes taut, the knot should push the head sharply to the right. Ideally gravity makes the rope jerk the body enough to break a spine in the neck, thus producing a hangman's fracture. In a classic hangman's fracture, the second cervical vertebra fractures its pedicles (see Figure 22.3), the pieces of bone on either side of the spinal cord attached to the vertebral body.*

* American hangmen also have placed the knot under the right ear hoping that the knot would crush the carotid arteries and jugular veins in the neck. The idea is to block blood flow and cause sudden loss of consciousness. Death is then supposed to occur within five minutes. But this is a purely theoretical proposition – death does not often happen so fast. People have been left dangling for almost half an hour before asphyxia finally becomes fatal.

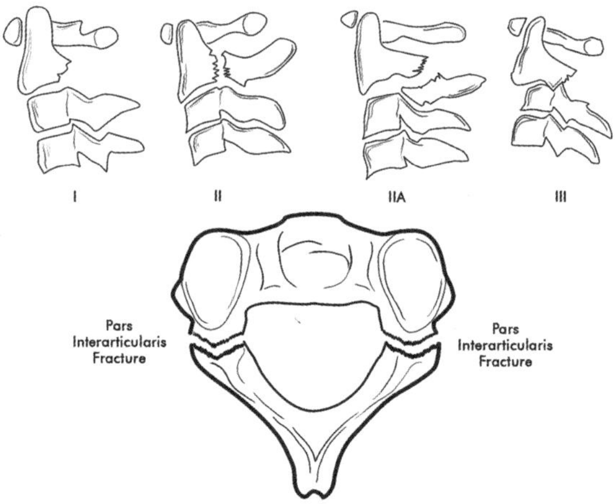

Figure 22.3: The so-called hangman's fracture. The images at the top show variants of the pars interarticularis fracture.

For a speedy death, the head and spine down to and including the second vertebra need to jerk forward, dislocating the spine. This movement crushes or tears the spinal cord between the second and third cervical vertebrae leading to neurogenic shock and sudden loss of consciousness. The body then hangs limply until death is finally declared by an attending physician.

The time before declaration of death varies. In 1993, the state of Washington hanged Westley Dodd. His death was pronounced four minutes after dropping through the trap door.[5] This is probably as fast as death could possibly be declared. Commonly, a longer time elapses before death becomes certain. In Delaware in 1996, Billy Bailey was not pronounced dead until 11 minutes after the trap door opened.[6]

History is replete with less than successful attempts to hang someone. Sometimes the knot in the rope's noose is too loosely tied. When the person drops through the trap door the noose unties, allowing the person to fall to the ground below. Since the rope never jerked around the neck death does not occur. The hanging must then be repeated with the rope more tightly knotted.

Another hanging mishap occurs with a rope that is too short or possibly too elastic. In that case the rope simply compresses the windpipe. It has no effect on the spine or spinal cord at all. The person hanging feels a lot of pain while the front of the windpipe is pressed against its back wall. Initially the hanging person remains conscious. Little, or possibly no, air will pass into the lungs.

Shortage of oxygen causes an increasingly panicky feeling. The person hanging starts to kick and jerk repeatedly. As seconds pass, the blood's oxygen level steadily decreases. Once their blood's oxygen saturation level drops below 55%, most of those hanging should lose consciousness.[7] Their bodies go limp. It may still take another 20 minutes for death from suffocation to be declared. That is a long time to die by hanging, but it does happen.

Decapitation

Beheading has been the preferred form of execution in many parts of the world throughout history. Even today, Islamic states, particularly Saudi Arabia, use beheading as the punishment for a number of crimes. Beheading was also quite common throughout European countries in centuries past, including Tudor England.

One of the most famous English beheadings was that of Mary Queen of Scots. On her appointed day Mary lay her head upon a block. The executioner then brought a blade's edge against the nape of Mary's neck. His first blow likely severed Mary's spinal cord. Loss of consciousness would have been instantaneous. The pain of Mary's death was probably momentary even though two more chops were needed to totally sever Mary's head from the rest of her body.[8]

At the time of French Revolution, watching the new-fangled guillotine execute aristocrats became a popular spectator sport for Jacobins in Paris. As many as 17,000 people are thought to have been guillotined during the period of Terror spawned by the revolution.[9] Throughout its reign speculation raged about the vitality of a severed head. Opinions about the length of time decapitated heads could live after their guillotining were based on the time eyelids could be seen to flicker.

A physician who watched a guillotining in 1905 made the following observations of a severed head in response to its name being called:

> Here, then, is what I was able to note immediately after the decapitation: the eyelids and lips of the guillotined man worked in irregularly rhythmic contractions for about five or six seconds. This

phenomenon has been remarked by all those finding themselves in the same conditions as myself for observing what happens after the severing of the neck …

I waited for several seconds. The spasmodic movements ceased. The face relaxed, the lids half closed on the eyeballs, leaving only the white of the conjunctiva visible, exactly as in the dying whom we have occasion to see every day in the exercise of our profession, or as in those just dead. It was then that I called in a strong, sharp voice: "Languille!" I saw the eyelids slowly lift up, without any spasmodic contractions — I insist advisedly on this peculiarity — but with an even movement, quite distinct and normal, such as happens in everyday life, with people awakened or torn from their thoughts. Next Languille's eyes very definitely fixed themselves on mine and the pupils focused themselves. I was not, then, dealing with the sort of vague dull look without any expression, that can be observed any day in dying people to whom one speaks: I was dealing with undeniably living eyes which were looking at me. After several seconds, the eyelids closed again, slowly and evenly, and the head took on the same appearance as it had had before I called out.

It was at that point that I called out again and, once more, without any spasm, slowly, the eyelids lifted and undeniably living eyes fixed themselves on mine with perhaps even more penetration than the first time. Then there was a further closing of the eyelids, but now less complete. I attempted the effect of a third call; there was no further movement — and the eyes took on the glazed look which they have in the dead.*

These are interesting observations.

It is almost certain there will never be studies on the lifespan of a severed human head. Nor will it ever become possible to measure the pain of a beheading. Were a coroner asked about the length of time before a decapitated head becomes unconscious, a safe reply would be "instantly." The brain's death follows a few minutes later, but its process of dying, while unconscious, is painless.

---

* Dr. Gabriel Beaurieux's observations of the severed head of Henri Languille right after it was guillotined on June 28, 1905. See https://www.guillotine.dk/pages/30sek.html

However, where the decapitation is slow or requires multiple cuts to sever the head from its body, dying is very painful. Cutting through the neck's skin produces pain to start with. More severe pain occurs when the muscles of the neck are cut. All muscles contain nerve endings that trigger pain when severed. Adjacent to both muscles at the front of the neck (the sternocleidomastoids), there are quite large nerves that, when cut, cause a lot of pain.

The human neck has identical structures on both sides. A brain only stops feeling pain when all nerves from both sides of the neck and the spinal cord are completely severed. Attempting decapitation from the front by slitting a person's throat first will always be painful for the victim. Try not to get into this with upset relatives. When nobody knows how a head was severed from its body, talk about a single cut and momentary, painless death.

The Middle East is the only place where state executions are likely to involve beheading nowadays. Most are in Saudi Arabia. This means that coroners will probably never have to deal with a judicially sanctioned beheading. Any beheadings that a coroner is likely to investigate are either criminal homicide or accidents.

Shooting

Countries that authorize execution by shooting do so in one of two ways. The simpler is a single shot in the back of the head. The more complicated method, virtually always used in military executions, requires a firing squad. In that case death arises from the result of a number of gunshot wounds. Some civilian jurisdictions, including the American state of Wyoming, do execute by gunshot. Coroners may investigate these deaths.

The single shot to the back of the head almost certainly causes an instantaneous loss of consciousness once it enters the brain. While death may not come for a few minutes, the dying person feels virtually no pain after being shot. A flash of discomfort while the bullet tore through the skin and bone, both of which contain nerve endings, would hardly have time to register in the brain because loss of consciousness would be instant. Fatal damage to the brain cells themselves is painless.

Should an executioner aim incorrectly and shoot into the neck or jaw, considerable discomfort results from shattered bones and nerves; the pain would continue until the person loses consciousness. Pain ceases if a second shot is delivered to the brain itself. Otherwise it might be a long, painful death. Most executions of this type take place in China, a country without coroners.

Death by firing squad makes it harder to estimate the pain of dying. The number of bullets used in an execution varies with the number of guns fired and the accuracy of the shooters. Soldiers on firing squads are usually trained to shoot for the chest, hoping to hit the heart. A good aim may result in an almost instant loss of consciousness. One prisoner condemned to execution by firing squad apparently had a monitor attached to his heart before he was executed. The monitor detected some sort of cardiac rhythm for 30 seconds after the shots entered his body. The existence of rhythm does not equate with consciousness, however.[10]

Of course, if shots go wildly askew, missing the heart, lungs or brain and simply hitting the condemned person's abdomen and limbs, death could be slow and painful as the wounded person bleeds to death. That won't happen in a judicial execution, but it could occur as part of death by torture carried out by gangsters. Shots that miss the heart only slightly pass through lungs, or possibly the aorta. In either case bleeding is massive and rapid. Loss of consciousness takes only seconds and brain death minutes.

Where a jurisdiction uses cardiac death as the standard for declaration of death by shooting, that determination can be made quite speedily. In Utah in 2010, Ronnie Lee Gardner was pronounced dead by a medical examiner two minutes after he was shot.[11] His heart had stopped working. One can assume that all his brain cells were not yet dead, however.

The Electric Chair

Only American coroners are likely to ever investigate a death after execution in an electric chair (see Figure 22.4). This device developed after competition between Edison and Westinghouse led to an electric method of execution that has never found favour outside the United

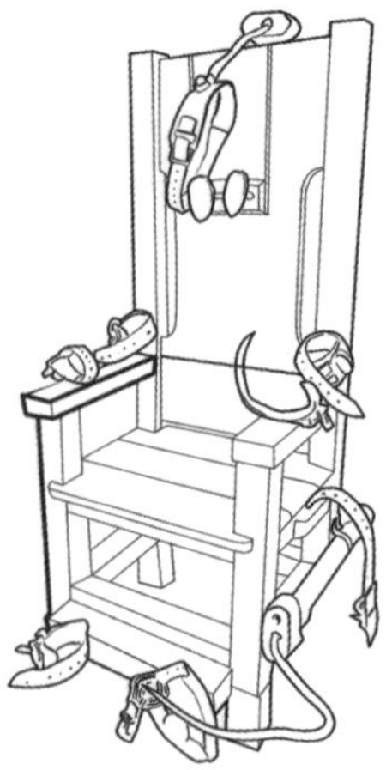

Figure 22.4: The electric chair is used for some executions in the United States.

States of America. In an electric chair the condemned person is subjected to around 1800 to 2000 volts (a high voltage) of electricity for a period of time that varies from 20 seconds to 90 seconds or more.

One jolt is not always enough to cause death. When this is the case, electrical shocks are delivered repeatedly until death finally happens. Requiring more than one dose of electricity is apparently not uncommon. In 1985 the Illinois execution of William Vandiver required three jolts of electricity before he could be declared dead. He took over 17 minutes to die.[12]

Electrocution does not always kill either. People are known to have survived the electric chair, usually because the current was improperly applied by the executioner. When the electricity in the chair does work, as is usual, the body's muscles go into spasm. That is usually visible to onlookers only as body stiffening because the condemned person is tightly strapped into the electric chair to prevent flailing limbs. Muscle spasms certainly cause pain while the person is conscious.

Electricity usually alters the heart's normal rhythm. When that change prevents the heart from pumping blood, loss of consciousness is immediate. The brain's nerve cells start to die, and five minutes or so later total brain death can be declared. This is the anticipated outcome of an electric chair execution. The heat produced by the electric current may create somewhat gruesome scenarios before this actually happens though.

Heat produced by an electric chair literally makes the blood boil. Boiling blood is a problem. It increases the pressure within the skull. When the intracranial pressure rises beyond what the skull can tolerate, the bones of the skull crack. Depending on the fracture type, pieces of bone, with or without scalp attached, may fly off the head. Losing this tissue does not kill the electrocuted person, but the heat transmitted to the brain prevents it from working properly and ends both breathing and heartbeat, ensuring a loss of consciousness in the remaining time before death.

It is not really possible to assure relatives of someone who has been electrocuted this way that the death was painless. It may have been, but it is equally possible it was not. Any conversation should focus on a possible speedy loss of consciousness. Observers cannot be certain how long the person being electrocuted remained conscious. Electrocution induces muscle spasm in jaw muscles that keep the mouth shut as long as electricity continues to flow. Breathing cannot be monitored either.

Gas Chamber

Execution in a gas chamber is carried out in two different ways. One uses a poisonous gas; the other deprives the condemned person of oxygen. Some American states still authorize death by gas chamber, so a coroner may investigate such a judicially sanctioned death, but these executions are rare nowadays.

The most common poisonous gas used for execution is hydrogen cyanide. This was the infamous Zyklon B used by the Nazis to carry out their slaughter in the Second World War death camps. This lethal gas is usually produced by mixing sodium cyanide pellets with sulphuric acid. That combination creates a cloud of hydrogen cyanide, a gas that is very poisonous and eventually kills anyone who inhales it. However, up to 18 minutes have been known elapse before a person could be certified dead after inhaling hydrogen cyanide.[13]

Death by hydrogen cyanide is not painless, although nobody alive actually knows what discomfort a person gassed with hydrogen cyanide feels while dying. Before losing consciousness, inhaled hydrogen cyanide may cause drooling, vomiting, convulsions and loss of control of urine and stool. These unpleasant symptoms are accompanied by the anxiety of increasing respiratory distress. If asked what a condemned person felt when executed with hydrogen cyanide, one should minimize the discomfort but not deny its existence.

An execution by oxygen deprivation may involve creating an atmosphere of carbon dioxide, carbon monoxide or pure nitrogen. In the first two of these cases, the gas chamber inhabitants develop an increasing air hunger, become restless, lose consciousness and then die after their brains are completely deprived of adequate oxygen for a few minutes. The actual time before death will depend on how long it takes to effectively remove oxygen from the gas chamber. With pure nitrogen dying follows a similar trajectory but with less discomfort and without any air hunger at the end.[14]

Lethal Injection

Lethal injection was introduced because it was expected to be a more humane form of execution than the more traditional methods. Drugs used for execution vary, but a common combination is something to relax or sedate to start the execution process, followed by a drug to stop breathing, and finally a drug to stop the heart from beating. These are usually drugs that are normally produced for medical uses, and some manufacturers have refused to supply drugs for executions. Refusals have required executioners to alter drug combinations used for executions. Forced drug substitution will likely continue in the future.

Sodium thiopental or some other short-acting barbiturate usually initiates the process. Anaesthetists have long used sodium thiopental to initiate sedation prior to surgery. An alternative that can replace sodium thiopental is midazolam. That drug might cause some people to lose consciousness. However, as many who have received midazolam before a colonoscopy know, it usually relaxes while consciousness remains.

Inappropriate drug use, along with technical difficulties in inserting needles into veins, have resulted in some executions using lethal drugs to be protracted rather than speedy. A lethal injection combination of midazolam, vercuronium and potassium chloride in Oklahoma in 2014 took 43 minutes to kill Clayton Lockett.[15] That was primarily because the paramedic who was starting the intravenous line was unable to do it properly. The same thing happened, in the same year, to Joseph Wood, who was executed in Arizona using simply midazolam and hydromorphone. It took two hours before his death could be declared.[16]

In an ideal lethal drug execution, death could be pronounced in about five minutes. In such an optimal case death might well be pain free, apart from the anxiety brought on by apprehension of impending death.

The first drug given, either a barbiturate (like sodium thiopental) or midazolam (a benzodiazepine), is supposed to induce a state close to unconsciousness. Administering this drug is painless. Then a second drug, like vercuronium bromide, paralyses all muscles, including the diaphragm, preventing movement or breathing. Once the person is unconscious, administration of this drug should not cause any symptoms. If the person is awake, a paralytic drug triggers great anxiety on discovering movement and breathing are impossible. That feeling cannot be transmitted because the paralysis prevents speech or any movement at all.

The third drug in the cocktail, potassium chloride, irritates veins on its way to causing cardiac death. Ventricular fibrillation follows and the heart first stops pumping and then stops beating. A conscious person injected with a potassium chloride solution feels burning at its injection site.

Garrotte

The garrotte was the state-sanctioned method of execution in Spain until the end of the Franco era (in 1975). Capital punishment was abolished in Spain in 1978. The last country where garrotting remained a legal method of execution was tiny Andorra. Andorra's legislature finally abolished garrotting in 1990.*

A garrotte is a ligature that is looped around the victim's neck and tightened with a winding mechanism that may simply be a peg attached to the ligature. The ligature rope or wire crushes the larynx and causes asphyxiation when it compresses one side of the windpipe

* Not that abolition made any difference. Nobody had been garrotted in Andorra for hundreds of years.

against the other. As the ligature tightens it will also eventually cut off blood flow to the brain. If the garrotting is quick the person being executed will feel a severe pain when the trachea is first compressed, but after air stops moving down to the lungs, unconsciousness should take but a minute and death three to five minutes more.

Coroners are unlikely to ever be confronted by a judicial execution using a garrotte. However, elite military units, such as the United Kingdom's SAS and the French Foreign Legion, are taught to silently kill guards by ligature compression using wire. This knowledge could find its way into civilian criminal gangs. If a gang executed an informer or enemy with garrotting, a coroner might be faced with such a criminal execution.

Stoning

Most people in the West think of stoning as a biblical punishment that is archaic and unlikely to happen nowadays. Not so. It still is carried out in Islamic countries such as Saudi Arabia and Somalia. The stoning can be done in at least a couple of ways. In one scenario, the woman (for it is usually a woman who is stoned) is buried in sand so that only her head is above the ground. Then invited stone throwers hurl rocks or hunks of concrete of varying size at her head until they are satisfied she is dead.

Alternatively, the woman to be stoned is trussed up with cord around her hands and feet before being put into a sack. She is left lying on the ground unable to see her executioners, who are readying the missiles with which they intend to stone her. Again, they pummel the sac with their rocks until movement stops and they hear no more breathing.

Most Islamic countries do not have coroners. A coroner will almost never investigate a stoning death unless the person killed by stoning is a citizen of the country where the coroner works, and the body is shipped home from the place of death. Only under special circumstances would a coroner be required to open an investigation into such an overseas death.

Stoning undoubtedly results in a horribly painful death. How long the pain lasts depends on the time until loss of consciousness. If one of the first stones strikes the woman's head, stunning her and then producing massive bleeding inside the skull, she might pass out quite rapidly. When that does not happen, the process of dying from multiple injuries is very painful and can take quite a long time.

A coroner faced with investigating a death that happened in a foreign country could not possibly estimate how long dying took or how much pain was involved in the execution. The family would almost certainly understand that and not ask those questions.

While information on executions may satisfy the professional curiosity of many coroners, it is likely to assist very few. This topic is included simply for completeness.

NOTES

1 Homer. *The Odyssey (A. S. Kline, Trans.) Book XXII, 433–501.* https://www.poetryintranslation.com/PITBR/Greek/Odyssey22.php#anchor_Toc90268922

2 Alamenciak, T. (2012, December 10). *The end of the rope: The story of Canada's last executions. Toronto Star. https://www.thestar.com/news/gta/2012/12/10/the_end_of_the_rope_the_story_of_canadas_last_executions.html*

3 Walton, G. (2019, April 8). *The executioner's rope of the 1700s and the 1800s.* https://www.geriwalton.com/the-executioners-rope-of-the-1700-and-1800s/

4 Trimble, M. (2019, July 30). The hanging judge's hangman discusses hanging. True West. https://truewestmagazine.com/hanging-judges-hangmen/

5 Associated Press. (1993, January 10). Coroner concludes murderer felt little pain when hanged. *The New York Times*, p. 23.

6 Associated Press. (1996, January 26). Delaware killer executed in 3rd U.S. hanging in 30 years. *Los Angeles Times.*

7 Bachus, E., Holm, H., Hamrefors, V., Melander, O., Sutton, R., Magnusson, M., & Fedorowski, A. (2018). Monitoring of cerebral oximetry during head-up tilt test in adults with history of syncopal orthostatic intolerance. *EP Eurospace, 20*(9), 1535–1542.

8 Charleston, L. J. (2019, February 16). The gruesome beheading of Mary Queen of Scots. New Zealand Herald. https://www.nzherald.co.nz/lifestyle/the-gruesome-beheading-of-mary-queen-of-scots/KT6ES7HXAEMBLTJQTSYBOYQMBU/

9 Linton, M. (2004). *The Terror in the French revolution.* https://www.academia.edu/5514345/The_Terror_in_the_French_Revolution

10 Wikipedia. (n.d.). *Execution by firing squad. https://en.wikipedia.org/wiki/Execution_by_firing_squad*

11 NBC News. (2015, March 25). *Firing squad to gas chamber: How long do executions take? https://www.nbcnews.com/news/us-news/firing-squad-gas-chamber-how-long-executions-take-n329371*

12 The Washington Post. (1985, October 17). Killer's electrocution takes 17 minutes in Indiana chair. https://www.washingtonpost.com/archive/politics/1985/10/17/killers-electrocution-takes-17-minutes-in-indiana-chair/3fd99ef4-8e72-4ab3-b35a-9f7635b17267/

13 Machelor, P. (1999, March 4). LaGrand:18 minutes to die. *Tucson Citizen.* http://tucsoncitizen.com/morgue2/1999/03/04/147996-lagrand-18-minutes-to-die/#:~:text=The%2037%2Dyear%2Dold%20killer,poisoning%20on%20April%206%2C%201992.

14 Shuler, J. (2015, March 20). Can executions be more humane? *The Atlantic.* https://www.theatlantic.com/politics/archive/2015/03/can-executions-be-more-humane/388249/#disqus_thread

15 Stern, J. E. (2015, June). The cruel and unusual execution of Clayton Lockett. *The Atlantic.* https://www.theatlantic.com/magazine/archive/2015/06/execution-clayton-lockett/392069/

16 Dart, T. (2014, August 2). Arizona inmate Joseph Wood was injected 15 times with execution drugs. *The Guardian.* https://www.theguardian.com/world/2014/aug/02/arizona-inmate-injected-15-times-execution-drugs-joseph-wood

Acknowledgements

There are a number of people to whom I must offer my most heartfelt thanks. Without their help and encouragement this book could not have been written. The first, and most important, contributor to this book is my wife, Joanne. She put up with a silent household for the first many months of the pandemic. Thank God she likes to knit and garden. Joanne had months of opportunity to practise her skills in both endeavours.

Secondly, I would like to thank the physicians who were kind enough to critique parts of the manuscript for me. Virbala Acharya, Yasmine Ayroud and Brian Johnston are pathologists with whom I had a long association as a coroner, and Maureen Grace and Kenneth Willis are clinical colleagues with whom I worked for years. Their assistance as reviewers is greatly appreciated.

My entry into the publishing world would have been impossible without the guidance of Magdalene Carson of New Leaf Publication Design. She explained to me what needed to be done to publish a book and then introduced me to Linda Jenkins of Red Pen Services, who graciously agreed to be my editor. Linda also explained the value of a proofreader. Thanks must be given to my wife, Joanne, who did the all-important final check.

Linda provided me with guidance chapter by chapter for months. She also helped me realize that publishing moves at a different pace from emergency medicine. Once this realization sank in the editing process became almost exciting, with the proposed changes for the next chapter an intriguing mystery to look forward to. The book was written with the intent to make it understandable for a non-medical reader, but the initial draft didn't quite achieve this. Linda located many instances of confusing medical jargon and suggested much more understandable English phrases as replacements.

Thanks must also be offered to Frances Curry, who created the index for the book. Until Magdalene told me that professional indexers exist, the task of creating an index seemed likely to fall onto my shoulders – a prospect that filled me with dread. Once Frances agreed to generate the book's index, she put her background as a nurse to good use. Frances is the reason why the index is so comprehensive.

Finally, I would like to thank John Rey Dado, the artist who created the book's illustrations from his atelier in the Philippines. John had to communicate with me in English, which is his second language. Nevertheless, we were able to understand each other. Our regular back and forth on the internet made it seem like John was emailing from the other side of town when in fact he was working half a world away. While the rest of the people I have thanked live in the Ottawa Valley, my dealings with John are an example of how much the internet contributes to globalization nowadays!

About the Author

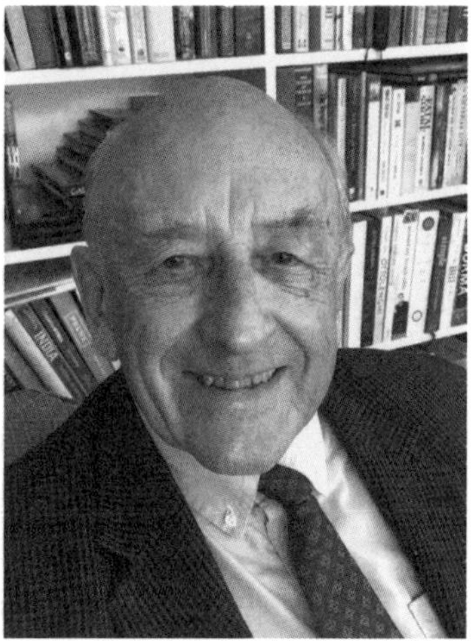

The author of this book, Gordon Watt, grew up in and has lived most of his life in Ottawa, Ontario, Canada. In 1960, he left Canada's capital to study medicine at Queen's University in Kingston, Ontario, for six years. After a 1966-67 internship at the Montreal General Hospital, Dr. Watt attended the University of Toronto Law School, graduating in 1970. Following the author's call to the Ontario Bar in 1972 he practised both law and medicine in tandem for more than a decade.

Dr. Watt initially practised law in Mississauga, Ontario. After 1975, he returned to Ottawa to continue legal practice in Ottawa firms. The Province of Ontario appointed Dr. Watt Queen's Counsel in recognition of his service to the Ontario legal profession. For five years, the author lectured in both the faculties of both Law and Medicine at the University of Ottawa. Dr. Watt's legal career ended in 1995 when he resigned his membership in the Law Society of Upper Canada (as it was then called). Thereafter the author confined himself to practising medicine and undertaking coroner's investigations. Dr. Watt continued both activities until his retirement in 2022.

The author worked as an emergency physician for thirty-five years - in both Toronto and Ottawa hospitals. Subsequently he practised acute care medicine in an Ottawa urgent care centre. The author has also provided occupational medical services to numerous Ottawa Valley employers. In 2015, Dr. Watt's peers in the Ottawa Academy of Medicine voted him "The Outstanding Physician in Ottawa." To earn that accolade, the author had used his best efforts to prevent deaths – most of the time successfully.

Not always though. As an emergency physician, the author frequently dealt with the dying and the dead. While witnessing many different types of deaths in the emergency room, Dr. Watt's sole objective had been to try to prevent them. That focus changed in 1981 once the province of Ontario appointed him a coroner, and the author began investigating deaths.

In the past forty years Dr. Watt has investigated thousands of deaths in and around Ottawa. He has presided over hundreds of inquests in towns throughout the Ottawa Valley. At one point before the author stopped holding inquests, he had presided at more inquests than any other coroner in Ontario. At the time of his retirement in 2022, Dr. Watt was a senior coroner, if not the longest-serving one, in the province.

Index*

* Images are denoted by *fig*; footnotes by *n*; tables by *t*.

B

R

S

V

W